Biowaste and Biomass in Biofuel Applications

This book reflects the new dimension of biofuel production from its introductory principles to the advancements from a future prospective. It summarizes the rationale for changes in liquid fuel utilization and the selection of new technologies to make biofuel cost-effective and move toward a carbon-neutral approach. It provides an evidence-based outline of how additives and nanotechnology chemically change biofuels' quality and effectiveness, including new and innovative approaches, such as nanomaterials and various nano-additives.

Features:

- It provides an overview of biowaste as a sustainable source in the field of biofuel production
- It includes effective conversion parameters of the biowaste feedstocks and their classification
- It summarizes current research into the development and exploitation of new biofuel sources
- It discusses the improvement of pilot scale scalability, chemical processing, and design flow
- It presents relevant and realistic global explanations of biowaste management techniques for biofuels

This book is aimed at senior undergraduate and graduate students, and researchers in bioprocessing, chemical engineering, and biotechnology.

Mathematical Engineering, Manufacturing, and Management Sciences

Series Editor
Mangey Ram
Professor, Assistant Dean (International Affairs),
Department of Mathematics, Graphic Era University, Dehradun, India

The aim of this new book series is to publish the research studies and articles that bring up the latest development and research applied to mathematics and its applications in the manufacturing and management sciences areas. Mathematical tool and techniques are the strength of engineering sciences. They form the common foundation of all novel disciplines as engineering evolves and develops. The series will include a comprehensive range of applied mathematics and its application in engineering areas such as optimization techniques, mathematical modelling and simulation, stochastic processes and systems engineering, safety-critical system performance, system safety, system security, high assurance software architecture and design, mathematical modelling in environmental safety sciences, finite element methods, differential equations, reliability engineering, etc.

Advances in Sustainable Machining and Manufacturing Processes
Edited by Kishor Kumar Gajrani, Arbind Prasad and Ashwani Kumar

Advanced Materials for Biomechanical Applications
Edited by Ashwani Kumar, Mangey Ram and Yogesh Kumar Singla

Biodegradable Composites for Packaging Applications
Edited by Arbind Prasad, Ashwani Kumar and Kishor Kumar Gajrani

Computing and Stimulation for Engineers
Edited by Ziya Uddin, Mukesh Kumar Awasthi, Rishi Asthana and Mangey Ram

Advanced Manufacturing Processes
Edited by Yashvir Singh, Nishant K. Singh and Mangey Ram

Additive Manufacturing
Advanced Materials and Design Techniques
Pulak M. Pandey, Nishant K. Singh and Yashvir Singh

Advances in Mathematical and Computational Modeling of Engineering Systems
Mukesh Kumar Awasthi, Maitri Verma and Mangey Ram

Biowaste and Biomass in Biofuel Applications
Edited by Yashvir Singh, Vladimir Strezov, and Prateek Negi

For more information about this series, please visit: www.routledge.com/Mathematical-Engineering-Manufacturing-and-Management-Sciences/book-series/CRCMEMMS

Biowaste and Biomass in Biofuel Applications

Edited by
Yashvir Singh, Vladimir Strezov, and Prateek Negi

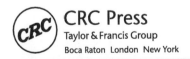

CRC Press is an imprint of the
Taylor & Francis Group, an **informa** business

Designed cover image: © Shutterstock

First edition published 2023
by CRC Press
6000 Broken Sound Parkway NW, Suite 300, Boca Raton, FL 33487–2742

and by CRC Press
4 Park Square, Milton Park, Abingdon, Oxon, OX14 4RN

CRC Press is an imprint of Taylor & Francis Group, LLC

© 2023 selection and editorial matter, Yashvir Singh, Vladimir Strezov, and Prateek Negi; individual chapters, the contributors

Reasonable efforts have been made to publish reliable data and information, but the author and publisher cannot assume responsibility for the validity of all materials or the consequences of their use. The authors and publishers have attempted to trace the copyright holders of all material reproduced in this publication and apologize to copyright holders if permission to publish in this form has not been obtained. If any copyright material has not been acknowledged please write and let us know so we may rectify in any future reprint.

Except as permitted under U.S. Copyright Law, no part of this book may be reprinted, reproduced, transmitted, or utilized in any form by any electronic, mechanical, or other means, now known or hereafter invented, including photocopying, microfilming, and recording, or in any information storage or retrieval system, without written permission from the publishers.

For permission to photocopy or use material electronically from this work, access www.copyright.com or contact the Copyright Clearance Center, Inc. (CCC), 222 Rosewood Drive, Danvers, MA 01923, 978–750–8400. For works that are not available on CCC please contact mpkbookspermissions@tandf.co.uk

Trademark notice: Product or corporate names may be trademarks or registered trademarks and are used only for identification and explanation without intent to infringe.

ISBN: 978-1-032-19358-8 (hbk)
ISBN: 978-1-032-20861-9 (pbk)
ISBN: 978-1-003-26559-7 (ebk)

DOI: 10.1201/9781003265597

Typeset in Times
by Apex CoVantage, LLC

Contents

Editor Biographies vii
List of Contributors ix
Preface xi

Chapter 1 Sustainability of Waste Cooking Oil for the Production of
Biodiesel and Its Tribological Applications: A Review 1

*Yashvir Singh, Erween Abd Rahim, Nishant Kumar Singh,
Abhishek Sharma, Amneesh Singla, and Arkom Palmanit*

Chapter 2 Application of Nanofluids in Solar Desalination
Process: A Review 19

*Avinash Yadav, Yashvir Singh, Erween Abd Rahim, Prateek
Negi, Wei-Hsin Chen, Nishant Kumar Singh, and Abhishek Sharma*

Chapter 3 Nanomaterials as Additives in Biodiesel 33

Anil Dhanola and Kishor Kumar Gajrani

Chapter 4 Challenges and Future Prospects of Biofuel Generations: An
Overview 49

*Amneesh Singla, Yashvir Singh, Erween Abd Rahim, Nishant
Kumar Singh, and Abhishek Sharma*

Chapter 5 A Comparative Study of Physicochemical Properties
and Performance Characteristics of Various Biodiesel
Feedstock: An Overview 63

*Harish Chandra Joshi, Waseem Ahmad, Neetu Sharma,
Vinod Kumar, Sanjeev Kimothi, and Bhawana*

Chapter 6 Chemical Processing Techniques Related to Bio-Waste for Their
Conversion to Biofuel 95

Harish Chandra Joshi, Nitika Grag, and Waseem Ahmad

vi   Contents

Chapter 7 The Effectiveness of *Balanites aegyptiaca* Oil Nanofluid
Augmented with Nanoparticles as Cutting Fluids during the
Turning Process 111

Nishant Kumar Singh, Yashvir Singh, Erween Abd Rahim,
Abhishek Sharma, Amneesh Singla, and P.S. Ranjit

Chapter 8 Lignocellulose Biomass Pyrolysis for Bio-Oil Production:
Biomass Pre-treatment Methods for Production of
Drop-In Fuels 123

Kumar, R., Strezov, V., Weldekidan, H., He, J., Singh, S.,
Kan, T., and Dastjerdi, B.

Chapter 9 Thermochemical Production of Bio-Oil: Downstream
Processing Technologies for Bio-Oil Upgrading, Production of
Hydrogen, and High Value-Added Products 197

Kumar, R. and Strezov, V.

Chapter 10 Free Fatty Acids and Their Role in CI Engines 267

P.S. Ranjit, Saravanan A., and Elumalai P.V.

Index 299

Editor Biographies

Dr Yashvir Singh is presently working as post-doctoral fellow in the Faculty of Mechanical and Manufacturing Engineering, Universiti Tun Hussein Onn Malaysia, Parit Raja, Batu Pahat, Johor, Malaysia. He is also an associate professor in the Department of Mechanical Engineering, Graphic Era Deemed to be University, Dehradun, Uttarakhand, India. He has more than 15 years of teaching experience. He has written over 100 research articles and published them in various peer-reviewed journals. He is also a reviewer and editorial board member of various journals. His specialization includes areas like tribology, biofuels, lubrication, manufacturing, and additive manufacturing. He has taught various subjects at UG and PG levels, such as non-conventional machining processes, advanced manufacturing processes, and additive manufacturing. He published various research papers in reputed journals and also reviewed various articles in the journals.

Prof Vladimir Strezov is a professor at the Department of Earth and Environmental Sciences, Faculty of Science and Engineering, Macquarie University, Australia. He holds a Ph.D. degree in chemical engineering and a B.E. degree in mechanical engineering. Before commencing academic work at Macquarie University in 2003, he was a researcher at the Department of Chemical Engineering, the University of Newcastle, and at BHP Research in Newcastle, Australia. Professor Strezov leads a research group at Macquarie University working on renewable and sustainable energy, industrial ecology, control of environmental pollution, and design of sustainability metrics of industrial operations. Professor Strezov was an advisory panel member for the Australian Renewable Energy Agency (ARENA) (2015–2020). He is a Fellow of the Institution of Engineers Australia and a Fellow of the Australian Institute of Energy. He is an editorial member for the journals *Sustainability, Environmental Progress & Sustainable Energy, International Journal of Sustainable Engineering*, and *International Journal of Chemical Engineering and Applications*. He is the author of ~300 publications and editor of four books: Biomass Processing Technologies, with T. J. Evans (2014), Antibiotics and Antibiotics Resistance Genes in Soils, with M. Z. Hashmi and A. Varma (2017), Renewable Energy Systems from Biomass: Efficiency, Innovation, and Sustainability with H.M. Anawar (2019) and Sustainable and Economic Waste Management: Resource Recovery Techniques with H.M. Anawar and Abhilash (2020).

Mr Prateek Negi is presently working as an assistant professor at the Department of Mechanical Engineering, Graphic Era Deemed to be University, Dehradun, Uttarakhand, India. His areas of specialization include thermal energy storage, energy technologies, and alternate fuels, and is currently working on the tribological analysis of bio-lubricants. Being a reviewer of some peer-reviewed journals, he has more than 20 journal and conference papers to his credit. He has taught various subjects at UG level, including heat and mass transfer, thermodynamics, non-conventional energy resources, computer-aided design, and manufacturing and operations research.

Contributors

Saravanan A.
Department of Mechanical Engineering,
  Aditya Engineering College
Surampalem, India

Waseem Ahmad
Department of Chemistry, Uttaranchal
  University
Dehradun, Uttarakhand, India

Bhawana
Department of Chemistry, Graphic Era
  deemed to be University
Dehradun, Uttarakhand, India

Wei-Hsin Chen
Department of Aeronautics and
  Astronautics, National Cheng Kung
  University
Tainan, Taiwan
Research Centre for Smart Sustainable
  Circular Economy
Tunghai, Taiwan
Department of Mechanical Engineering,
  National Chin-Yi University of
  Technology
Taichung, Taiwan

B. Dastjerdi
School of Natural Sciences, Faculty of
  Science & Engineering, Macquarie
  University
Sydney, NSW, Australia

Anil Dhanola
University Institute of Engineering,
  Department of Mechanical Engineering,
  Chandigarh University
Mohali, Punjab, India

Kishor Kumar Gajrani
Department of Mechanical
  Engineering, Indian Institute of
  Information Technology, Design and
  Manufacturing
Kancheepuram, Chennai,
  Tamil Nadu, India
Centre for Smart Manufacturing,
  Indian Institute of Information
  Technology, Design and
  Manufacturing
Kancheepuram, Chennai,
  Tamil Nadu, India

Nitika Grag
Department of Chemistry, RKGIT
Ghaziabad, Uttar Pradesh, India

J. He
School of Natural Sciences, Faculty of
  Science & Engineering, Macquarie
  University
Sydney, NSW, Australia

Harish Chandra Joshi
Department of Chemistry, Graphic Era
  deemed to be University
Dehradun, Uttarakhand, India

T. Kan
School of Natural Sciences, Faculty of
  Science & Engineering, Macquarie
  University
Sydney, NSW, Australia

Sanjeev Kimothi
Research & Development Division,
  Uttaranchal University
Dehradun, Uttarakhand, India

x   Contributors

R. Kumar
School of Natural Sciences, Faculty of
Science & Engineering, Macquarie
University
Sydney, NSW, Australia

Vinod Kumar
Department of Life Science, Graphic
Era deemed to be University
Dehradun, Uttarakhand, India

Prateek Negi
Department of Mechanical Engineering,
Graphic Era Deemed to be University
Dehradun, Uttarakhand, India

Arkom Palmanit
Energy System Research Institute,
Prince of Songkla University
Hat Yai Songkhla, Thailand

Elumalai P.V.
Department of Mechanical Engineering,
Aditya Engineering College
Surampalem, India

Erween Abd Rahim
Faculty of Mechanical and
Manufacturing Engineering,
Universiti Tun Hussein Onn Malaysia
Parit Raja, Batu Pahat, Johor, Malaysia

P.S. Ranjit
Department of Mechanical Engineering,
Aditya Engineering College
Surampalem, India

Abhishek Sharma
Department of Mechanical Engineering,
G L Bajaj Institute of Technology
and Management
Greater Noida, Uttar Pradesh, India

Neetu Sharma
Department of Chemistry, Graphic Era
deemed to be University
Dehradun, Uttarakhand, India

Nishant Kumar Singh
Department of Mechanical
Engineering, Harcourt Butler
Technical University
Kanpur, Uttar Pradesh, India

S. Singh
Department of Organic and
Petrochemical Technology,
School of Chemical Engineering,
Hanoi University of Science and
Technology
1 Dai Co Viet, Hanoi, Vietnam

Yashvir Singh
Faculty of Mechanical and
Manufacturing Engineering,
Universiti Tun Hussein Onn
Malaysia
Parit Raja, Batu Pahat, Johor,
Malaysia
Department of Mechanical Engineering,
Graphic Era Deemed to be
University
Dehradun, Uttarakhand, India

Amneesh Singla
Department of Mechanical Engineering,
University of Petroleum and Energy
Studies
Dehradun, Uttarakhand, India

V. Strezov
School of Natural Sciences, Faculty of
Science & Engineering, Macquarie
University
Sydney, NSW, Australia

Avinash Yadav
Department of Mechanical
Engineering, Graphic Era Deemed to
be University
Dehradun, Uttarakhand, India
Department of Mechanical
Engineering, College of Engineering
Roorkee
Roorkee, Uttarakhand, India

Preface

Biofuels are renewable alternatives to conventional fuels obtained from biomass, which can be plant or animal waste. Biofuels can be cost-effective and sustainable options for petroleum and other conventional energy sources, especially with the continuous increase in petroleum prices and adverse impacts on our environment. The global energy demand is expected to keep on developing, and it is broadly perceived that alternative, sustainable solutions should be discovered to address the associated environmental and economic issues. Biofuels can play a significant role in future energy creation because of their favorable and sustainable properties in response to the current challenges. The purpose of this book is to serve as a compilation of cutting-edge research in the field of biofuels. Eminent specialists have written chapters in the field focusing on several aspects of biofuels, from raw materials to production technologies. With expanding interest in energy around the world, alongside the exhaustion of conventional petroleum product reserves, there is developing worldwide interest in creating alternative sources of energy. Concern has likewise been communicated in developing economies about energy security. The book will summarize the most recent cutting-edge data on the status of biofuel production and related aspects of biofuel technologies.

The major features of this book, which make it unique, are as follows: (1) Fuel, from conventional to non-conventional; (2) Role of vegetable oil in biofuel production; (3) Chemical processing techniques related to biomass for their conversion to biofuels; (4) Biomass feedstocks and discussion of chemical processing routes for conversion to biofuels; (5) Recent advances, methods, and issues related to the production of biofuels from various sources; (6) The use of additives and nanomaterials for sustainable production of biofuels; (7) Production and optimization of biofuels using green nanomaterials; (8) Forthcoming trends and outlooks in biofuels production; and (8) Solar energy application for processing routes related to nanofluids.

The book will be an edited compendium of new research and case studies on advancements in biofuel production, presented by scholars, academics, and field practitioners on several approaches to the sustainable production of green fuels, deeply aligned and grouped into segments of topics. This book provides an evidence-based outline of how those additives and nanotechnology have chemically changed the quality and effectiveness of biofuels. Due to a large range of applications, and a carbon-neutral approach using bio-waste/biomass, biofuel production is becoming a major new technological development in the automobile sector. This book will address a wide range of new and innovative approaches, such as nanomaterials and various nano-additives, which will be a sure step toward our sustainable and bright future.

Yashvir Singh
Vladimir Strezov
Prateek Negi

1 Sustainability of Waste Cooking Oil for the Production of Biodiesel and Its Tribological Applications
A Review

Yashvir Singh[1,2], Erween Abd Rahim[1],
Nishant Kumar Singh[3], Abhishek Sharma[4],
Amneesh Singla[5], and Arkom Palmanit[6]

1 Department of Mechanical and Manufacturing
   Engineering, Universiti Tun Hussein Onn Malaysia,
   Parit Raja, Batu Pahat, Johor, Malaysia
2 Department of Mechanical Engineering, Graphic Era
   Deemed to be University, Dehradun, Uttarakhand, India
3 Department of Mechanical Engineering, Harcourt Butler
   Technical University, Kanpur, Uttar Pradesh, India
4 Department of Mechanical Engineering, G L
   Bajaj Institute of Technology and Management,
   Greater Noida, Uttar Pradesh, India
5 Department of Mechanical Engineering,
   University of Petroleum and Energy Studies,
   Dehradun, Uttarakhand, India
6 Energy System Research Institute, Prince of
   Songkla University, Hat Yai Songkhla, Thailand

CONTENTS

1.1 Introduction 2
1.2 Biodiesel and Its Production 4
1.3 Waste Cooking Oil and Its Conversion to Biodiesel 5
    1.3.1 Feedstocks for Waste Cooking Oil 6

DOI: 10.1201/9781003265597-1

Biowaste and Biomass in Biofuel Applications

	1.3.2	Waste Cooking Oil Properties	7
		1.3.2.1 Cetane Number	7
		1.3.2.2 Density	7
		1.3.2.3 Viscosity	7
		1.3.2.4 Calorific Value	7
		1.3.2.5 Value of Saponification	7
		1.3.2.6 Acid Value	8
	1.3.3	Comparison of Waste Cooking Oil with Other Feedstocks	8
1.4	Aspects of Biodiesel for Tribological Applications		8
	1.4.1	Friction and Wear of Biodiesel	9
	1.4.2	Biodiesel Corrosion	10
1.5	Role of Additives in Biodiesel		11
1.6	Conclusions and Suggestions		12
References			13

1.1 INTRODUCTION

Rapid, cost-effective globalization, population progress, and development have increased the consumption of petroleum products, leading to increased greenhouse gas discharges and enormous carbon deposition in the air, which carelessly elevates the worldwide temperature, resulting in environmental change. Increased requirement for energy has encouraged countries to expand their energy portfolios to decrease their reliance on fossil fuels and strengthen their energy security. Biofuels originating as viable causes and possessing the necessary chemical properties have gained popularity [1]. Depending on the crops used and the population supply, first-generation biofuels derived from edible crops may directly affect the food cycle. As a result, the energy industry is refocusing its efforts on substitute fuel resources. The second generation of biofuels is a concept that emphasizes the orderly and efficient utilization of remaining waste, including waste cooking oil (WCO). WCO contains accrued free fatty acids, making it a feasible feedstock for biofuel transformation [2,3]. It is also readily available and inexpensive because of its diverse origins, including restaurants, food processing firms, quick food shops, and households. Additionally, because WCO is manufactured globally, it reduces the struggle amongst oil assets and edible oil-based food crops and may be responsible for a sustainable substitute for biofuel change [4].

Cooking oil is mostly derived from edible oil plants. Due to economic concerns, it is frequently normal to reuse the same oil during continuous frying. Because lipid browning increases the oil's acidity and the production of a disagreeable odor, recycling WCO is also hazardous to human consumption. Additionally, damaged old cooking oil includes excessive free fatty acid and water, resulting in a low economic value [5,6]. Due to population growth and increased food consumption, the WCO dumping problem is becoming a global concern. Illegal dealers have been observed reselling WCO and drain oil as conventional cooking oil, raising worries about food safety and related health hazards [7]. As a result of these concerns, politicians have begun to impose restrictions on WCO disposal and recycling methods while supporting innovative approaches to value-added product production. In recent years, the rounded low-cost concept has emphasized repurposing waste materials and closing the raw material cycle to maintain value through consumption optimization. WCO has emerged as a leading candidate, with considerable interest in recycling and repurposing WCO for biofuel generation [8].

WCO biodiesel is non-toxic and biodegradable, containing no or very little sulfur. It can be utilized in CI engines with little adjustments. Biodiesel exploration is not thorough until it is experienced in CI engines, as CI engines were not specifically established to use biodiesel fuel. Except for NOx and smoke emissions, engines fueled by a blend of biodiesel and gasoline contribute to reducing greenhouse gas emissions and volatile organic compounds (VOCs) [9].

Additionally, mixtures of biodiesel and diesel improved fuel efficiency, thermal brake efficiency, engine torque, and braking power [10]. On the other hand, continuous use of the biodiesel–diesel blend may result in the leakage of blended biofuel into the engine compartment as a result of damage to bearings, cams, piston rings, cylinder liners, valve stem seals, or gaskets, polluting the lubricating oil, and so forth. In most circumstances, contaminated lubricating oil increases wear on critical components, reduces the frequency of oil changes, and degrades the engine compartment's durability. As a result, it is vital to understand how contamination from biofuel impacts lubricating oil. Lubricating oil aims to lessen the frictional force generated by moving surfaces or parts in the engine, reducing wear and power loss while improving engine performance and reducing fuel consumption. Additionally, engine oil functions as a detergent, removing sludge and impurities from engine components and depositing and transferring them to an oil filter, preventing metal deposit adhesion.

Additionally, engine oil acted as a rust inhibitor and sealed between the piston and the cylinder. As a result, the qualities of engine oil play a vital role in determining engine performance. Because it is necessary to maintain the thickness of the lubricating film, viscosity is one of the most critical properties determining the lubricating oil's quality. Additionally, the lubricating oil must enable proper engine oil flow at lower temperatures in the engine components. As a result, various researchers have examined biodiesel's lubricity properties. For instance, Zulkifli et al. [11] investigated the wear resistance of a trimethylolpropane (TMP) ester derived from palm oil in combination with lubricating oil. The wear properties of palm oil-based TMP ester blends with lubricating oil were investigated using a four-ball machine (1%, 3%, 5%, 7%, and 11% palm oil-based TMP ester). The results indicated that 3% of TMP could support the greatest weight (223 kg), while 7% of TMP might reduce friction by 52%. Mosarof et al. [12] conducted a comparison of the friction and wear parameters of palm biodiesel and Calophylluminophyllum (CIME) (POME). This study combined CIME and POME with diesel fuel and tested it in a four-ball machine without the addition of lubricating oil. CIME and POME were blended at 10% and 20% with diesel fuel, respectively. Adding diesel fuel to pure CIME and POME increased the friction coefficient by 27.4% and 22.8%. Oxidation and metal concentration are decreased in PB10 and PB20. PB20 reduced the wear scar diameter compared to other fuels studied, indicating enhanced lubrication performance due to the high lubricating film. Xiao et al. [13] studied the wear behavior of soybean biodiesel with petrodiesel at volume ratios of 20%, 40%, 60%, and 80% of soybean biodiesel (HFRR). They reported that by incorporating biodiesel into the mix, they could minimize the diameter of wear scars on steel–steel contact by 24.7%. The combination of WC biodiesel and ethylene glycol (EG) results in dioleoyl ethylene glycol ester (biolubricant) that meets the ISO VG68 viscosity grade standards [14]. Sesame seed oil, safflower oil, soyabean oil, castor bean oil, chicken fat, and *Litseacubeba* kernel oil are the oils having the majority of research on the lubricity and wear properties of the oils biodiesel [15].

1.2 BIODIESEL AND ITS PRODUCTION

Biodiesel is made from feedstocks like non-edible, edible, and waste oil converted into methyl or ethyl esters from having long-chain fatty acids. The physicochemical characteristics of biodiesel are equivalent to regular diesel fuel, making it an excellent fuel for diesel engines. It is an enticing renewable fuel for the energy sector because of its unique properties, such as its lack of sulfur, more cetane number and flash point, less toxicity, and supportability to the environment. The lack of sulfur in the fuel enhances the engine's life. Because biodiesel has a higher flash point than regular diesel, it may be safely stored [16]. Because biodiesel emits less harmful emissions than diesel, it is better for the environment. Pollutants in engine exhaust are detrimental to people's health. Exhaust emissions cause headaches, fatigue, respiratory troubles, and other health problems. The European Academies Science Advisory Council (EASAC) categorized biodiesels based on the feedstock style. Biodiesel is divided into four groups: Feedstocks like edible, non-edible, and derived from waste are the first, second, and third generations, respectively. Solar biodiesel feedstocks are artificial biotic technology-based fourth-generation biodiesel feedstocks. This method augments the biodiesel class by increasing photon to fuel conversion efficiency (PFCE). The study of feedstocks in the fourth generation is still in its early phases because their manufacturing is relatively costly; third-generation biodiesel feedstocks are the most encouraging causes of biodiesel fabrication. Table 1.1 shows the different third-generation biodiesel feedstocks and their main reasons, oil outputs, and noteworthy producing countries.

TABLE 1.1

Third-Generation Fuel Sources with Feedstocks, Oil Yield Percentage, and Their Noteworthy Producing Countries.

Feedstock	Origin	Yield (%)	Major producing countries	References
Waste cooking oil	Used oil from restaurants and hostel mess	26–29	Japan, Europe, Malaysia, China, USA	[17]
Waste oil	Biomass, plastic waste	38–42	Japan, China	[18]
Tallow oil	Fat from beef and pig	42–55	China, Australia, Malaysia	[7]
Algae oil	Sea, ponds	25–75	Israel, USA, Japan, Taiwan	[19]
Grease oil	Homes, schools, restaurants, apartments	60–70	Russia, USA, China	[20]

1.3 WASTE COOKING OIL AND ITS CONVERSION TO BIODIESEL

Manufacturers think of their struggles in employing low-cost feedstock, such as waste oils [21]. Waste oils are manufactured in significant quantities in every country, and if a proper disposal system is not in place, they might damage water resources. Waste oils can come from various sources, including food, non-food, restaurant, and household waste. Biodiesel can be made from non-food feedstocks such as waste tire oil, waste plastic oils, etc. To generate biodiesel from these feedstocks, the pyrolysis method is typically utilized. WCO is a waste product that can be used to create biodiesel. It is made from various culinary oils. In 2020–21, worldwide edible oil consumption will reach 193.25 MMT. The most popular edible oils are soybean, coconut, cottonseed, sunflower, rapeseed, and other vegetable oils. The percentage of these oils in worldwide edible oil consumption is depicted in Figure 1.1.

Biodiesel is a viable substitute for viable diesel because the characteristics are comparable, and low-volume blends do not require any significant modifications to existing compression ignition engines. Some major fuel standards, such as EN590, limit biodiesel consumption in diesel fuel blends to retain the fuel's low-temperature performance and lessen the impact on sealing materials. These are well-known issues with biodiesel use. Biodiesel has several advantages over commercial diesel, including lower CO, HCs, and soot emissions, while some studies have found a small increase in NOx emissions and brake-specific fuel consumption. The fatty acid concentration or degree of unsaturation of the feedstock corresponds with the

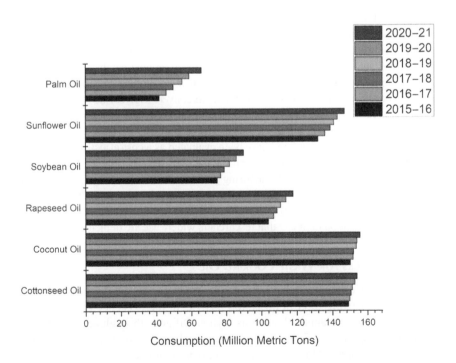

FIGURE 1.1 Oil consumption of edible oils globally during different years.

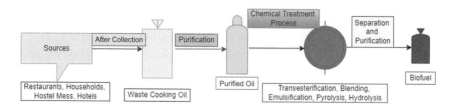

FIGURE 1.2 Process of collection of waste cooking oil and its conversion process to biofuel.

fuel characteristics of biodiesel. The biodiesel fuel characteristics must meet ASTM D6751 or EN 14214 requirements to be qualified as a diesel alternative and used in ground transportation [22–24].

Transesterification is traditionally catalyzed by a base catalyst, improving reaction efficiency and yielding high-purity biodiesel. However, the transesterification process can only be carried out with low free fatty acid (FFA) content feedstock since excessive levels of FFA will react with the base catalyst and result in saponification. Due to catalyst degradation and saponification-induced triacylglycerol hydrolysis, the yield of fatty acid methyl esters (FAME) is low [25,26]. Before biofuel manufacturing, it is critical to know the oil characteristics in the case of WCO. This is due to variations in WCO characteristics produced by frying mode and parameters such as frying time, oil re-use, and the type of fried meals in terms of sugar and protein content, which can result in polymers dimers, oxidized triglycerides, and free fatty acids. As a result, determining if the WCO contains a high acid value is critical for improving the output and efficiency of biodiesel synthesis. A two-step biodiesel synthesis method is frequently used to minimize the acid value of high-FFA oils. The first stage is the esterification process, which converts FFA into biodiesel and is often catalyzed by an acid catalyst such as H_2SO_4 or HCl as a pre-treatment. The classic transesterification procedure is frequently catalyzed by a base catalyst such as KOH or NaOH to convert triglyceride and alcohol into FAME and glycerol. In addition to traditional acid and base catalysts, non-conventional catalysts such as enzymes, industrial waste, and biologically derived catalysts can be utilized to catalyze the process and have been evaluated as a cost-effective and environmentally beneficial technique. Aside from the catalyst, the reaction can be sped up or slowed down by changing the manufacturing procedures [25,27]. The goal is to increase the mixability of the solvents to speed up the response and create more biodiesel, even though the methods differ in reaction mechanism and conditions. The complex procedures for the purification of WCO that researchers widely use are depicted in Figure 1.2.

1.3.1 Feedstocks for Waste Cooking Oil

For frying, edible oils are widely used in food manufacturing and fast food industries. The process of heating food in oil at 160–220 °C in the existence of antioxidants, moisture, and pro-oxidants is known as frying. Oil goes through several reactions during the frying process, including oxidation, hydrolysis, breakdown, polymerization, and isomerization. Once the frying process is complete, these oils are reflected in waste and can be used to generate biodiesel. Edible oils, including canola, corn,

Sustainability of Waste Cooking Oil

palm, canola, cottonseed, mustard, and others, are used to manufacture biodiesel once used for frying or cooking. The leading WCO manufacturers are the United States, China, the European Union, Malaysia, and Japan [7,28–30].

1.3.2 WASTE COOKING OIL PROPERTIES

While vegetable oil is used for frying, it undergoes physical and chemical changes. Oil volatility declines, and molecular weight upsurges as oligomeric molecules are formed during frying. Oleic acid (43.78%) and linoleic acid (43.78%) make up the majority of WCO (36.12%). When the FFA profile of biodiesel changes, the physicochemical properties of the fuel change. The number of double or unsaturated bonds and the carbon chain length influence the fatty acid profile. Carbon atoms tend to bond to as many hydrogen atoms as possible in these chains. Straight-chain fatty acids like stearic acid don't have double bonds. Linoleic acid is categorized as an unsaturated fatty acid due to double bonds. The carbon atom does not attach the maximal amount of hydrogen atoms due to double bonds in the unsaturated fatty acid chain. Changes in physicochemical characteristics affect the performance of biodiesel in CI engines. WCO's transesterified biodiesel has more viscosity, poor combustion features, and a great carbon residue Conradson. Table 1.2 summarizes the physicochemical characteristics of WCO biodiesel and diesel fuel.

1.3.2.1 Cetane Number

The cetane number of gasoline determines its explosion superiority (CN). When the CN of the fuel is high, the ignition delay is shortened. The most versatile CN range is between 44 and 64. WCO biodiesel has a CN ranging from 46.3 to 58.7. There is a difference because biodiesel is generated from WCO, which originates from various food oils, such as palm, canola, and rapeseed.

1.3.2.2 Density

The maximum density of biodiesel allowed at 15 °C is 890 kg/m^3. There are various standards for identifying density, like ASTM D 1298 and EN ISO 12185/3675.

1.3.2.3 Viscosity

The highest restraining value of viscosity, according to ASTM standards, is 6.0 mm^2/s. The kinematic viscosity of WCO is very more in value. Fuel atomization is poor due to the high viscosity, and engine performance decreases. The transesterification procedure reduces this quantity.

1.3.2.4 Calorific Value

Except for algae-based biodiesel, biodiesel fuels have a lower calorific value (LCV) than diesel fuel. WCO biodiesel has an LCV ranging from 39.26 to 42.56 MJ/kg. The brake-specific fuel consumption was low, and the thermal efficiency was good due to the higher LCV.

1.3.2.5 Value of Saponification

With arise in FFA and moisture content, the saponification value (SV) rises. More soap is formed when the oil contains a high level of FFA and water. In the frying of

TABLE 1.2
Comparison Between Properties of Waste Cooking Oil and Diesel Fuel.

Properties	Units	Diesel	WCO biodiesel	References
Higher calorific value	MJ/kg	43.18	38.92	[30]
Density @ 15 °C	kg/m³	834–876	892–897	[18]
Flash point	°C	72	156	[31]
Pour point	°C	5.4	6.8	[7]
Self-ignition temperature	°C	262	-	[29]
Free fatty acids	(% wt.)	-	0.82	[32]
Saponification value	(mg KOH/g)	-	208	[33]
Iodine number	(1 g/100g)	87	4–9	[34]

edible oils, this value for waste oil increases. The SV for waste oil biodiesel is 208 mg KOH/g (Table 1.2).

1.3.2.6 Acid Value

The biodiesel acid number (AN) measures the content of fuel-free fatty acid (FFA). Because of the frying operation, the acid number of waste oil increases. Most standards set a maximum value allowed for acid number at 0.60 mg KOH/g, except for the GB/T 20828 standards (0.80 mg KOH/g).

1.3.3 COMPARISON OF WASTE COOKING OIL WITH OTHER FEEDSTOCKS

The majority of waste oils come from first-generation feedstocks. Non-edible sources are used to make some waste oils, such as waste tire oil and waste plastic oil. Due to the frying process, WCO has different physicochemical properties than parent vegetable oils. The frying procedure alters the physicochemical characteristics of the food due to hydrolysis and oxidation reactions. These reactions raise the FFA and moisture content of the WCO in the biodiesel synthesis process, resulting in soap production. If the water content in WCO biodiesel is too high, engine parts may degrade. WCO also causes engine wear with a high FFA level. WCO must be pre-treated before the transesterification reaction for these reasons. The moisture content is reduced to less than 0.27%, and the acid number (AN) is less than 1 mg KOH/g throughout the pre-treatment process. Waste oils are a better option for biodiesel production since they are less expensive than first-generation feedstocks. WCO is a more cost-effective feedstock than jatropha, Karanja, mahua, algae, and other second- and third-generation feedstocks.

1.4 ASPECTS OF BIODIESEL FOR TRIBOLOGICAL APPLICATIONS

The study of analyzing two moving bodies or surface interactions while in motion relative to each other is called tribology. Friction, lubrication, wear, corrosion, metal surface deprivation, engine lifespan, and loss of energy are all issues that must be

Sustainability of Waste Cooking Oil

considered. Because these processes waste a lot of energy, reducing and eliminating friction and wear losses is vital.

Even though biodiesel has highlighted several environmental and fossil fuel depletion concerns, tribologists face significant obstacles. One of the most crucial difficulties is car material compatibility with biodiesel fuel. When using biodiesel, essential components like the cylinder, piston, piston rings, bearings, and so on are extremely important. Biodiesel is now blended with conventional diesel in various percentages, including B10 (10% biodiesel and 90% conventional gasoline), B20, B40, and B50 (10% biodiesel and 50% conventional fuel). Wear and friction, corrosion, and tribo-corrosive are some of the material compatibility difficulties of biodiesel, discussed in this study [30].

1.4.1 Friction and Wear of Biodiesel

Tribologists are putting forth a lot of effort to overwhelm the issues with engine parts and fuel contact. The fuel approaches various parts, like fuel tank, filter, piston and piston rings, connecting rods, liners, and connecting rods. As a result, numerous experiments involving different diesel-biodiesel blends have been carried out in demand to recognize the better friction and wear mechanism in fuels with diesel engine applications. Fazal et al. [35] performed a four-ball test on diverse blends for 1 hour with a fixed load and variable speeds and discovered that the percentage of biodiesel in the mix was increased, resulting in decreased wear. According to the research, the wear scar diameter diminishes as the number of biodiesel increases. The same pattern was observed in the case of the coefficient of friction. As the proportion of biodiesel in the blend grows, the friction coefficient decreases. Kumar et al. [36] discovered a small shift in the trend, with B40 wear scar value of 0.62 mm and B100 of 0.68 mm, respectively. In their experiment, increasing the amount of biodiesel from 40% to 100% augmented the wear scar diameter. Under a load of 60 kg, the drift in coefficient of friction for B40 and B100 followed a similar pattern. Sorate et al. [37] investigated the wear of piston rings. As a long-term usage test, a diesel and biodiesel engine was run for 512 hours. The uppermost piston ring lost the greatest weight when exposed to the highest temperature. Afterward, the initial ring, the compression ring, was found to have larger bulk damage. The oil ring had the smallest weight loss. Biodiesel resulted in a greater overall weight loss. Figure 1.3 shows the loss of weight in piston rings having blends.

Kalam and Masjuki [38] investigated the effects of material wear in biodiesel and diesel in an experiment. They used a 300-hour engine with 15% palm biodiesel and 85% diesel. The engine wore down less with B15 than with diesel fuel because there were fewer wear elements in oil samples. Agarwal et al. [39] tested a B20 blend for 500 hours and reported less wear. Agarwal et al. [40] discovered that biodiesel caused less harm in another field test. For 512 hours, two identical engines were run, one with B20 and the other with standard diesel fuel. According to the data, the carbon deposited on the system tested with B20 was 40% less than a diesel-powered engine. A diesel-fueled system injector tip had more carbon deposition after 200 hours than a B20-fueled system injection after 512 hours. Several researchers used biodiesel in engines for 2–4 years [41–43]. Their findings revealed engine wear nearly identical to that caused by diesel fuel.

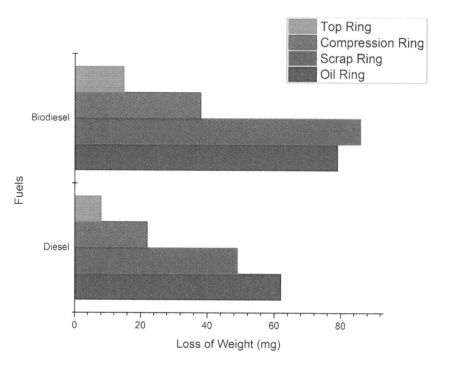

FIGURE 1.3 Loss of weight for a pin during different fuels.

The data suggest that while biodiesel reduces friction and wear in the near term, long-term use is still a concern. Based on these data, it may be concluded that biodiesel has a higher lubricity and, thus, less wear than regular diesel in short-term experiments. On the other hand, long-term testing reveals biodiesel loses lubricity with time and wears out similarly to diesel fuel. This is due to biodiesel's tendency to auto-oxidize. When exposed to oxygen, biodiesel undergoes auto-oxidation, which is increased by high temperatures. When biodiesel is kept or even cycled in an engine, it oxidizes. This is because biodiesel has more unsaturated fatty acids and more carbon-to-carbon double bonds in its chemical composition. Auto-oxidation reduces viscosity, cloud point, flash point, and density, impairing engine performance and life by increasing wear, corrosion, and tribo-corrosion [44–46].

1.4.2 Biodiesel Corrosion

Many engine parts come into contact with fuel, including fuel injectors, pumps, rings, filters, and bearings. According to investigations, carbon steel, aluminum, and stainless steel materials are moderately friendly with biodiesel. Zinc, lead, tin, copper, bronze, and brass are all incompatible with biodiesel. These materials damage biodiesel's steadiness and make it more acidic [47–49].

A number of factors cause the corrosiveness of biodiesel. Biodiesel has a higher hygroscopicity than regular diesel fuel. Moisture and water content build in biodiesel

Sustainability of Waste Cooking Oil

after long storage, hastening the breakdown of ester bonds. The formation of free fatty acids (FFA) increases corrosiveness [50,51]. Auto-oxidation, microbial attack, residual pollutants after the trans-esterification process, and light and temperature contribute to biodiesel's corrosiveness.

Sgroi et al. [52] used sintered bronze filters at 70°C to test bronze in biodiesel for 10 hours. On the surface, they noticed pitting corrosion. Static immersion studies for copper and leaded bronze in B0, B50, and B100 were done by Haseeb et al. [53]. They submerged these materials for 2640 hours in the abovementioned fuels at room temperature. According to their research, copper is more prone to corrosion in biodiesel than leaded bronze. Several different scientists have looked into the causes of biodiesel corrosion. In a static immersion test, Kaul et al. [54] employed non-edible biodiesels *Jatrophacurcas*, *Salvadoraoleoides*, *Madhuca indica*, and *Pongamiaglabra*. They immersed cut engine parts, such as piston metal and piston liner, in fuels at room temperature for 300 days. All biodiesel samples lost weight in the piston liner scenario; however, none of the test materials produced gum. Geller et al. [55] corrosion investigations corroborate these findings. Copper, aluminum, brass, bronze, and zinc have also been proposed as incompatible metals for biodiesel. Fazal et al. [35] conducted immersion experiments on copper surfaces in palm biodiesel. They discovered microscopic pits on a copper surface that had been dipped for 200 hours. As the biodiesel immersion time is increased, these pits appear to progress. As the oxygen concentration in the water enriched with time spent immersed, these pits grew larger. The corrosion rate of mild steel increased as the temperature was raised for both diesel and biodiesel fuel. At room temperature, it was discovered that the corrosion rates for diesel and biodiesel are 0.046 and 0.052 mpy, respectively. The corrosion rate in diesel lowers to 0.05 mpy and 0.059 mpy in biodiesel when the temperature is raised to 80 °C. As a result, biodiesel is more corrosive than conventional diesel.

As biodiesel fuel degrades, its properties change. Changes in the TAN number, viscosity, density, cetane number, flash point, and other factors promote corrosion. Furthermore, the feedstock affects the corrosiveness of biodiesel [56]. Non-edible Jatrophacurcas, Pongamiaglabra (Karanja), Madhucaindica (Mahua), and Salvadoraoleoides (Pilu) oils were studied by Kaul et al. [54]. Biodiesel from Zuleta et al. [57] showed clear deterioration on both metal parts of the diesel engine compared to regular diesel fuel; however, biodiesel from other oils exhibited little or no damage.

Because biodiesel is more prone to oxidation than regular diesel, several studies have concluded it is more corrosive. The corrosiveness of biodiesel is typically investigated using static immersion tests. As the percentage of biodiesel in the blend increases, the rate of biodiesel corrosion increases. Corrosion happens even with a small percentage of 2–5% biodiesel in the blend [58–60]. Additional research is needed to make biodiesel more compatible with engine materials and alleviate the corrosion problem.

1.5 ROLE OF ADDITIVES IN BIODIESEL

Biodiesel has problems with oxidation and thermal and storage constancy. Because bonds have a saturated form, biodiesel is easily oxidized and loses its endurance.

Jayadas et al. [61] tested the oxidative stability of Karanja biodiesel over a lengthy period and discovered that as the peroxide value and viscosity grew, so did the oxidative stability. Refining biodiesel and adding additives early in production is a very productive and cost-effective solution to overcome biodiesel stability and use problems. The use of alkaline catalysts in the synthesis of biodiesel, such as sodium hydroxide (NaOH), potassium hydroxide (KOH), and sodium and potassium methoxides (CH_3ONa and CH_3OK), results in a larger biodiesel yield, but it also promotes soap formation. As a result, refining biodiesel is crucial. Membrane technology, a new way of refining and purifying biodiesel, has simplified and improved the process. Biodiesel can be purified and refined to improve its lubricity and compatibility with engine parts. Chemicals added to fuels to improve efficiency and fuel economy are additives [62,63]. Adding additives to biodiesel has been shown to increase lubrication. They also assist the gasoline in meeting environmental emission restrictions while improving engine performance.

Adding additives to the emissions and performance of a biodiesel-diesel blend engine is a straightforward and effective procedure. Antioxidants, for example, slow biodiesel degradation considerably. Under accelerated controlled conditions, Dunn [64] investigated the effects of oxidation on methyl Soyate (SME) fuel characteristics. The tests were conducted at temperatures of up to 150 °C. He discovered that the antioxidants TBHQ and tocopherol effectively reduced oxidative damage under these conditions. The antioxidant pyrogallol (PY) was the most effective on metal-contaminated biodiesel/diesel blends utilizing Jatropha biodiesel by Jain et al. [65]. Sarin et al. [66] investigated the oxidation stability of the extremely stable Palm methyl ester (PME) in the presence of metal pollutants at 110 °C with different antioxidant dosages. The antioxidant TBHQ was discovered to be the most effective of them all. After testing biodiesel blends and antioxidant additives, Karavalakis et al. [67] found that PG, PA, and TBHQ were the most effective in simple methyl esters, while BHA and BHT were the least effective. A similar conclusion was reached in another investigation by Sarin et al. [68], in which the effects of natural and synthetic antioxidants on non-edible biodiesel oxidation stability were analyzed. Natural and synthetic antioxidants both enhanced biodiesel OS, but synthetic antioxidants outperformed natural antioxidants. Artificial additives such as PG, BHT, PY, and others are widely used. Wear and friction are improved by adding chemicals. They enhance the performance of automobile engines by preventing biodiesel auto-oxidation [62,69–71].

1.6 CONCLUSIONS AND SUGGESTIONS

The current review study brings together the most current knowledge on WCO biodiesel production and its use in CI engines. WCO is a biofuel that belongs to the third generation of biofuels. Around 30% of edible oil consumption per capita is wasted. WCO reduces the cost of producing biodiesel while simultaneously easing the burden on waste disposal facilities. WCO is generated from fried edible oils. Food processing industries, restaurants, and private houses can all provide WCO. This WCO contains a lot of water and FFA. Pre-treatment of oil is required before biodiesel production to reduce these values.

Sustainability of Waste Cooking Oil

With characteristics like biodegradability, environmental friendliness, renewability, and enhanced lubrication, biodiesel generated from spent cooking oil is a viable alternative to standard diesel fuel. Still, it poses significant wear, friction, and injection pin clogging risks to engine components. Storage, high temperatures, moisture absorption, and metal contamination can all affect the characteristics of biodiesel. While the qualities of biodiesel, when obtained, fulfill the stated requirements, they can vary as it degrades. According to literature studies, biodiesel from WCO has been shown to minimize wear and friction when used for a short length of time. When using biodiesel for a long time, the wear and friction are comparable to diesel. Because WCO biodiesel is more corrosive than regular diesel, it poses significant issues to vehicle engine components.

When stored for a long time, WCO biodiesel is hygroscopic, absorbing moisture from the air. It also oxidizes at higher temperatures, increasing the free water amount even more. As a result, the characteristics of WCO biodiesel deteriorate. The oxidation stability of biodiesel is harmed by exposure to certain metals and pollutants. Metal impurities reduce the induction time (IP) of biodiesel while increasing the water content, acid value (AV), and peroxide value of the fuel (PV). However, more research is needed to assess its potential for separating and purifying biodiesel mixtures. Furthermore, additives improve the oxidation stability of plain biodiesels, indicating that they should be used.

While significant research has been done on improving biodiesel stability, additional research, development, and commercialization are still needed to reduce the negative impacts of the constituents that cause biodiesel instability and fuel deterioration. To reduce the corrosiveness of biodiesel and stabilize its oxidation process, more research on the best anti-corrosion and antioxidant additives is needed.

REFERENCES

[1] Veljković, V. B., S. H. Lakićević, O. S. Stamenković, Z. B. Todorović, and M. L. Lazić, "Biodiesel production from tobacco (Nicotiana tabacum L.) seed oil with a high content of free fatty acids," *Fuel*, vol. 85, pp. 2671–2675, 2006/12/01.

[2] Palash, S., M. Kalam, H. Masjuki, B. Masum, I. R. Fattah, and M. Mofijur, "Impacts of biodiesel combustion on NOx emissions and their reduction approaches," *Renewable and Sustainable Energy Reviews*, vol. 23, pp. 473–490, 2013.

[3] Fangsuwannarak, K., and K. Triratanasirichai, "Improvements of palm biodiesel properties by using nano-TiO$_2$ additive, exhaust emission and engine performance," *Romanian Review of Precision Mechanics, Optics & Mechatronics*, vol. 43, pp. 111–118, 2013.

[4] Naresh Kumar Reddy, S., and M. Marouf Wani, "Engine performance and emission studies by application of nanoparticles as additive in biodiesel diesel blends," *Materials Today: Proceedings*, vol. 43, pp. 3631–3634, 2021/01/01.

[5] Zhang, Y., M. Dube, D. McLean, and M. Kates, "Biodiesel production from waste cooking oil: 2. Economic assessment and sensitivity analysis," *Bioresource Technology*, vol. 90, pp. 229–240, 2003.

[6] Juan, J. C., D. A. Kartika, T. Y. Wu, and T.-Y. Y. Hin, "Biodiesel production from Jatropha oil by catalytic and non-catalytic approaches: An overview," *Bioresource Technology*, vol. 102, pp. 452–460, 2011/01/01.

[7] Dhanasekaran, R., S. Ganesan, B. Rajesh Kumar, and S. Saravanan, "Utilization of waste cooking oil in a light-duty DI diesel engine for cleaner emissions using bio-derived propanol," *Fuel*, vol. 235, pp. 832–837, 2019/01/01.

[8] Ağbulut, Ü., M. K. Yeşilyurt, and S. Sarıdemir, "Wastes to energy: Improving the poor properties of waste tire pyrolysis oil with waste cooking oil methyl ester and waste fusel alcohol–A detailed assessment on the combustion, emission, and performance characteristics of a CI engine," *Energy*, vol. 222, p. 119942, 2021.

[9] Silitonga, A. S., H. H. Masjuki, H. C. Ong, F. Kusumo, T. M. I. Mahlia, and A. H. Bahar, "Pilot-scale production and the physicochemical properties of palm and Calophyllum inophyllum biodiesels and their blends," *Journal of Cleaner Production*, vol. 126, pp. 654–666, 2016/07/10.

[10] Dharma, S., H. C. Ong, H. Masjuki, A. Sebayang, and A. Silitonga, "An overview of engine durability and compatibility using biodiesel–bioethanol–diesel blends in compression-ignition engines," *Energy Conversion and Management*, vol. 128, pp. 66–81, 2016.

[11] Zulkifli, N., M. Kalam, H. Masjuki, M. Shahabuddin, and R. Yunus, "Wear prevention characteristics of a palm oil-based TMP (trimethylolpropane) ester as an engine lubricant," *Energy*, vol. 54, pp. 167–173, 2013.

[12] Mosarof, M., M. Kalam, H. Masjuki, A. Alabdulkarem, M. Habibullah, A. Arslan, et al., "Assessment of friction and wear characteristics of Calophyllum inophyllum and palm biodiesel," *Industrial Crops and Products*, vol. 83, pp. 470–483, 2016.

[13] Xiao, H., H. Zou, S. Liu, and C. Li, "An investigation of the friction and wear behavior of soybean biodiesel," *Tribology International*, vol. 131, pp. 377–385, 2019.

[14] Mariod, A. A., M. E. Saeed Mirghani, and I. Hussein, "Chapter 3—Cassia obtusifolia (Senna or Sicklepod Seed)," in *Unconventional Oilseeds and Oil Sources*, A. A. Mariod, M. E. Saeed Mirghani, and I. Hussein, Eds. Academic Press, pp. 13–19, 2017.

[15] Silitonga, A., H. Masjuki, T. Mahlia, H. Ong, W. Chong, and M. Boosroh, "Overview properties of biodiesel diesel blends from edible and non-edible feedstock," *Renewable and Sustainable Energy Reviews*, vol. 22, pp. 346–360, 2013.

[16] Farooq, A., S. S. Lam, G. H. Rhee, J. Lee, M. A. Khan, B.-H. Jeon, *et al.*, "Technical benefits of using methane as a pyrolysis medium for catalytic pyrolysis of Kraft Lignin," *Bioresource Technology*, p. 127131, 2022.

[17] Hamze, H., M. Akia, and F. Yazdani, "Optimization of biodiesel production from the waste cooking oil using response surface methodology," *Process Safety and Environmental Protection*, vol. 94, pp. 1–10, 2015.

[18] Dabai, M., F. Owuna, M. Sokoto, and A. Abubakar, "Assessment of quality parameters of ecofriendly biolubricant from waste cooking palm oil," *Asian Journal of Applied Chemistry Research*, pp. 1–11, 2018.

[19] Haik, Y., M. Y. E. Selim, and T. Abdulrehman, "Combustion of algae oil methyl ester in an indirect injection diesel engine," *Energy*, vol. 36, pp. 1827–1835, 2011/03/01.

[20] He, Q., A. Li, Y. Guo, S. Liu, and L. Kong, "Effect of nanometer silicon dioxide on the frictional behavior of lubricating grease," *Nanomaterials and Nanotechnology*, vol. 7, p. 1847980417725933, 2017.

[21] Subramonian, W., T. Y. Wu, and S.-P. Chai, "An application of response surface methodology for optimizing coagulation process of raw industrial effluent using Cassia obtusifolia seed gum together with alum," *Industrial Crops and Products*, vol. 70, pp. 107–115, 2015/08/01.

[22] Mahalingam, A., Y. Devarajan, S. Radhakrishnan, S. Vellaiyan, and B. Nagappan, "Emissions analysis on mahua oil biodiesel and higher alcohol blends in diesel engine," *Alexandria Engineering Journal*, pp. 2627–2631, 2017/08/30.

[23] Pandit, P. R., and M. H. Fulekar, "Egg shell waste as heterogeneous nanocatalyst for biodiesel production: Optimized by response surface methodology," *Journal of Environmental Management*, vol. 198, pp. 319–329, 2017/08/01.

[24] Damanik, N., H. C. Ong, W. T. Chong, and A. S. Silitonga, "Biodiesel production from Calophyllum inophyllum–palm mixed oil," *Energy Sources, Part A: Recovery, Utilization, and Environmental Effects*, vol. 39, pp. 1283–1289, 2017/06/18.

[25] Elkelawy, M., S. E.-D. H. Etaiw, M. I. Ayad, H. Marie, M. Dawood, H. Panchal, et al., "An enhancement in the diesel engine performance, combustion, and emission attributes fueled by diesel-biodiesel and 3D silver thiocyanate nanoparticles additive fuel blends," *Journal of the Taiwan Institute of Chemical Engineers*, pp. 369–380, 2021/02/26.

[26] Sunil, S., B. S. Chandra Prasad, S. Kakkeri, and Suresha, "Studies on titanium oxide nanoparticles as fuel additive for improving performance and combustion parameters of CI engine fueled with biodiesel blends," *Materials Today: Proceedings*, vol. 44, pp. 489–499, 2021/01/01.

[27] Joshi, H. C., N. Grag, S. Kumar, and W. Ahmad, "Influence of the catalytic activity of MgO catalyst on the comparative studies of Schlichera oleosa, Michelia champaca and Putranjiva based biodiesel and its blend with ethanol-diesel," *Materials Today: Proceedings*, vol. 38, pp. 18–23, 2021/01/01.

[28] Katre, G., S. Raskar, S. Zinjarde, V. Ravi Kumar, B. D. Kulkarni, and A. Ravi Kumar, "Optimization of the in situ transesterification step for biodiesel production using biomass of Yarrowia lipolytica NCIM 3589 grown on waste cooking oil," *Energy*, vol. 142, pp. 944–952, 2018/01/01.

[29] Singh, P., and V. Goel, "Effect of bio-lubricant on wear characteristics of cylinder liner-piston ring and cam-tappet combination in simulated environment," *Fuel*, vol. 233, pp. 677–684, 2018/12/01.

[30] Abbas Ali, S., S. Hunagund, S. Sameer Hussain, and A. Hussain Bagwan, "The effect of nanoparticles dispersed in waste cooking oil (WCO) biodiesel on thermal performance characteristics of VCR engine," *Materials Today: Proceedings*, vol. 43, pp. 888–891, 2021/01/01.

[31] Kataria, J., S. Mohapatra, and K. Kundu, "Biodiesel production from waste cooking oil using heterogeneous catalysts and its operational characteristics on variable compression ratio CI engine," *Journal of the Energy Institute*, vol. 92, pp. 275–287, 2019.

[32] Milano, J., H. C. Ong, H. H. Masjuki, A. S. Silitonga, W.-H. Chen, F. Kusumo, et al., "Optimization of biodiesel production by microwave irradiation-assisted transesterification for waste cooking oil-Calophyllum inophyllum oil via response surface methodology," *Energy Conversion and Management*, vol. 158, pp. 400–415, 2018.

[33] Hajjari, M., M. Tabatabaei, M. Aghbashlo, and H. Ghanavati, "A review on the prospects of sustainable biodiesel production: A global scenario with an emphasis on waste-oil biodiesel utilization," *Renewable and Sustainable Energy Reviews*, vol. 72, pp. 445–464, 2017/05/01.

[34] Wang, E., X. Ma, S. Tang, R. Yan, Y. Wang, W. W. Riley, et al., "Synthesis and oxidative stability of trimethylolpropane fatty acid triester as a biolubricant base oil from waste cooking oil," *Biomass and Bioenergy*, vol. 66, pp. 371–378, 2014/07/01.

[35] Fazal, M., A. Haseeb, and H. H. Masjuki, "Investigation of friction and wear characteristics of palm biodiesel," *Energy Conversion and Management*, vol. 67, pp. 251–256, 2013.

[36] Kumar, Varun N., and S. Chauhan, "Analysis of tribological performance of biodiesel," *Proceedings of the Institution of Mechanical Engineers, Part J: Journal of Engineering Tribology*, vol. 228, pp. 797–807, 2014.

[37] Sorate, K. A., and P. V. Bhale, "Biodiesel properties and automotive system compatibility issues," *Renewable and Sustainable Energy Reviews*, vol. 41, pp. 777–798, 2015.

[38] Kalam, M. A., and H. H. Masjuki, "Emissions and deposit characteristics of a small diesel engine when operated on preheated crude palm oil," *Biomass and Bioenergy*, vol. 27, pp. 289–297, 2004/09/01.

[39] Agarwal, D., S. Sinha, and A. K. Agarwal, "Experimental investigation of control of NOx emissions in biodiesel-fueled compression ignition engine," *Renewable Energy*, vol. 31, pp. 2356–2369, 2006/11/01.

[40] Agarwal, D., L. Kumar, and A. K. Agarwal, "Performance evaluation of a vegetable oil fuelled compression ignition engine," *Renewable Energy*, vol. 33, pp. 1147–1156, 2008/06/01.

[41] Jain, A., A. P. Singh, and A. K. Agarwal, "Effect of split fuel injection and EGR on NOx and PM emission reduction in a low temperature combustion (LTC) mode diesel engine," *Energy*, vol. 122, pp. 249–264, 2017.

[42] Agarwal, H., S. V. Kumar, and S. Rajeshkumar, "A review on green synthesis of zinc oxide nanoparticles–An eco-friendly approach," *Resource-Efficient Technologies*, vol. 3, pp. 406–413, 2017.

[43] Patel, C., N. Tiwari, and A. K. Agarwal, "Experimental investigations of Soyabean and Rapeseed SVO and biodiesels on engine noise, vibrations, and engine characteristics," *Fuel*, vol. 238, pp. 86–97, 2019/02/15.

[44] Ren, S., J. Meng, J. Wang, J. Lu, and S. Yang, "Tribo-corrosion behaviors of Ti_3SiC_2/Si_3N_4 tribo-pair in hydrochloric acid and sodium hydroxide solutions," *Wear*, vol. 274–275, pp. 8–14, 2012/01/27.

[45] Araghi, A., and M. H. Paydar, "Wear and corrosion characteristics of electroless Ni–W–P–B4C and Ni–P–B4C coatings," *Tribology—Materials, Surfaces & Interfaces*, vol. 8, pp. 146–153, 2014/09/01.

[46] Ahmadi Ashtiani, A., S. Faraji, S. Amjad Iranagh, and A. H. Faraji, "The study of electroless Ni–P alloys with different complexing agents on Ck45 steel substrate," *Arabian Journal of Chemistry*, vol. 10, pp. S1541–S1545, 2017/05/01.

[47] Tewari, P., E. Doijode, N. Banapurmath, and V. Yaliwal, "Experimental investigations on a diesel engine fuelled with multiwalled carbon nanotubes blended biodiesel fuels," *International Journal of Emerging Technology and Advanced Engineering*, vol. 3, pp. 72–76, 2013.

[48] Hossain, A., M. Ouadi, S. Siddiqui, Y. Yang, J. Brammer, A. Hornung, et al., "Experimental investigation of performance, emission and combustion characteristics of an indirect injection multi-cylinder CI engine fuelled by blends of de-inking sludge pyrolysis oil with biodiesel," *Fuel*, vol. 105, pp. 135–142, 2013.

[49] Khalid, A., N. Tamaldin, M. Jaat, M. F. M. Ali, B. Manshoor, and I. Zaman, "Impacts of biodiesel storage duration on fuel properties and emissions," *Procedia Engineering*, vol. 68, pp. 225–230, 2013.

[50] Kafuku, G., and M. Mbarawa, "Alkaline catalyzed biodiesel production from moringa oleifera oil with optimized production parameters," *Applied Energy*, vol. 87, pp. 2561–2565, 2010/08/01.

[51] Brunet, R., E. Antipova, G. Guillén-Gosálbez, and L. Jiménez, "Reducing the environmental impact of biodiesel production from vegetable oil by use of a solar-assisted steam generation system with heat storage," *Industrial & Engineering Chemistry Research*, vol. 51, pp. 16660–16669, 2012.

[52] Sgroi, M., G. Bollito, G. Saracco, and S. Specchia, "BIOFEAT: Biodiesel fuel processor for a vehicle fuel cell auxiliary power unit: study of the feed system," *Journal of Power Sources*, vol. 149, pp. 8–14, 2005.

[53] Haseeb, A. S. M. A., S. Y. Sia, M. A. Fazal, and H. H. Masjuki, "Effect of temperature on tribological properties of palm biodiesel," *Energy*, vol. 35, pp. 1460–1464, 2010.

[54] Kaul, S., R. Saxena, A. Kumar, M. Negi, A. Bhatnagar, H. Goyal, et al., "Corrosion behavior of biodiesel from seed oils of Indian origin on diesel engine parts," *Fuel Processing Technology*, vol. 88, pp. 303–307, 2007.

[55] Geller, D. P., T. T. Adams, J. W. Goodrum, and J. Pendergrass, "Storage stability of poultry fat and diesel fuel mixtures: specific gravity and viscosity," *Fuel*, vol. 87, pp. 92–102, 2008.

[56] Surana, A. R., Y. Singh, V. H. Rajubhai, K. Suthar, and A. Sharma, "Development of mahua oil as a lubricant additive and its tribological characteristics," *Materials Today: Proceedings*, vol. 25, pp. 724–728, 2020.

[57] Zuleta, E. C., L. A. Rios, and P. N. Benjumea, "Oxidative stability and cold flow behavior of palm, sacha-inchi, Jatropha and castor oil biodiesel blends," *Fuel Processing Technology*, vol. 102, pp. 96–101, 2012.

[58] Alviso, D., G. Artana, and T. Duriez, "Prediction of biodiesel physico-chemical properties from its fatty acid composition using genetic programming," *Fuel*, vol. 264, p. 116844, 2020.

[59] Singh, N. K., Y. Singh, A. Sharma, and E. A. Rahim, "Prediction of performance and emission parameters of Kusum biodiesel based diesel engine using neuro-fuzzy techniques combined with genetic algorithm," *Fuel*, vol. 280, p. 118629, 2020/11/15.

[60] Karagoz, M., C. Uysal, U. Agbulut, and S. Saridemir, "Exergetic and exergoeconomic analyses of a CI engine fueled with diesel-biodiesel blends containing various metal-oxide nanoparticles," *Energy*, vol. 214, p. 118830, 2021.

[61] Jayadas, N., K. P. Nair, and G. Ajithkumar, "Tribological evaluation of coconut oil as an environment-friendly lubricant," *Tribology International*, vol. 40, pp. 350–354, 2007.

[62] Li, W., S. Zheng, B. Cao, and S. Ma, "Friction and wear properties of ZrO_2/SiO_2 composite nanoparticles," *Journal of Nanoparticle Research*, vol. 13, pp. 2129–2137, 2011/05/01.

[63] Habibullah, M., H. H. Masjuki, M. A. Kalam, N. W. M. Zulkifli, B. M. Masum, A. Arslan, et al., "Friction and wear characteristics of Calophyllum inophyllum biodiesel," *Industrial Crops and Products*, vol. 76, pp. 188–197, 2015/12/15.

[64] Dunn, R. O., "Effect of antioxidants on the oxidative stability of methyl soyate (biodiesel)," *Fuel Processing Technology*, vol. 86, pp. 1071–1085, 2005.

[65] Jain, M., U. Chandrakant, V. Orsat, and V. Raghavan, "A review on assessment of biodiesel production methodologies from Calophyllum inophyllum seed oil," *Industrial Crops and Products*, vol. 114, pp. 28–44, 2018/04/01.

[66] Sarin, A., R. Arora, N. P. Singh, R. Sarin, and R. K. Malhotra, "Blends of biodiesels synthesized from non-edible and edible oils: Influence on the OS (oxidation stability)," *Energy*, vol. 35, pp. 3449–3453, 2010/08/01.

[67] Karavalakis, G., D. Hilari, L. Givalou, D. Karonis, and S. Stournas, "Storage stability and ageing effect of biodiesel blends treated with different antioxidants," *Energy*, vol. 36, pp. 369–374, 2011.

[68] Sarin, A., R. Arora, N. Singh, M. Sharma, and R. Malhotra, "Influence of metal contaminants on oxidation stability of Jatropha biodiesel," *Energy*, vol. 34, pp. 1271–1275, 2009.

[69] Hernández Battez, A., R. González, J. L. Viesca, J. E. Fernández, J. M. Díaz Fernández, A. Machado, et al., "CuO, ZrO_2 and ZnO nanoparticles as antiwear additive in oil lubricants," *Wear*, vol. 265, pp. 422–428, 2008/07/31.

[70] Choi, Y., C. Lee, Y. Hwang, M. Park, J. Lee, C. Choi, et al., "Tribological behavior of copper nanoparticles as additives in oil," *Current Applied Physics*, vol. 9, pp. e124–e127, 2009.

[71] Ganesh, D., and G. Gowrishankar, "Effect of nano-fuel additive on emission reduction in a biodiesel fuelled CI engine,"*2011 International Conference on Electrical and Control Engineering*, pp. 3453–3459, 2011.

2 Application of Nanofluids in Solar Desalination Process
A Review

Avinash Yadav[1], Yashvir Singh[1,2], Erween Abd Rahim[2], Prateek Negi[1], Wei-Hsin Chen[3,4,5], Nishant Kumar Singh[6], and Abhishek Sharma[7]

1 Department of Mechanical Engineering, Graphic Era (Deemed to be) University, Dehradun, India
2 Faculty of Mechanical and Manufacturing Engineering, Universiti Tun Hussein Onn Malaysia, Parit Raja, Batu Pahat, Johor, Malaysia
3 Department of Aeronautics and Astronautics, National Cheng Kung University, Tainan, Taiwan
4 Research Centre for Smart Sustainable Circular Economy, Tunghai, Taiwan
5 Department of Mechanical Engineering, National Chin-Yi University of Technology, Taichung, Taiwan
6 Department of Mechanical Engineering, Harcourt Butler Technical University, Kanpur, Uttar Pradesh, India
7 Department of Mechanical Engineering, G L Bajaj Institute of Technology and Management, Greater Noida, Uttar Pradesh, India

CONTENTS

2.1	Introduction	20
2.2	Principle of Solar Desalination	20
2.3	Classification of Solar Desalination	21
2.4	Active Solar Desalination/Distillation System	22
2.5	Passive Solar Still	24
2.6	Use of Nanoparticles in Solar Distillation System	25
2.7	Conclusion	29
References		29

DOI: 10.1201/9781003265597-2

2.1 INTRODUCTION

Fresh water is not only the need of humans but also the need of industries and agriculture. The paucity of fresh water creates problems for human life. As we know, about 71% of the earth is water, but only about 3% of water is available on the earth in pure form. Out of which, 1% is hardly available for our use. The rest 2% is stored in glaciers, ice caps, atmosphere, and soils. The change in climate, increase in pollution on the rivers and lakes, and overconsumption create the scarcity of fresh water. The change in demographic structure and the growth of industrialization increases the demand for fresh water.

History has proven the importance of water for the sustainability of human life and development. Energy and water cannot be separated because they provide the stability of human life and helps civilization. As we know, all historical civilizations have developed on the brink of rivers. Energy is as important as water because it helps the sustainability of life. Two thousand years ago, energy was developed from the water by using its force. Further, this energy is used for the grinding of grain [1].

The Greeks were the first to study energy and water behavior and provide many notions. In the fourth century (384–322 BC), one of the greatest philosophers and scientists of antiquity, Aristotle, provided the idea to convert seawater into a sweet form. They suggested that the vaporization process can help to convert the saline water into a useful form. He also conducted the experiment and proved it [2].

The ocean is the only source of water through which the demand for water can be fulfilled. But the major drawback, however, is their high salinity. Desalinization is the process of removing salt from saline water. The world health organization (WHO) recommends the limit of salinity in water is 500 ppm, and for special cases, it is about 1000 ppm. The water available on the earth has a salinity of about 10,000 ppm, and seawater has a salinity of about 35,000–45,000 ppm. An excessive amount of salinity restricts the direct use of saline water. Its harmful effect can be observed on the human body.

Desalination is the process in which seawater, supply water, and brackish water can be converted into a useful form. This process requires a high amount of energy to achieve the separation of salt from impure water. If the desalination process is done by conventional sources of energy such as fossil fuels, the cost increase will be observed, and the pollution on the environment will also increase [2].

Rainwater is the source of pure water, and the solar desalination process can also be observed in the ecosystem. The solar radiation falling on the ocean is absorbed by the water, the vaporization takes place with the help of the wind, the vapor moves, and the condensation process takes place (up to its dew point). After condensation, the water participates as rain.

2.2 PRINCIPLE OF SOLAR DESALINATION

Solar desalination is the process that removes unnecessary and harmful particles from the water and converts it into a pure form. The advantage of solar desalination over other processes is that it is cost-effective. This process is one of the oldest technology for converting impurities or aquatic water into fresh form.

Application of Nanofluids in Solar Desalination Process

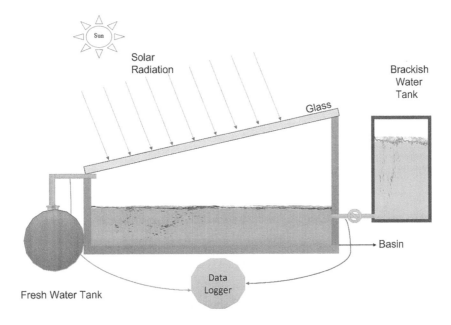

FIGURE 2.1 Solar desalination system.

The main components in the solar desalination process are basin (black), transparent glass cover, and the collection tank, as shown in Figure 2.1. The basin holds the saline water and absorbs solar energy (radiation). The vaporized water condenses on the underside of the glass cover, runs on the trough, and is collected into the tanks. The solar radiation falls on the unit of distillation. Some amount of solar radiation is absorbed and reflected by the glass cover, and the remaining amount of energy is absorbed by the blackened surface (basin). Both the conduction and convection process takes place inside the unit. The thermal energy is convected to the water mass, and the remaining energy is exhausted into the atmosphere by the conduction process.

The water gets heated due to the energy transfer by the convection, and the temperature of the water mass is higher than the glass cover temperature. The vaporization process takes place inside the unit. Water gets evaporated and sticks to the glass cover. Further, it moves toward the collection tank. The inclination of the glass cover plays an important role. Here, the gravity action takes place as well as sufficient surface tension is provided so that the water cannot drop into the basin. The collected water can be used for further operations. Both internal and external heat transfer takes place during this operation.

2.3 CLASSIFICATION OF SOLAR DESALINATION

As time passed, modifications in the solar distill unit and mode of operation have been observed. Solar desalination can be classified between Active solar desalination

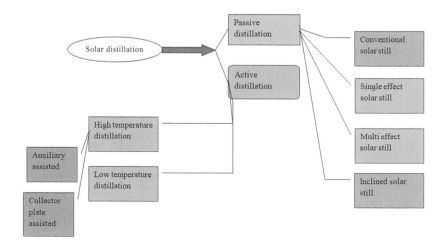

FIGURE 2.2 Classification of solar distillation systems [3].

and Passive solar desalination. Figure 2.2 shows the classification of the solar distillation system.

A detailed study on active solar desalination or passive solar desalination is given below.

2.4 ACTIVE SOLAR DESALINATION/DISTILLATION SYSTEM

Solar energy is available in huge amounts. It provides the best solution for the distillation of water in rural areas or where the availability of fresh water is very less. Solar distillation is a cost-effective method compared to the other methods.

The efficiency of solar still cannot be predicted because the intensity of radiation, the velocity of wind, and ambient temperature cannot be controllable. Only the angle of inclination, depth of the basin, use of material (fabrication), and thickness of the insulation can be controlled. In the active solar distillation system, with the help of external equipment, thermal energy is fed into the still unit to increase the efficiency of the solar still unit. The active solar distillation system can be divided into (i) high-temperature distillation, (ii) pre-heated water application, and (iii) nocturnal production [4].

In high-temperature distillation, the basin is contained with hot water. A constant flow of hot water is maintained in the basin in pre-heated water application, whereas once a day, hot water is supplied in the basin in nocturnal production [5]. The additional solar collector helps to increase the temperature of the basin from 20–50 °C to 70–80°C [6]. There are two modes of circulation of water in the solar distill, that is, natural circulation and forced circulation. The flat plate solar collector coupled with the solar still produces high temperatures and can be used in both circulation methods.

In the forced circulation method, an external device, such as a pump, is used to circulate the water from the basin to the basin via a flat plate collector. A comparative study between coupled and uncoupled flat plate collectors using the forced circulation method was first done by Rai and Tiwari [7] they reported, the distillation rate became 24% higher in the coupled solar collector. In another study, salt is taken into consideration. It enhances the surface tension but decreases the evaporation rate. In another research, the black dye was used as a supplement in the water, and blackened jute cloth was floating over the water in the basin. The result shows an increase in the distillation rate by 30% [8].

Tiwari and Dhiman [9] reported that with an increase in effective area, conventional solar performance is still high. In an active solar distillation system, the insulation in the bottom becomes an important design parameter. In their experimental study, the heat exchanger length increases from 6 m to 12m. They found the yield of the system increased by 12% and the system's overall efficiency increased from 15% to 19%. The study is done for New Delhi climate conditions to observe annual high yield. The flat plate collector has been used in the distilling unit. The study suggested that the angle of inclination for the collector is 20° and that of the glass cover is 15° [10]. Kumar and Tiwari [11] suggested that an increase in the number of solar collectors increases the yield, while with an increase in the area of the basin, a reduction in temperature and loss of thermal efficiency has been observed.

In the natural circulation method, the system uses the thermosyphon modestem because of cost-effectiveness, simplicity, and reliability over the forced circulation method. The comparative study is done by Yadav [12] using a flat plate collector in the solar unit. The result shows that the forced circulation method provides a 5–10% higher yield than the natural circulation method. The solar still is connected with the two flat plate collectors, and the comparative study was done by Tiris et al. [13]. The result shows an increase in 100% yield compared to the ordinary basin solar still unit. In natural circulation mode, the double slope active solar is still used and compared with the passive solar still having a double slope. The result shows active solar still provides a 51% higher yield [14].

The thermosyphon mode is used in active regenerative solar still while considering the climate conditions of New Delhi. The water was floated over the glass cover, enhancing the still's overall performance. Whereas enhancement in output is not observed, and the efficiency is much lower than the passive solar still because active solar still was functioning at higher temperatures [15]. In the regenerative solar still, the increase in solar collector area will decrease the thermal efficiency of the still [16].

Table 2.1 depicts the comparative study and various modes with various types of active solar stills. Many more studies have been conducted over the last decade to analyze and improve the performance of active solar stills. Because it is required in rural and tribal areas where water is scarce or the salinity of the water is high.

In the active solar still, the basin liner is generally made up of aluminum, GI sheet, GRP, FRP, and other materials. But it can be replaced by composite material, and a study should be made on this. The efficiency of active solar stills can be improved by using natural circulation modes in the still, which eliminates the need for electricity.

TABLE 2.1
Study of Active Solar Still Having Different Type and Operation.

Author (s)	Type of still (Active)	Type of solar still	Conclusion
Kumar and Sinha [17]	Regenerative type solar still using concentrator	Double slope	The higher yield is observed due to regeneration
Tiwari and Sinha [18]	Solar still with regeneration	Single basin	Comparative result shows higher yield from flat plate collectors
Tiwari et al. [19]	Pre-heated water solar still	Single basin	It provides high rate of production compared to simple solar still
Voropoulos et al. [20]	Hybrid	Green house	It provides hot water and distilled water simultaneously
Hiroshi et al. [21]	Heat pipe is added into the still	Vertical multiple effect	Best option for high production
Velmurgan et al. [22]	Solar pond coupled with still	Stepped solar still	Suitable for industries. Puzzling construction and payback time about 1 year
Rai et al. [23]	Coupled with flat plate collector (forced circulation)	Single basin	50% higher compared to thermosyphon mode
Badran and Al-Tahaineh [24]	Coupled with flat plate collector (natural circulation)	Single basin	36% higher output than simple solar basin but productivity rate is slow compared with forced circulation

2.5 PASSIVE SOLAR STILL

Solar distillation is the way to purify the saline water into the form that can be used. The distillate output's driving force is the temperature difference between the glass and the surface of the water. The researchers have examined numerous designs for passive solar and improved techniques, designs, and methods over time. The passive solar still study is examined in greater detail below.

The productivity of water is investigated in the traditional solar still by adding dye to the basin. The addition of a die increases the still's productivity [25–29]. In the conventional solar distillation system, the solar's thermal efficiency is still investigated. The results show that the system achieved a thermal efficiency of 60% [30]. Sodha et al. [31] conducted a comparison study of single-basin solar still and double-basin solar still. The researcher observed a 36% increase in production when compared to a single solar still.

The corrugated (blackened) shaped youth jute wick and a swelling sheet of polystyrene was studied by Al Karaghuouli [32]. The comparison with the solar-type basin is still made. The result shows the production increase. The Mc Cracken Porta solar still system, having an area of 8.18 m^2 and insulated at the bottom, was created by Porta et al. [33]. The results show a decrease in overall production

Application of Nanofluids in Solar Desalination Process 25

but an increase in overnight production because of the larger thermal inertia. For routine laboratory work, the solar still, having a size of 60″ × 48″, was constructed by Balladin et al. [34]. The distilled water can be utilized at a lower scale and is also cost-effective.

The comparative study is done between shallow horizontal still and still have a black color aluminum sheet at the top surface, and the bottom is thermally insulated. The experimental setup of aluminum provides higher efficiency [35]. Solars still built by Ward J [36] are obtained by plastic at an environmental temperature of 35°, or approximately 1000 w/m², and observed a distillate output of up to 91 m². Muller-Holst et al. [37] designed a pilot solar multi-effect humidification desalination system. They suggested this type of solar still can be useful in rural areas because of the high quality of drinking water.

Many of the researchers made a theoretical method to examine the performance of the solar still. The productivity of solar still has been examined by floating the water over the glass cover uniformly because it decreases the temperature of the glass cover; hence, the solar's productivity still increases. For this study, the transient performance has still been done on the single solar basin [38]. Lawerence and Tiwari [39] derived an expression to calculate the heat loss during evaporation, and they considered the still in open cycle mode. The expression made by them satisfied with actual. The conventional solar still is taken for the study to derive the expression to calculate the efficiency of the still. They concluded that the system's efficiency increases as the water's mass decreases, whereas other parameters have a fixed value [40].

Many theoretical and experimental studies have been done on passive solar still. The various works over solar distill are listed in Table 2.2.

The researchers perpetually adopt many methods and designing techniques to enhance the performance of the solar still. A new fabrication method can also be adapted to enhance the performance of the solar still.

Nanomaterials can also use to enhance the performance of the solar still. The nanoparticles are continuously adopted due to favorable thermos-physical characteristics. A detailed study on the use of nanoparticles has been studied in the succeeding section.

2.6 USE OF NANOPARTICLES IN SOLAR DISTILLATION SYSTEM

The addition of nanoparticles improves solar distillate systems' overall performance. Because of their beneficial characteristics, nanoparticles are frequently employed. Different criteria such as form, size, content, origin, and the categorization of nanoparticles play an important role [38]. The nanomaterials as Zero, 1-dimensional, 2-dimensional, and 3-dimensional were categorized on the basis of the structure of Sanjay and Pandey [39]. Nanomaterials can be categorized as follows [39]:

Organic: Quants, polymers, liposomes, and dendrimers.
Inorganic: Magnetic and non-magnetic metals and alloys, semiconductors, metal oxide, composite, and various structures of carbon.

TABLE 2.2
Review of Solar Still.

Author (s)	Aim of work	Conclusion
Garg [41], Morse [42], and Cooper [43]	Ambient temperature effect on still performance	As the ambient temperature falls below 26.7°C, decrease in output is observed
Baibutaev et al. [44]	Effect of salt concentration	The distillate output decreased as salt concentration increased beyond the saturation point in the distillation water
El-Wify and Metias [45]	L-type solar still having aspect ratio 2 with glass cover angle of 25°	An increased in productivity is observed
Bannat [46]	Shell and tube module type, an inclination angle of 19°, and an area of 0.98 × 0.98 m	Because of the shell and tune membrane, the salt concentration is negligible
Velmurgan et al. [47]	From a basin type solar still the reflection in radiation from the outer reflector is calculated	For a smaller increase in summer, solar still productivity has been increased and reflector benefits have been increased less in the summer
Prakash and Kavanthekar [48]	Analyzed regenerative type solar still	They discovered that the daily output was approximately 7.5 lm^{-2}
Tiwari and Madhuri [49]	The depth of water has been analyzed using transient method	A strong function of the temperature of the basin in the basin was dependent upon the yield and increased for the initial temperature of basin≤45°C and decreased as the temperature of the basin decreased below 40°C

Nanomaterials are much more to be classified. Nanoparticles enhance the thermophysical characteristics of the basic fluid. The thermal potential of the nanoparticles depends on many factors. Many scientists found the possibility of improving solar energy performance using different nanoparticles. The thermal conductivity and the cost of nanoparticles are summarized in Table 2.3.

The change in heat conductivity and cost are shown in Table 2.1. Thus it can be deduced from the table that the various nanomaterials have differing thermal conductivity, and some cost extremely high, such that they cannot be yet afforded in solar.

The thermal performance monitoring of single solar was still conducted. PCM is a nanoparticle composed of Al_2O_3 and Paraffin Wax (Phase Change Material). Under the baseline and partition where saline water accumulates, the PCM layer is placed. Productivity is compared with PCM and without PCM. The study reveals a 66% improvement in daily efficiency via PCM. Figure 2.1 shows the variation in daily efficacy of solar still with PCM, without PCM, and PCM with nanomaterial [50]. Al_2O_3's nanopowders were utilized on three solar plates using PCM to monitor the thermal activity. When adding thermometer storing materials with Al_2O_3 nanopowder, the experimental findings demonstrate that solar efficiency is still improving. Improvements were found at a water depth of 0.04 m [51].

TABLE 2.3
Thermal Conductivity and Cost of Various Nanoparticles. [40].

Nanopowders	Thermal conductivity (W/m/K)	Quantity	Cost (Indian rupees)
Aluminum oxide (Al_2O_3)	40	25 g	2000
Zinc oxide (ZnO)	29	100 g	1500
Tin oxide (SnO_2)	36	25 g	1500
Iron oxide (Fe_2O_3)	7	25 g	1750
Gold nanopowder (Au)	315	1 g	35,029
Titanium dioxide (TiO_2)	8.5	100 g	12,859
Copper oxide (CuO)	76	5 g	3111
Carbon nanotubes	3000–6000	250 mg	19,521
Zirconium (IV) oxide (ZrO_2)	2	100 mL	10,611
Silicon nitride (Si_3N_4)	29–30	25 g	11,434
Boron nitride (BN)	30–33	50 g	4911
Aluminum nitride (AlN)	140–180	50 g	5193
Diamond nanopowder (C)	900	1 g	8755
Silver nanopowder (Ag)	424	5 g	12,917

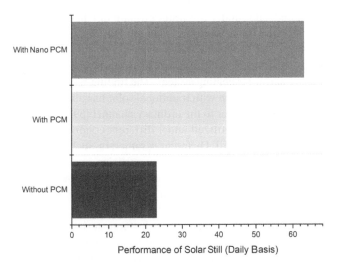

FIGURE 2.3 Daily efficiency of solar still performed.

Kabeel et al. [52] employed graphite nanostructure (hybrid storage material) and paraffin wax for effective distillation monitoring in their solar still experimental setup. The investigation showed that the daily efficacy of solar products was still enhanced by 94.5% and 65.13% at nanoparticular graphite concentrations by 20%. Figure 2.3 shows the daily efficiency of solar still.

In order to calculate the solar-radio absorbent radiation-absorptive nature, a solar distillation system is covered with a blend of black color and TiO_2 nanoparticles. Water depths are 1,2,3, and 3.5 cm throughout the system. In comparison with those without solar coating, researchers reported a 6.1% higher efficiency [53]. Sain and Kumawat [54] have yet to analyze solar performance. The still size is 1 m^2 basin area and isolated from a thermocolate thickness of 50 mm. The combination of Al_2O_3 and black paint is employed for the solar still. The researchers observed that the solar still basin temperature continually increases, improving water efficiency and yield rate. For this analysis, the size of nanoparticles ranged from 50 nm to 100 nm [55]. Thermally insulated coated material made up of 1% SiO_2 and 6% PVF with unsaturated polyester resin was used in solar still. The result showed that as the water's depth increases, the yield capacity decreases, whereas the distillate productivity of water increases by 35% [56].

The changes in the Nusselt number, convective heat transfer, and production rate in distilled water were studied by Sahota et al. [57] utilizing double slope hybrid solar still. The inclination angle is 30° of the glass, which is linked to the heat exchanger and N PV/T solar thermal collector. The research found improved nanofluids H_2O/Al_2O_3, CuO, and TiO_2 mixed with water in the basin under varied climatic conditions and showed an improvement in the number of Nusselt water and the water production and thermal conductivity. Sathyamurthy et al. [58] conducted an experimental trial to examine the maximal yield of nanofluids MgO and TiO_2 under the water climate of Chennai (India). The highest yields for MgO and TiO_2 were 61.89% and 41.05%, respectively, at 0.2% of concentrations.

Cooper oxide nanoparticles are utilized in drum-type solar still linked by an external condenser and solar heating system. The finding reveals that productivity is still 350% higher. A comparison with traditional solar has also been carried out. The solar drum is still much superior to the ordinary channel [59].

Many methods have been utilized under different conditions for years to evaluate the performance of solar still. Different parameters, such as the size of nanomaterial particles, structure, the concentration of particles, and many more properties, become the key function to enhancing the productivity and yield of solar still. Table 2.4 helps find the efficiency of solar still with the use of different types of nanomaterials.

The investigators continue to employ Nobel nanomaterials to further improve the solar's overall performance. The usage of nanofluids continuously increased the total solar performance. In order to examine solar performance, the properties of nanofluids should be analyzed. The researchers should be more concerned with the exergy analysis and the economic-environmental behavior of various materials. There is still a need to study design factors under diverse solar forms such as V-shaped, Wick-type, Tubular, and hemispheric solar.

As the rural area is filled with water scarcity, the distillation system can easily be constructed and utilized there to resolve the problem. The solar systems' efficiency generally varies with the area's latitude, so that the nanoparticles can be added as an additive to enhance the system's overall performance.

TABLE 2.4
Nanomaterials and Its Effect on Yield Performance.

Author (s)	Nanoparticles	Size (nm)	System efficiency
Sain and Kumawat [60]	Al_2O_3	50–100	Thermal efficiency 12.18%
Sharshir et al. [61]	CB and CuO	40	Thermal efficiency with CB 64.15% and with CuO 61%
Abdullah et al. [62]	CuO	10–14	Daily efficiency 85.5%
Safai et al. [63]	GO	-	Yield enhancement by 25%
Kabeel et al. [64]	Graphite	-	Daily efficiency 65.13% at 20% concentration
Muraleedharan et al. [65]	Al_2O_3	-	Daily average thermal efficiency 53.55% at 0.1% concentration

2.7 CONCLUSION

Solar energy technology and its usage are very important for human life. The solar distillation system is one of the best renewable energy sources. The solar distillation system can be used in rural areas or where the scarcity of fresh water. The efficiency of solar distillation can be enhanced by using different types of solar collectors, which enhance the system's heating capacity so that the rate of evaporation will increase. The use of nanomaterials will also enhance the yield capacity and production rate. The investigators continue to employ Nobel nanomaterials to further improve the solar's overall performance. The usage of nanofluids continuously increased the total solar performance.

In order to examine solar performance, the properties of nanofluids should be analyzed. The researchers should be more concerned with the exergy analysis and the economic-environmental behavior of various materials. There is still a need to study design factors under diverse solar forms such as V-shaped, Wick-type, Tubular, and hemispheric solar. It is also observed that the cost of the nanomaterials is too high, so the production rate can be analyzed, and it should be compared with the conventional channel.

As the rural area is filled with water scarcity, the distillation system can easily be constructed and utilized there to resolve the problem. The solar systems' efficiency generally varies with the area's latitude so that the nanoparticles can be added as an additive to enhance the system's overall performance.

REFERENCES

[1] Major JK. Water wind and animal power. In: McNeil, J. (Ed.), *An Encyclopedia of the History of Technology*. Great Britain, Bungay: Rutledge, R. Clay Ltd, 1990; pp. 229–270.

[2] Kalogirou S. Seawater desalination using renewable energy sources. *Progress in Energy and Combustion Science* 2005;31(3):242–281.

[3] Balan R, Chandrasekaran J, Shanmugan S, Janarthanan B, Kumar S. Review on passive solar distillation and water treatment. *Desalination and Water Treatment* 2011;28(1–3):217–238.

[4] Tiwari GN, Tiwari AK. *Solar Distillation Practice for Water Desalination Systems.* New Delhi: Anamaya Publishers, 2008.

[5] Kumar S, Tiwari GN, Singh HN. Annual performance of an active solar distillation system. *Desalination* 2000;127:79–88.

[6] Sampathkumar K, Arjunan VT, Pitchandi P, Senthilkumar P. Active solar distillation-A detailed review. *Renewable ad Sustainable Energy Reviews* 2010;14:1503–1526.

[7] Rai SN, Tiwari GN. Single basin solar still coupled with flat plate collector. *Energy Conversion and Management* 1983;23(3):145–149.

[8] Rai SN, Dutt DK, Tiwari GN. Some experimental studies of single basin solar still. *Energy Conversion and Management* 1990;30(2):149–153.

[9] Tiwari GN, Dhiman NK. Performance study of a high temperature distillation system. *Energy Conversion and Management* 1991;32(3):283–291.

[10] Kumar S, Tiwari GN, Singh HN. Annual performance of an active solar distillation system. *Desalination* 2000;127:79–88.

[11] Kumar S, Tiwari GN. Optimization of collector and basin areas for a higher yield for active solar stills. *Desalination* 1998;116:1–9.

[12] Yadav YP. Analytical performance of a solar still integrated with a flat plate solar collector: thermosiphon mode. *Energy Conversion and Management* 1991;31(3):255–263.

[13] Tiris C, Tiris M, Erdalli Y, Sohmen M. Experimental studies on a solar still coupled with a flat plate collector and a single basin still. *Energy Conversion and Management* 1998;39(8):853–856.

[14] Dwivedi VK, Tiwari GN. Experimental validation of thermal model of double slope active solar still under natural circulation mode. *Desalination* 2010;250(1):49–55.

[15] Singh AK, Tiwari GN. Thermal evaluation of regenerative active solar distillation under thermosyphon mode. *Energy Conversion and Management* 1993;34(8):697–706.

[16] Tiwari GN, Kumar S, Sharma PB, Emran Khan M. Instantaneous thermal efficiency of an active solar still. *Applied Thermal Engineering* 1996;16(2):189–192.

[17] Kumar S, Sinha S. Transient model and comparative study of concentrator coupled regenerative solar still in forced circulation mode. *Energy Conversion and Management* 1996;37(5):629–636.

[18] Tiwari GN, Sinha S. Parametric studies of active regenerative solar still. *Energy Conversion and Management* 1993;34(3):209–218.

[19] Tiwari GN, Madhuri Garg HP. Effect of water flow over the glass cover of a single basin solar still with an intermittent flow of waste hot water in the basin. *Energy Conversion and Management* 1985;25(3):315–322.

[20] Voropoulos K, Mathioulakis E, Belessiotis V. A hybrid solar desalination and water heating system. *Desalination* 2004;164:189–195.

[21] Tanaka H, Nakatake Y, Tanaka M. Indoor experiments of the vertical multiple effect diffusion type solar still coupled with a heat pipe solar collector. *Desalination* 2005;177:291–302.

[22] Velmurugan V, Pandiarajan S, Guruparan P, Subramanian H, David Prabaharan C, Srithar K. Integrated performance of stepped and single basin solar stills with mini solar pond. *Desalination* 2009;249(3):902–909.

[23] Rai SN, Dutt DK, Tiwari GN. Some experimental studies of single basin solar still. *Energy Conversion and Management* 1990;30(2):149–153.

[24] Badran OO, Al-Tahaineh HA. The effect of coupling a flat plate collector on the solar still productivity. *Desalination* 2005;183:137–142.

[25] Sodha MS, Kumar A, Tiwari GN, Pandey GC. Effect of dye on the thermal performance of solar still. *Applied Energy* 1980a;7(1–3):147–162.

Application of Nanofluids in Solar Desalination Process 31

[26] Akash BA, Mohsen MS, Osta O, Elayan Y. Experimental evaluation of a single-basin solar still using different absorbing materials. *Renewable Energy* 1998;14(1–4):307–310.

[27] Al. Hayak, I, Badran OO. The effect of using different design of solar stills on water distillation. *Desalination* 2004;169:121–127.

[28] Cooper PI. Some factors affecting the absorption of solar radiation in solar stills. *Solar Energy* 1972;13(4):373–381.

[29] Garg HP, Mann HS. Effect of climatic, operational and design parameters on the year round performance of single sloped and double sloped solar stills under Indian Arid Zone conditions. *Solar Energy* 1976;18:159–164.

[30] Cooper PI. The maximum efficiency of single effect solar still. *Solar Energy* 1973;15:205–217.

[31] Sodha MS, Nayak JK, Tiwari GN, Kumar A. Double basin solar still. *Energy Convers Manage* 1980b;20(1):23–32.

[32] Al-Karaghouli AA, Minasian AN. A floating-wick type solar still. *Renewable Energy* 1995;6(1):77–79.

[33] Porta MA, Chargoy N, Fernandez JL. Extreme operating conditions in shallow solar stills. *Solar Energy* 1997;61(4):279–286.

[34] Balladin DA, Headley O, Roach A. Evaluation of concrete solar still. *Renewable Energy* 1999;17:191–206.

[35] Rahim NHA. New method to store heat energy in horizontal solar desalination still. *Renewable Energy* 2003;28:419–433.

[36] Ward J. A plastic solar water purifier with high output. *Solar Energy* 2003;75:433–437.

[37] Muller-Holst H, Engelhardt M, Scholkopf W. Small-scale thermal seawater desalination simulation and optimization of system design. *Desalination* 1999;122:255–262.

[38] Tiwari GN, Rao VSVB. Transient performance of a single basin solar still with water flowing over the glass cover. *Desalination* 1984;49:231–241.

[39] Lawrence SA, Tiwari GN. Theoretical evaluation of solar distillation under natural circulation with heat exchanger. *Energy Conversion and Management* 1990;30(3):205–213.

[40] Tiwari GN, Thakur K. An analytical expression for efficiency of solar still. *Energy Conversion and Management* 1991;32(6):595–598.

[41] Garg HP, Mann HS. Effect of climatic, operational and design parameters on the year round performance of single sloped and double sloped solar stills under Indian Arid Zone conditions. *Solar Energy* 1976;18:159–164.

[42] Morse RN, Read WRW. A rational basis for the engineering development of a solar still. *Solar Energy* 1968;12(1):5–17.

[43] Cooper PI. Some factors affecting the absorption of solar radiation in solar stills. *Solar Energy* 1972;13(4):373–381.

[44] Baibutaev KB, Achilov BM, Kamaeva G. Effect of salt concentration on the evaporation process in solar stills. *Geliotekhnika* 1970;6(2):83–85.

[45] El-Wify ME, Metias MZ. Analysis of double exposure solar still. *Renew Energy* 2002;26:531–547.

[46] Bannat F, Jumah R, Garaibeh M. Exploitation of solar energy collected by solar stills for desalination by membrane distillation. *Renew Energy* 2002;25:293–305.

[47] Velmurugan, V, Pandiarajan S, Guruparan P, Subramanian LH, Prabaharan CD, Srithar K. Integrated performance of stepped and single basin solar stills with mini solar pond. *Desalination* 2009a;249(3):902–909.

[48] Prakash J, Kavanthekar AK. Performance prediction of a regenerative solar still. *International Journal of Solar and Wind Technology* 1986;3:119–128.

[49] Tiwari GN, Madhuri. Effect of water depth on daily yield of still. *Desalination* 1987;6(1):67–75.

[50] Buzea C, Blandino IIP, Robbie K. Nanomaterials and nanoparticles: sources and toxicity. *Biointerphases* 2007;2(4). https://doi.org/10.1116/1.2815690.

[51] Sanjay SS, Pandey AC. A brief manifestation of nanotechnology. EMR/ESR/EPR spectroscopy for characterization of nanomaterials. *Advanced Structured Materials* 2017;62. https://doi.org/10.1007/978-81-322-3655-9_2

[52] Elango T, Kannan A, Murugavel KK. Performance study on single basin single slope solar still with different water nanofluids. *Desalination* 2015;360:45–51.

[53] Rajasekhar G, Eswaramoorthy M. Performance evaluation on solar still integrated with nano–composite phase change materials. *Applied Solar Energy* 2015;51(1):15–21.

[54] Thakkar H, Panchal H. Performance investigation on solar still with PCM and nano–composites: experimental investigation. *International Journal of Innovation Science and Research* 2016;3(1):334–339.

[55] Kabeel AE, Sathyamurthy R, Sharshir SW, Muthumanokar A, Panchal H, Prakash N, et al. Effect of water depth on a novel absorber plate of pyramid solar still coated with TiO_2 nano black paint. *Journal of Cleaner Production* 2019;213:185–191.

[56] Sain MK, Kumawat G. Performance enhancement of single slope solar still using nano–particles mixed black paint. *Advanced Nanoscience and Technology An International Journal* 2015;1(1):55–65.

[57] Balachandran GB, David PW, Vijayakumar ABP, Kabeel AE, Athikesavan MM, Sathyamurthy R. Enhancement of PV/T–integrated single slope solar desalination still productivity using water film cooling and hybrid composite insulation. *Environmental Science and Pollution Research* 2019. https://doi.org/10.1007/s11356-019-06131-9.

[58] Sahota L, Gupta VS, Tiwari GN. Analytical study of thermo–physical performance of nanofluid loaded hybrid double slope solar still. *Journal of Heat Transfer* 2018. https://doi. org/10.1115/1.4040782.

[59] Sathyamurthy R, Kabeel AE, El–Agouz, E, Rufus D, Panchal H, Arunkumar T, Manokar AM, Winston DGP. Experimental investigation on the effect of MgO and TiO_2 nanoparticles in stepped solar still. *International Journal of Energy Research* 2019. https://doi.org/10.1002/er.4460.

[60] Sain MK, Kumawat G. Performance enhancement of single slope solar still using nano–particles mixed black paint. *Advanced Nanoscience and Technology An International Journal* 2015;1(1):55–65.

[61] Sharshir SW, Kandeal AW, Ismail M, Abdelaziz GB, Kabeel AE, Yang N. Augmentation of a pyramid solar still performance using evacuated tubes and nanofluid: experimental approach. *Applied Thermal Engineering* 2019;160:113997.

[62] Abdullah AS, Essa FA, Omara ZM, Rashid Y, Hadj-Taieb L, Abdelaziz GB, et al. Rotating–drum solar still with enhanced evaporation and condensation techniques: comprehensive study. *Energy Convers Manage* 2019;199:112024.

[63] Safaei MR, Goshayeshi HR, Chaer I. Solar still efficiency enhancement by using Graphene oxide/Paraffin nano–PCM. *Energies* 2019;12:2002. https://doi.org/10.3390/en12102002.

[64] Kabeel AE, Abdelgaied M, Eisa A. Effect of graphite mass concentrations in a mixture of graphite nanoparticles and paraffin wax as hybrid storage materials on performances of solar still. *Renew Energy* 2019;132:119–128.

[65] Muraleedharan M, Singh H, Udayakumar M, Suresh S. Modified active solar distillation system employing directly absorbing Therminol 55–Al_2O_3 nano heat transfer fluid and Fresnel lens concentrator. *Desalination* 2019;457:32–38.

3 Nanomaterials as Additives in Biodiesel

Anil Dhanola[1] and Kishor Kumar Gajrani[2,3]

1 University Institute of Engineering, Department of Mechanical Engineering, Chandigarh University, Mohali, Punjab, India

2 Department of Mechanical Engineering, Indian Institute of Information Technology, Design and Manufacturing, Kancheepuram, Chennai, Tamil Nadu, India

3 Centre for Smart Manufacturing, Indian Institute of Information Technology, Design and Manufacturing, Kancheepuram, Chennai, Tamil Nadu, India

CONTENTS

3.1 Introduction 33
3.2 Biodiesel: Aneco-Friendly Transportation Fuel 35
3.3 Nanomaterials for Biodiesel Production 37
    3.3.1 Impact of Nanoparticles on Biodiesel Fuel Properties 37
    3.3.2 Impact of Nanomaterials on Engine Performance and Emission Attributes 38
3.4 Key Challenges and Limitations of Nano-Based Biodiesel 42
3.5 Conclusions and Future Outlook 43
3.6 Acknowledgment 45
References... 45

3.1 INTRODUCTION

In the present era, fossil energy is a key energy source, accounting for about 80% of total energy consumption, with the transport industry contributing 58% [1]. These fossil fuel and oil reserves are rapidly decreasing and have been recognized as a primary source of hazardous gas emissions. Hazardous gases have adverse consequences such as glacier retreat, biodiversity loss, global warming, rising sea levels, and so on [2]. The transportation sector is vital to the country's economic growth [3]. Diesel engines may now be found in various modern transportation vehicles, including passenger cars and public transportation, power generators, commercial heavy-duty machinery, and agricultural machinery [4]. Despite the fact that diesel engines provide excellent performance and fuel efficiency, the smoke from a diesel engine is

DOI: 10.1201/9781003265597-3

the main cause of air pollution and poses substantial cancerous serious threats to human health. Also, the widespread usage of diesel engines leads to uninterrupted fuel consumption, raising concerns about fuel supplies and their pace of depletion. With a growth rate of 1.3%, global diesel consumption reached 27,955 million barrels per day in 2019 [5]. Diesel as a transportation fuel is expected to rise significantly in the next years. Due to the ecological issues that emerged from the burning of petroleum products, researchers have been encouraged to discover alternative, cost-effective, sustainable, green, and efficient energy sources. Till now, a large number of renewable energy sources have been successfully investigated to restrict fossil fuel usage and decline the adverse effects imposed by greenhouse gas emissions emitted by fossil fuel consumption.

Biofuels like biodiesel and ethanol are the most viable alternative for the transportation industry as they are renewable and emit low emissions, which are likely to contribute to global climate change [6]. Biodiesel has received much attention from researchers as a promising alternative fuel to petroleum diesel [7,8]. Biodiesel is a sustainable and ecologically friendly substitute for petroleum-based diesel, emitting less smoke, unburned hydrocarbons, and carbon monoxide [9,10]. Plant/animal-based sources, like vegetable oils (edible and non-edible) and animal fats, can be used to make biodiesel [11]. Waste cooking oils may also be used to make biodiesel [11]. Biodiesel's life cycle is represented in Figure 3.1 [12]. Biodiesels are monoalkyl

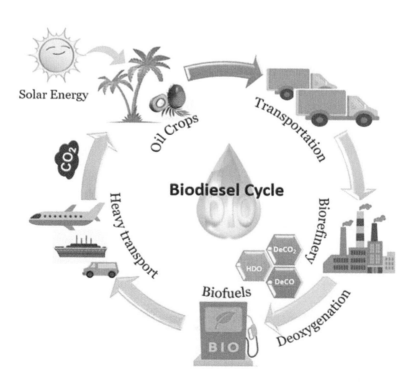

FIGURE 3.1 The life cycle of biodiesel [12].

Nanomaterials as Additives in Biodiesel   35

esters of long-chain fatty acids having a number of other advantages, including less emission of harmful gases, biodegradability, absence of sulfur, intrinsic lubrication attribute, positive energy balance, conformity with current fuel distribution infrastructure, sustainability, etc. [13,14]. Biodiesel is not extensively employed owing to several flaws. Its drawbacks include larger density, minor heating value, less cetane number, lower flash point, higher fuel consumption, increased nitrogen oxides (NO_x), and bad solubility, which are especially noticeable in winter seasons/ cold places [6].

Recent research has suggested many approaches to address these concerns, including adding fuel additives, which might improve engine performance and decrease harmful emissions [15,16]. According to a recent study, adding nanomaterials as additives in liquid and hydrocarbon further enhances the engine's performance and emissions properties [4]. Nanomaterials offer extraordinary properties such as a large surface area, larger surface energy, etc., which give a large dynamic surface for chemical reactions in biodiesel's production [17]. This chapter summarizes the recent advancements in nanoparticle-based biodiesel and the influence of different nanomaterials on diesel engines' performance, combustion efficiency, exhaust properties, and fuel properties. Also, challenges associated with nanoparticle-based biodiesel have been discussed.

3.2   BIODIESEL: AN ECO-FRIENDLY TRANSPORTATION FUEL

Biodiesel is growing rapidly as a competitive alternate fuel to petroleum-based fuel for vehicles. The biodiesel industry is still developing today, and it is firmly established in over 60 countries across the world like Indonesia: B20, the USA: up to B10 in some states, Colombia: B2-B10, Argentina: B10, Brazil: B10, France: B8 and Malaysia: B10 [18]. Biodiesels are petroleum products made from long-chain alkyl (methyl, ethyl, or propyl) esters and made from vegetable oil or animal fat. They are non-toxic, non-explosive, biodegradable, and non-flammable. Vegetable oils (both edible and non-edible), waste-cooking oils, animal fats (tallow, yellow grease, lard, chicken fat, etc.), and omega-3 fatty acids from fish oil are the major feedstocks for biodiesel synthesis [19]. Palm oil accounts for 31% of global biodiesel production, followed by soybean oil (27%) and rapeseed oil (20%). Countries utilize different feedstocks depending on their abundance. Table 3.1 lists the principal feedstocks considered in biodiesel synthesis in numerous countries [19]. Biodiesel synthesis from food-based crops, such as palm oil, soyabean oil, and sunflower oil, is not generally preferred due to the scarcity of edible oil and the hike in oil prices. Due to the usage of feedstock (palm oil) in biodiesel production, the price of edible palm oil increased by 70% in Malaysia [20]. As a result, using non-edible oils (like pongamia oil, castor bean, jojoba, mahua, and Jatropha) as biodiesel feedstocks is extremely important for lowering biodiesel costs [21]. Many studies have suggested that non-edible oils might be a viable biodiesel option. Some popular processes for producing biodiesel from vegetable oils include pyrolysis/cracking, dilution with hydrocarbons, mixing, emulsification, and transesterification [22]. The steps for transesterification process for producing biodiesel are represented in Figure 3.2 [23].

TABLE 3.1
Available Feedstocks for the Biodiesel Synthesis in Different Countries [19].

Name of country	Feedstock
Argentina	Soybean
Australia	*Jatropha curcas*; Pongamia pinnata; Waste cooking oil; Animal fat
Bangladesh	Rubber seed; *Pongamia pinnata*
Brazil	Soybean; Palm oil; Castor oil; Cotton oil
China	*Jatropha curcas*; Waste cooking oil; Rapeseed oil
Canada	Rapeseed oil; Animal fat; Soybean oil
France	Rapeseed oil; Sunflower oil
Germany	Rapeseed oil
India	*Jatropha curcas*; *Pongamia pinnata*; Soybean oil; Rapeseed oil; Sunflower oil
Italy	Rapeseed oil; Sunflower oil
Iran	Palm oil; *Jatropha curcas*; Castor oil; Algae oil
Japan	Waste cooking oil
Malaysia	Palm oil
New Zealand	Waste cooking oil; Tallow
Norway	Animal fat
Pakistan	Jatropha oil
Philippines	Coconut oil; Jatropha oil
Spain	Linseed oil; Sunflower oil
Sweden	Rapeseed oil
Turkey	Sunflower oil; Rapeseed oil
Thailand	Palm oil; Jatropha oil; Coconut oil
UK	Rapeseed oil; Waste cooking oil
USA	Soybean; Waste oil; Peanut oil

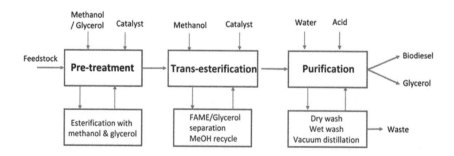

FIGURE 3.2 Block diagram of biodiesel synthesis [23].

Nanomaterials as Additives in Biodiesel

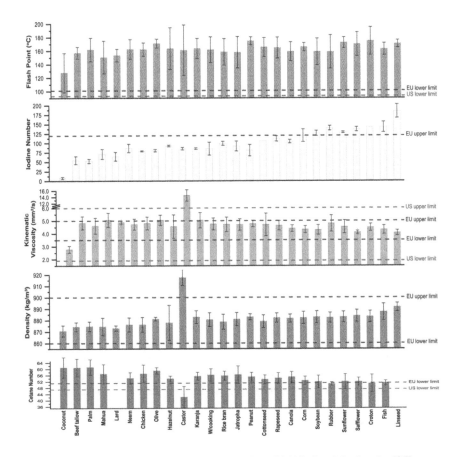

FIGURE 3.3 Comparative illustration of properties of 26 biodiesel feedstocks [25].

The transesterification process is the most popular of these techniques. The transesterification process allows for the adoption of a range of feedstocks to generate a biofuel that is similar in quality to standard diesel. Oil/fat (triglycerides) is transformed into alkyl esters with viscosity equivalent to diesel fuel [24]. For effective biodiesel production, important factors, for instance, the molar ratio of alcohol to oil, type/concentration of catalyst, reaction temperature and time, reaction medium, and type/relative number of solvents [24]. Giakoumis [25] studied the comparative study of physicochemical properties of 26 different feedstocks for biodiesel synthesis. A comparison study is depicted in Figure 3.3.

3.3 NANOMATERIALS FOR BIODIESEL PRODUCTION

3.3.1 Impact of Nanoparticles on Biodiesel Fuel Properties

Additives play an essential part in satisfying worldwide fuel requirements as well as the real-time issues that come with biodiesel. A key purpose of additives is to enhance the fuel properties and engine performance and decrease exhaust emissions. The addition of additives into biodiesel also overcomes a number of technical issues that previously limited biodiesel's acceptance as an alternative fuel in all circumstances. Fuel additives are used in low contents, ranging from 100–1000 parts per million. Antioxidants, cetane enhancers, anti-knocking elements, anti-freezing agents, stability enhancers, corrosion inhibitors, cold-flow enhancers, fuel-borne catalysts, anti-wear elements, and so on are some of the fuel additives [26]. The addition of antioxidants helps to escape biodiesel auto-oxidation. Antioxidants such as BHT (Butylated hydroxytoluene), TBHQ (Tert-butyl hydroquinone), BHA (Butylated hydroxyanisole), PG (Propyl gallate), and PA (Pyrogallol) are added in biodiesel [27]. Oxygenated additives are added to improve the burning properties of the fuel. Ethanol, methanol, biodiesel, dimethyl ether, dimethyl carbonate, di-ethylene glycol diethyl ether, sorbitan monooleate, and so on are applied as oxygenated additives [27]. For improving the cold flow properties of biodiesel ethylene vinyl acetate copolymer, glycerol ketals, glycerol acetates, phthalimide, and succinimide copolymers are commonly used [27]. Cetane number plays an important role in affecting fuel properties. Fuel having high cetane value (45) provides better performance with respect to compression ignition engine. Additives like nitrates, nitro alkanes, nitro carbonates, and peroxides are used for improving biodiesel cetane value [27].

Previous research has shown that adding metal and metal oxide-based nanomaterials as additives to biodiesels improves engine performance and physicochemical properties of biodiesels while lowering emissions. These nanoadditives increase the oxidation process during combustion without changing the chemical constitution of the biodiesel [28]. In literature, nanomaterials like Titanium oxide (TiO_2), zinc oxide (ZnO), copper oxide (CuO), aluminum oxide (Al_2O_3), iron oxide (Fe_3O_4), carbon nanotubes (CNTs), ferric oxide (Fe_2O_3), nickel oxide (NiO), cerium oxide (CeO_2), cobalt oxide (CO_3O_4), magnalium (Al-Mg), and silicon dioxide (SiO_2), have been shown to have an important effect on diesel engine performance/emissions due to their distinct physicochemical features, including as optical, electrical, and magnetic capabilities, as well as antibacterial qualities [26,29]. Further, nanomaterials have received a lot of interest as biodiesel catalysts due to their large specific surface area, strong catalytic activity, good stiffness, and great resistance to saponification [30]. They improve transesterification reactions and result in a high yield of biodiesel [30]. Table 3.2 depicts the impact of mixing various proportions of nanomaterials into biodiesel on fuel characteristics.

3.3.2 Impact of Nanomaterials on Engine Performance and Emission Attributes

A diesel engine is commonly used in commercial applications because of its high performance and efficient energy conversion mechanism. Biofuel has established itself as a potential rival to diesel fuel. On the other hand, biofuel has several technical problems, like a low calorific value and limited cold flow qualities. Biofuels' performance may be altered by adding various nanomaterials to address these issues, with nanomaterials resulting in significant increases in thermo-physical properties and making them competitive with conventional diesel fuel. This section discusses

TABLE 3.2

Influence of Addition of Different Nanomaterials with Different Concentrations to Biodiesel on Fuel Properties.

Biodiesel	Nanomaterials	Concentration (ppm)	Density (Kg/m³)	Viscosity (Cst)	Flash point (°C)	Calorific value (mJ/kg)	Cetane number	References
Jatropha curcas	Al_2O_3	0	895	5.25	85	38.88	53	[31]
		25	896	5.31	84	39.22	54	
		50	897	5.35	82	39.53	56	
Jatropha curcas 20% + Diesel 70% + Ethanol 10%	Al_2O_3	25	837.2	2.57	22	39.137	54	[32]
Palm	Al_2O_3	0	-	4.8	130	38.49	51	[33]
		25		4.76	160	38.52	55	
		50		4.74	168	38.56	59	
		75		4.73	172	38.58	62	
		100		4.73	180	38.59	63	
Ruber seed B20	Al_2O_3	10	-	4.1	-	42	-	[34]
		20		4.2		41		
		30		4.2		41		
Mustard	TiO_2	100	-	4.34	-	37.85	54	[35]
		200		4.38		37.65	57	
C. inophyllum B20	TiO_2	40	844.5	3.72	-	41.93	53.94	[36]
Canola	TiO_2	0	915	4.8			42	[37]
		300	840	3.4			56	
	TiO_2	0	-	3.12	60.49	40.42	47	[38]
Algae	SiO_2	50	817	3.03	62.45	42.60	48	
		100	817	3.01	63.61	44	48	
Mahua methyl ester 20%+Diesel 80%	CuO	50	840	4.3	60	43.1	-	[21]

recent progress in biodiesel containing nanomaterials and effects of nanomaterials on various engine and emission performance characteristics.

Radhakrishnan et al. [39] evaluated the impact of Al_2O_3 nanoparticles added to cashew nutshell biodiesel on diesel engine emissions and performance. In contrast to diesel fuel, the experimental findings indicate that emission characteristics like carbon monoxide (CO), hydrocarbons (HC), NOx, and smoke were reduced by 5.3%, 7.4%, 10.23%, and 16.1% using BD100 and 8.8%, 10.1%, 12.4%, and 18.4% using B100 A, sequentially. In comparison to diesel fuel, the brake thermal efficiency (BTE) decreased by 1.1% and 2.3% at full load, while the brake-specific fuel consumption (BSFC) increased by 3.8% and 5.1% using B100 A and B100, respectively. Mirzajanzadeh et al. [40] investigated the effect of CeO_2 and multiwall carbon nanotube (MWCNT) nanoparticles coupled with B5 and B10 diesel on engine performance. According to the data, there was a 7.81% gain in power and 4.91% rise in torque, as well as an improvement in combustion and a considerable reduction in exhaust gas discharge. The BSFC is lowered by 4.50% when using B20 with 90 ppm nanoparticles in the solution. Furthermore, in comparison with B20 fuel, HC, CO, and NO_x emissions are reduced by 26.3%, 71.4%, and 18.9%, respectively. Khalife et al. [41] studied the impact of CeO_2 nanomaterials in biodiesel on the performance/ exhaust characteristics of diesel engines in an experimental investigation. The nano-biofuel improved the burning quality, as per the findings. The BSFC of B5 oil with 3% water and 90 ppm CeO_2 was clearly determined to be 5% and 16% lower than pure B5. Furthermore, CO, HC, and NO_x emissions remarkably declined. EL-Seesy et al. [42] claimed that filling of jatropha methyl ester containing graphene oxide in a one-cylinder AC-DICI diesel engine significantly increased efficiency metrics and a substantial decrease in exhaust emissions with biodiesel containing graphene oxide (50 mg/L). Attia et al. [43] studied the engine properties like performance/ combustion/emissions using B20-Jojoba methyl ester and diesel blends with Al_2O_3 nanoadditives added in different concentrations (10 mg/L to 50 mg/L). As compared to neat diesel, the BSFC was reduced by up to 6%, while the thermal efficiency was raised by 7%. When compared to biodiesel, NO_x is reduced by up to 70%, CO is decreased by 75%, unburn hydrocarbon (UBHC) is reduced by up to 55%, and smoke opacity is reduced by 5%. Prabhu Arockiasamy et al. [44] used Jatropha biodiesel with Al_2O_3 and CeO_2 nanomaterials to investigate engine performance and other features. The ultrasonication procedure was used to add nanoadditions to biodiesel, and the additives were stable for up to 48 hours. For both samples, BTE rose by up to 5%. In comparison to plain biodiesel, JBD30A exhibited a 9% decrease in NO_x, a 33%deduction in UBHC, a 20%deduction in CO, and a 17%deduction in smoke opacity. In comparison to plain biodiesel, JBD30C demonstrated a 7% decrease in NO_x, a 28% reduction in UBHC, a 20% reduction in CO, and a 20% reduction in smoke opacity. The engine behavior of mahua biodiesel containing Al_2O_3 nanoparticles was studied by Aalam and Saravanan [45]. MME with a 100 ppm Al_2O_3 nanoparticles mix enhanced engine performance while also lowering emissions. The addition of nanoparticles raised the cylinder pressure along with the heat release rate. BSFC decreased by up to 7.66% when B20ANP100 was compared to the B20 mix. BTE increased faster than diesel in all B20 nano mixtures. In all B20 mixtures, HC and CO emissions were lower than in plain diesel; nevertheless, NO_x emissions were greater. Karthikeyan et al. [46] studied the performance/emission characteristics of a fourstroke CI engine utilizing a biodiesel blend containing ZnO_2 nanoadditives. As compared to biodiesel, the BSFC of blends containing ZnO additives dropped. In comparison to biodiesel, BTE rose for ZnO mixes. CO and HC emissions were less in ZnO-added blends than in B20. Shaafi et al. [47] published a review study that explored the impact of adding different nanoadditives to various biodiesels on various characteristics such as performance/combustion/emission characteristics. Results concluded that engine performance did not increase proportionally with nanoadditive concentration. Gavhane et al. [48] mixed SiO_2 nanoparticles with soybean biodiesel to enhance the diesel engine's performance and emission characteristics. Compared to B25, they found a maximum 6.39% rise in BTE and 9.88% rise in BSFC, as well as a maximum of 17.5%, 27.5%, and 23.54% decrease in CO, HC, and smoke emissions, respectively. Sateesh et al. [49] discovered engine performance/emission characteristics using dairy scum methyl ester biodiesel containing Al_2O_3 nanoadditives. Biodiesel with Al_2O_3 nanoadditives exhibited improved BTE by 11.5%, 23.2% reduction in smoke, 21.4% decrease in HC and CO emissions, and 32.6% higher NO_x levels at % load than biodiesel without nanoadditives, according to the findings. Krupakaran et al. [33] operated a single-cylinder four stroke diesel engine with nano-based palm biodiesel (including 25 ppm Al_2O_3 nanoadditives) under varied loads. At maximum load, results indicated a 33.3% decrease in CO, a 16% decrease in HC, and a 29% decrease in NO_x. Hosseini et al. [50] investigated waste cooking oil biodiesel containing alumina, which resulted in reduced BSFC for B5AL90, B10AL90, and B10AL60 fuels better than diesel of around 16%, 15%, and 15%, respectively, due to secondary atomization of injected fuels and better combustion of fuel. Prabu [51] analyzed jatropha biodiesel mixed with Al_2O_3 and CeO_2 nanoadditives and reported a 30% reduction in NO_x emissions as nanoadditives have the capacity to convert nitric oxide to N_2 and O_2. Srinivasa Rao et al. [52] reported that a jatropha oil biodiesel mix doped with Al_2O_3 nanoadditives decreased smoke by 25% due to the catalytic activity of nanoadditives and a larger surface area-to-volume ratio resulting in the complete combustion process. Recently, the effects of mixing various quantities of Al_2O_3 nanoparticles to castor oil biodiesel on diesel engine characteristics were studied numerically and practically by Al-Dawody and Edam [53]. The results revealed (Figure 3.4) that adding Al_2O_3 (25 ppm, 50 ppm, and

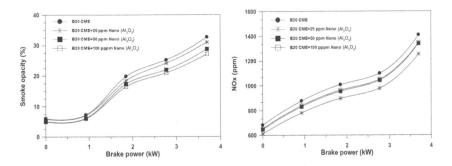

FIGURE 3.4 Variation of smoke capacity and NO_x with brake power [53].

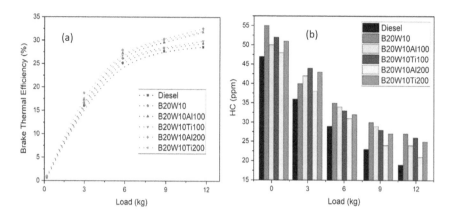

FIGURE 3.5 (a) Brake thermal efficiency vs. load; (b) hydrocarbon emission vs. load [54].

100 ppm) to 20% of castor methyl ester reduced smoke opacity by 5.2%, 12%, and 17.0%, respectively. The highest deduction in NO_x is seen at 25 ppm Al_2O_3, with a drop of 11%, along with 4.89% and 4.32% drop at 50 ppm and 100 ppm, sequentially.

Kautkar and Premkartikkumar [54] studied the single-cylinder engine performance and other engine characteristics using cotton seed nano emulsified biodiesel fuel blending with different nanoadditives Al_2O_3 and TiO_2. The maximum BTE produced for B20W10Al200 at maximum load was determined to be 32.59%, which is roughly 13.69% greater than the pure diesel operation. Further, the lowest HC was observed for the same sample, and it was around 55.35% lower than engines fueled with diesel fuel (Figure 3.5).

Najafi [55] studied the influence of silver (Ag)/CNT nanoadditive-based biodiesel-diesel blended fuel on engine performance/emission characteristics. Results stated that the new fuel blend boosts peak pressure rise and heat release rates by up to 23.33% and 28%, respectively. Also, he observed that, as compared with neat diesel fuel, CO and HC were reduced, whereas CO_2 and NO_x were raised (shown in Figure 3.6). Further, the author identified reasons for variation in different emissions characteristics using different nano-based biodiesel blends (shown in Table 3.3).

3.4 KEY CHALLENGES AND LIMITATIONS OF NANO-BASED BIODIESEL

According to the research examined, nanomaterials have been shown to increase engine performance and combustion characteristics and lower diesel engine emissions rates. However, significant obstacles restrict the application of nano-based biodiesel fuels as an alternate to traditional diesel. The introduction of nanoparticles into liquid fuel causes issues with the blend's stability. Nanomaterials have a substantial surface area and surface activity, which causes them to quickly agglomerate and coagulate. Nanomaterials with smaller surface areas usually provide higher stability.

Nanomaterials as Additives in Biodiesel 43

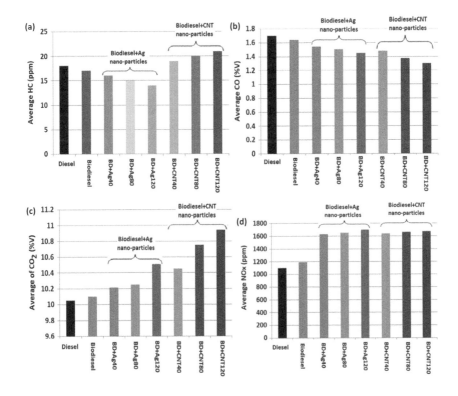

FIGURE 3.6 Variation of different emission characteristics with respect to various nano-biodiesel-diesel fuel blends [55].

Aside from that, the stirring method, correct mixing proportions, suitable surfactant, etc., can further improve the stability. Furthermore, the problem observed during the utilization of nano-based biodiesel at the industrial scale is greater production costs, which require future research. Biodiesel's use as a commercial fuel for transportation and other energy sectors is hindered by supply limits, food security, and pricing concerns. Adding nanomaterials such as CeO_2, Al_2O_3, and others to biodiesel dramatically reduces HC and CO emissions. However, such nanomaterials might be expelled into the emissions and pollute the environment.

3.5 CONCLUSIONS AND FUTURE OUTLOOK

In this chapter, the recent progress of nano-based biodiesel as a sustainable fuel is discussed. Studies presented in this chapter clearly reveal that nanomaterials have an important role in enhancing biodiesel fuel's thermo-chemical properties and combustion characteristics, along with overall engine performance/emissions reduction. Biodiesel infused with nanomaterials like Al_2O_3, TiO_2, CNT, and CeO_2 seems to have the capability to improve the performance of the engine and has shown to be effective as an additive in biodiesel. Nevertheless, substantial experimental studies

TABLE 3.3
Primary Causes in CI Engine Emissions with Utilizing Nano-Based Biodiesel Blends [55].

CI engine performance parameters variation	Reasons
Increase in NO_x	• The effect of oxygenated additives improves combustion with longer ignition delay caused by the mixture of biodiesel and additives, resulting in quicker premixed combustion, which leads to greater combustion temperatures and higher NO_x emissions. • Nanomaterials may offer oxygen for CO oxidation, and through a second mode of action, they may also reduce NO_x formation.
Reduction in pollution	• Nanomaterials can deliver an oxygen molecule in a chain reaction that results in full combustion of unburned HC and CO_2, lowering pollution levels.
Reduction in emissions	• The CNTs utilized served as a catalyst, accelerating the combustion rate and efficiency, which results in lower emissions and more power and receive more complete combustion.
Reduction in hydrocarbon/smoke emissions	• CNTs act as a catalyst to enhance the burning process, consequently a light ignition time and a faster peak heat release. • CNT's activation energy operates to burn carbon deposits in the engine cylinder under wall temperature, preventing the deposition of non-polar chemicals on the cylinder wall, resulting in a considerable reduction in hydrocarbon and smoke emissions.
Cleaner combustion	• Cleaner combustion yields less CO_2 and NO_x emissions, and researchers are using the increased range of tools made accessible to them by breakthroughs in nanotechnology to develop innovative fuel additives that seek to increase combustion cleanliness in engine.
Decomposition of unburned HCs and soot	• CNTs added to gasoline can aid in the breakdown of unburned HCs and soot, lowering the quantity of these pollutants produced in the exhaust and lowering the amount of fuel consumed.
Reduction in overall temperature	• Adding nanomaterials to fuel lowers the pressure in the combustion chamber, making combustion reactions more efficient and reducing NO_x production. Additives also act as a heat sink within the combustion chamber, lowering the overall temperature, avoiding hotspots, and lowering NOx production.

are necessary to explore the effect of nanomaterials on biodiesel combustion characteristics under varied operating settings. The stability of nanofuels is still a key challenge for the production of stable nano-based biofuels. Therefore, the stability aspects of nano-based biodiesel fuels under various operating settings, and the effective selection of surfactants should be considered. The performance/emission characteristics of a diesel engine are also influenced by the type, shape, and size of nanomaterials. As a result, additional study is needed in this area. Nanomaterials in biodiesel production may help supply a low-cost, clean energy source in the coming years and become a significant global industry.

3.6 ACKNOWLEDGMENT

Authors are thankful to the publishers for providing copyright permission to all figures and Tables 3.1 and 3.3 in the current chapter.

REFERENCES

[1] Escobar, J.C., Lora, E.S., Venturini, O.J., Yáñez, E.E., Castillo, E.F. and Almazan, O., 2009. Biofuels: environment, technology and food security. *Renewable and Sustainable Energy Reviews*, *13*(6–7), pp. 1275–1287.

[2] Gaurav, N., Sivasankari, S., Kiran, G.S., Ninawe, A. and Selvin, J., 2017. Utilization of bioresources for sustainable biofuels: a review. *Renewable and Sustainable Energy Reviews*, *73*, pp. 205–214.

[3] Lenin, A.H., Ravi, R. and Thyagarajan, K., 2013. Performance characteristics of a diesel engine using mahua biodiesel as alternate fuel. *Iranica Journal of Energy & Environment*, *4*(2), pp. 136–141.

[4] Hoang, A.T., 2021. Combustion behavior, performance and emission characteristics of diesel engine fuelled with biodiesel containing cerium oxide nanoparticles: a review. *Fuel Processing Technology*, *218*, p. 106840.

[5] BP, 2020. Primary energy – BP Statistical Review of World Energy 2020.

[6] Mofijur, M., Rasul, M.G., Hyde, J. and Bhuyia, M.M.K., 2015. Role of biofuels on IC engines emission reduction. *Energy Procedia*, *75*, pp. 886–892.

[7] Demirbas, A., 2009. Progress and recent trends in biodiesel fuels. *Energy conversion and management*, *50*(1), pp. 14–34.

[8] Hoang, A.T., 2021. Prediction of the density and viscosity of biodiesel and the influence of biodiesel properties on a diesel engine fuel supply system. *Journal of Marine Engineering & Technology*, *20*(5), pp. 299–311.

[9] Meng, Y.L., Tian, S.J., Li, S.F., Wang, B.Y. and Zhang, M.H., 2013. Transesterification of rapeseed oil for biodiesel production in trickle-bed reactors packed with heterogeneous Ca/Al composite oxide-based alkaline catalyst. *Bioresource Technology*, *136*, pp. 730–734.

[10] Salinas, D., Araya, P. and Guerrero, S., 2012. Study of potassium-supported TiO_2 catalysts for the production of biodiesel. *Applied Catalysis B: Environmental*, *117*, pp. 260–267.

[11] Hoang, A.T., Pham, V.V. and Nguyen, X.P., 2021. Use of biodiesel fuels in the diesel engines, in: O. Konur (Ed.), *Handbook of Biodiesel and Petrodiesel Fuels: Science, Technology, Health, and Environment*, CRC Press, Boca Raton, FL.

[12] Jin, W., Pastor-Pérez, L., Villora-Pico, J.J., Pastor-Blas, M.M., Sepúlveda-Escribano, A., Gu, S., Charisiou, N.D., Papageridis, K., Goula, M.A. and Reina, T.R., 2019. Catalytic conversion of palm oil to bio-hydrogenated diesel over novel N-doped activated carbon supported Pt nanoparticles. *Energies*, *13*(1), p. 132.

[13] Singh, I. and Taggar, M.S., 2014. Recent trends in biodiesel production—an overview. *International Journal of Applied Engineering Research*, *9*(10), pp. 1151–1158.

[14] Hajjari, M., Ardjmand, M. and Tabatabaei, M., 2014. Experimental investigation of the effect of cerium oxide nanoparticles as a combustion-improving additive on biodiesel oxidative stability: mechanism. *RSC Advances*, *4*(28), pp. 14352–14356.

[15] Prabu, A. and Anand, R.B., 2014. Influence of oxygenate additives on the performance and emission characteristics of Jatropha fuelled direct injection diesel engine. *Biofuels*, *5*(6), pp. 667–672.

[16] Sajeevan, A.C. and Sajith, V., 2013. Diesel engine emission reduction using catalytic nanoparticles: an experimental investigation. *Journal of Engineering*, *2013*.

[17] Rodríguez-Couto, S., 2019. Green nanotechnology for biofuel production, in: *Sustainable Approaches for Biofuels Production Technologies* (pp. 73–82), Springer, Cham.

[18] Yusoff, M.N.A.M., Zulkifli, N.W.M., Sukiman, N.L., Chyuan, O.H., Hassan, M.H., Hasnul, M.H., Zulkifli, M.S.A., Abbas, M.M. and Zakaria, M.Z., 2021. Sustainability of palm biodiesel in transportation: a review on biofuel standard, policy and international collaboration between Malaysia and Colombia. *Bioenergy Research*, *14*(1), pp. 43–60.

[19] Changmai, B., Vanlalveni, C., Ingle, A.P., Bhagat, R. and Rokhum, L., 2020. Widely used catalysts in biodiesel production: a review. *RSC Advances*, *10*(68), pp. 41625–41679.

[20] Ali, A.M. and Alias, M.H., 2014. Impact of biodiesel blend mandate (810) on the Malaysian palm oil industry. *Jurnal Ekonomi Malaysia*, *48*(2), pp. 29–40.

[21] Chandrasekaran, V., Arthanarisamy, M., Nachiappan, P., Dhanakotti, S. and Moorthy, B., 2016. The role of nano additives for biodiesel and diesel blended transportation fuels. *Transportation Research Part D: Transport and Environment*, *46*, pp. 145–156.

[22] Atabani, A.E., Mahlia, T.M.I., Masjuki, H.H., Badruddin, I.A., Yussof, H.W., Chong, W.T. and Lee, K.T., 2013. A comparative evaluation of physical and chemical properties of biodiesel synthesized from edible and non-edible oils and study on the effect of biodiesel blending. *Energy*, *58*, pp. 296–304.

[23] Dimian, A.C. and Kiss, A.A., 2019. Eco-efficient processes for biodiesel production from waste lipids. *Journal of Cleaner Production*, *239*, p. 118073.

[24] Gebremariam, S.N. and Marchetti, J.M., 2017. Biodiesel production technologies. *Aims Energy*, *5*(3), pp. 425–457.

[25] Giakoumis, E.G., 2013. A statistical investigation of biodiesel physical and chemical properties, and their correlation with the degree of unsaturation. *Renewable Energy*, *50*, pp. 858–878.

[26] Dey, S., Reang, N.M., Deb, M. and Das, P.K., 2021. Experimental investigation on combustion-performance-emission characteristics of nanoparticles added biodiesel blends and tribological behavior of contaminated lubricant in a diesel engine. *Energy Conversion and Management*, *244*, p. 114508.

[27] Venkatesan, H., Sivamani, S., Sampath, S., Gopi, V. and Kumar, D., 2017. A comprehensive review on the effect of nano metallic additives on fuel properties, engine performance and emission characteristics. *International Journal of Renewable Energy Research (IJRER)*, *7*(2), pp. 825–843.

[28] EL-Seesy, A.I., Kosaka, H., Hassan, H. and Sato, S., 2019. Combustion and emission characteristics of a common rail diesel engine and RCEM fueled by n-heptanol-diesel blends and carbon nanomaterial additives. *Energy Conversion and Management*, *196*, pp. 370–394.

[29] Bidir, M.G., Millerjothi, N.K., Adaramola, M.S. and Hagos, F.Y., 2021. The role of nanoparticles on biofuel production and as an additive in ternary blend fuelled diesel engine: A review. *Energy Reports*, *7*, pp. 3614–3627.

[30] Rengasamy, M., Anbalagan, K., Mohanraj, S. and Pugalenthi, V., 2014. Biodiesel production from pongamia pinnata oil using synthesized iron nanocatalyst. *International Journal of ChemTech Research*, *6*(10), pp. 4511–4516.

[31] Sadhik Basha, J. and Anand, R.B., 2013. The influence of nano additive blended biodiesel fuels on the working characteristics of a diesel engine. *Journal of the Brazilian Society of Mechanical Sciences and Engineering*, *35*(3), pp. 257–264.

[32] Venu, H. and Madhavan, V., 2016. Effect of Al_2O_3 nanoparticles in biodiesel-diesel-ethanol blends at various injection strategies: performance, combustion and emission characteristics. *Fuel*, *186*, pp. 176–189.

[33] Krupakaran, R.L., Hariprasasd, T., Gopalakrishna, A. and Babu, P., 2016. The performance and exhaust emissions investigation of a diesel engine using γ- Al_2O_3 nanoparticle additives to biodiesel. *Carbon Management*, *7*(3–4), pp. 233–241.

[34] Mahalingam, S. and Ganesan, S., 2020. Effect of nano-fuel additive on performance and emission characteristics of the diesel engine using biodiesel blends with diesel fuel. *International Journal of Ambient Energy, 41*(3), pp. 316–321.

[35] Yuvarajan, D., Babu, M.D., Beem Kumar, N. and Kishore, P.A., 2018. Experimental investigation on the influence of titanium dioxide nanofluid on emission pattern of biodiesel in a diesel engine. *Atmospheric Pollution Research, 9*(1), pp. 47–52.

[36] Praveen, A., Rao, G.L.N. and Balakrishna, B., 2018. Performance and emission characteristics of a diesel engine using Calophylluminophyllum biodiesel blends with TiO_2 nanoadditives and EGR. *Egyptian Journal of Petroleum, 27*(4), pp. 731–738.

[37] Nithya, S., Manigandan, S., Gunasekar, P., Devipriya, J. and Saravanan, W.S.R., 2019. The effect of engine emission on canola biodiesel blends with TiO_2. *International Journal of Ambient Energy, 40*(8), pp. 838–841.

[38] Karthikeyan, S. and Prathima, A., 2017. Microalgae biofuel with CeO_2 nano additives as an eco-friendly fuel for CI engine. *Energy Sources, Part A: Recovery, Utilization, and Environmental Effects, 39*(13), pp. 1332–1338.

[39] Radhakrishnan, S., Munuswamy, D.B., Devarajan, Y. and Mahalingam, A., 2018. Effect of nanoparticle on emission and performance characteristics of a diesel engine fueled with cashew nut shell biodiesel. *Energy Sources, Part A: Recovery, Utilization, and Environmental Effects, 40*(20), pp. 2485–2493.

[40] Mirzajanzadeh, M., Tabatabaei, M., Ardjmand, M., Rashidi, A., Ghobadian, B., Barkhi, M. and Pazouki, M., 2015. A novel soluble nano-catalysts in diesel–biodiesel fuel blends to improve diesel engines performance and reduce exhaust emissions. *Fuel, 139*, pp. 374–382.

[41] Khalife, E., Tabatabaei, M., Najafi, B., Mirsalim, S.M., Gharehghani, A., Mohammadi, P., Aghbashlo, M., Ghaffari, A., Khounani, Z., Shojaei, T.R. and Salleh, M.A.M., 2017. A novel emulsion fuel containing aqueous nano cerium oxide additive in diesel–biodiesel blends to improve diesel engines performance and reduce exhaust emissions: Part I–Experimental analysis. *Fuel, 207*, pp. 741–750.

[42] EL-Seesy, A.I., Hassan, H. and Ookawara, S.J.E.C., 2018. Performance, combustion, and emission characteristics of a diesel engine fueled with Jatropha methyl ester and graphene oxide additives. *Energy Conversion and Management, 166*, pp. 674–686.

[43] Attia, A.M., El-Seesy, A.I., El-Batsh, H.M. and Shehata, M.S., 2014, November. Effects of alumina nanoparticles additives into jojoba methyl ester-diesel mixture on diesel engine performance, in: *ASME International Mechanical Engineering Congress and Exposition* (Vol. 46521, p. V06BT07A019), American Society of Mechanical Engineers, Montreal, Quebec, Canada.

[44] Arockiasamy, P. and Anand, R.B., 2015. Performance, combustion and emission characteristics of a DI diesel engine fuelled with nanoparticle blended jatropha biodiesel. *Periodica Polytechnica Mechanical Engineering, 59*(2), pp. 88–93.

[45] Aalam, C.S. and Saravanan, C.G., 2017. Effects of nano metal oxide blended Mahua biodiesel on CRDI diesel engine. *Ain Shams Engineering Journal, 8*(4), pp. 689–696.

[46] Karthikeyan, S., Elango, A. and Prathima, A., 2014. Performance and emission study on zinc oxide nano particles addition with pomolion stearin wax biodiesel of CI engine. *Journal of Scientific and Industrial Research, 73*, pp. 187–190.

[47] Shaafi, T., Sairam, K., Gopinath, A., Kumaresan, G. and Velraj, R., 2015. Effect of dispersion of various nanoadditives on the performance and emission characteristics of a CI engine fuelled with diesel, biodiesel and blends—a review. *Renewable and Sustainable Energy Reviews, 49*, pp. 563–573.

[48] Gavhane, R.S., Kate, A.M., Soudagar, M.E.M., Wakchaure, V.D., Balgude, S., Rizwanul Fattah, I.M., Nik-Ghazali, N.N., Fayaz, H., Khan, T.M., Mujtaba, M.A. and Kumar, R., 2021. Influence of silica nano-additives on performance and emission characteristics of Soybean biodiesel fuelled diesel engine. *Energies, 14*(5), p. 1489.

[49] Sateesh, K.A., Yaliwal, V.S., Soudagar, M.E.M., Banapurmath, N.R., Fayaz, H., Safaei, M.R., Elfasakhany, A. and EL-Seesy, A.I., 2022. Utilization of biodiesel/Al_2O_3 nanoparticles for combustion behavior enhancement of a diesel engine operated on dual fuel mode. *Journal of Thermal Analysis and Calorimetry, 147*(10), pp. 5897–5911.

[50] Hosseini, S.H., Taghizadeh-Alisaraei, A., Ghobadian, B. and Abbaszadeh-Mayvan, A., 2017. Effect of added alumina as nano-catalyst to diesel-biodiesel blends on performance and emission characteristics of CI engine. *Energy, 124*, pp. 543–552.

[51] Prabu, A., 2018. Nanoparticles as additive in biodiesel on the working characteristics of a DI diesel engine. *Ain Shams Engineering Journal, 9*(4), pp. 2343–2349.

[52] Rao, M.S. and Anand, R.B., 2016. Performance and emission characteristics improvement studies on a biodiesel fuelled DICI engine using water and AlO (OH) nanoparticles. *Applied Thermal Engineering, 98*, pp. 636–645.

[53] Al-Dawody, M.F. and Edam, M.S., 2022. Experimental and numerical investigation of adding castor methyl ester and alumina nanoparticles on performance and emissions of a diesel engine. *Fuel, 307*, p. 121784.

[54] Kautkar, N.U. and Premkartikkumar, S.R., 2022. An impact of emulsified cottonseed biodiesel with Nano additives on low heat rejection engine. *Environment, Development and Sustainability*, pp. 1–20.

[55] Najafi, G., 2018. Diesel engine combustion characteristics using nano-particles in biodiesel-diesel blends. *Fuel, 212*, pp. 668–678.

4 Challenges and Future Prospects of Biofuel Generations
An Overview

Amneesh Singla[1], Yashvir Singh[2,3],
Erween Abd Rahim[2], Nishant Kumar
Singh[4], and Abhishek Sharma[5]

1 Department of Mechanical Engineering, University of Petroleum & Energy Studies, Dehradun, India

2 Faculty of Mechanical and Manufacturing Engineering, Universiti Tun Hussein Onn Malaysia, Parit Raja, Batu Pahat, Johor, Malaysia

3 Department of Mechanical Engineering, Graphic Era Deemed to be university, Dehradun, Uttarakhand, India

4 Department of Mechanical Engineering, Harcourt Butler Technical University, Kanpur, Uttar Pradesh, India

5 Department of Mechanical Engineering, G L Bajaj Institute of Technology and Management, Greater Noida, Uttar Pradesh, India

CONTENTS

4.1 Introduction 50
4.2 Different Biofuel Generations 51
    4.2.1 First Generation 51
    4.2.2 Second Generation 52
    4.2.3 Third Generation 55
4.3 Sustainability Considerations and Economic Factors 56
4.4 Future Prospect and Conclusion 56
References 57

DOI: 10.1201/9781003265597-4

4.1 INTRODUCTION

Alternative, renewable fuels are being studied and developed in order to meet future energy requirements and satisfy existing and future sustainability due to the global overuse of fossil fuels and rising emissions of greenhouse gases (GHGs). According to BP and Shafiee, some fossil fuels could deplete within the next 50 years, and severe ecological damages affected by climate, rising temperatures, urban pollution, and acid rain could occur [1,2]. This has incited governments and international associations to target cutbacks in carbon pollutants into the atmosphere [3,4].

Crops, wildlife, wastes, and microorganisms are among the primary sources of biofuels [5]. Solid, gas, and liquid biofuels can all be found in biomass, which is made up of organic matter. Biomass can be used to produce them [6,7]. It is possible to use biomass in a variety of ways to generate alternative energy. For example, biofuels in transhipment, the oil sector, and economic modeling have all been addressed [8]. Another major concern is the biofuel supply chain, which is riddled with uncertainties. In Ref. [9], the development of biofuels and the main components of the biofuel supply chain have been discussed in detail. There have been certain studies that have exclusively looked at one kind of biofuel in particular. As an illustration, analyzed the present scenarios for glycerol generation and its international economies in the biodiesel business [10]. A previous research discussed biodiesel development possibilities, residues, oil extraction, and biogas generation [11]. Biodiesel's advantages over fossil fuels have also been examined, as have the fuel's possible sources, which include waste plastic and cooking oil [12].

There are numerous advantages to using liquid biofuels over solid biofuels when it comes to renewable energy sources. Compared to fossil fuels, they may reduce CO_2 emissions, toxic elements, and particulates by up to 50% [13]; by up to 35% [14]; by up to 35% [15]; and by up to 35% [16] by helping countries differentiate their energy sources [17,18].

Research into the prospective supply and demand of biofuels is common. Existing research on biofuel potentials and current methods of biofuel conversion was examined. Bioenergy and biofuels were examined in terms of their past, present, and potential future [19,20]. In terms of the international energy market and forthcoming energy supply, just a few studies focus on biofuels [21]. Discussing how much biofuels and fossil fuels should be used in our daily lives is crucial because both are essential for future generations. The cost of essential items, such as oil, has risen sharply. In this case, biofuels are the best option to meet the human need for energy in a time of crisis [22]. Replacement for fossil fuels and their dwindling store of fossil fuels. As a result, a sustainable and dependable energy source is created to mitigate the effects of global warming. Because they are constantly replenished, biofuels are a long-lasting and renewable resource. Our deep earth is depleted of fossil fuels since it takes millions of years for them to create [23]. As a result, it is the general public's responsibility to restore them so that they do not have to deal with problems caused by a shortage of storage. The availability of biofuel as a replacement is a miracle of modern science. As a result, we believe that a greater understanding of these various biofuels and their comparative analysis is necessary to pique the attention of a wider audience in this critical issue, which could have a profound impact on the future of our planet. All those who are working on this subject may find this review useful in highlighting the necessity for a holistic approach. In addition, we hope that this assessment will educate and inspire individuals who are new to the field and start making their own valuable contributions to this captivating and fast-changing area.

Challenges and Future Prospects of Biofuel Generations

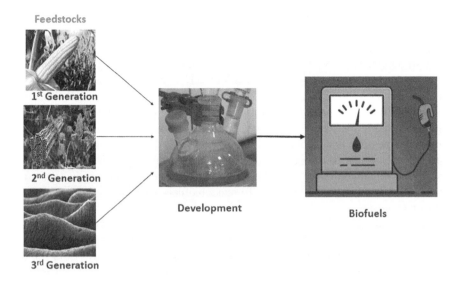

FIGURE 4.1 Feedstocks for biofuels of various generations.

4.2 DIFFERENT BIOFUEL GENERATIONS

Biofuels are those fuels that are produced through a biological process. Fossil fuels, on the other hand, are the result of geological processes such as the production of fossil fuels. Firewood, woody biomass, pellets, and organic matter are the most common primary biofuels used for burning, food, and power generation. Figure 4.1 represents the basic feedstocks required for all generations. Liquid biofuels derived from cultivated biomass and widely used in transportation and various industrial purposes are termed secondary biofuels. Biofuel generation and its merits and disadvantages were thoroughly examined in this article. We also compared and contrasted each other.

4.2.1 FIRST GENERATION

A biofuel's basic structure doesn't really vary much over time, but rather its particular source of origin. In the first generation of biofuel feedstock, food crops such as corn, wheat, soybeans, vegetable oils, and sugar cane made up the majority [24,25]. First-generation biofuels include ethanol from sugar & corn, starch-based biodiesel, and pure plant oils. Sugar, starch, oil-bearing crops, and animal fats are commonly used to produce first-generation biofuels. Some of these can be used as food and feed, while others are made from waste food that has been processed using standard methods such as fermentation, esterification, and distillation. Scientifically, these methods are well-established and have been used for centuries in various applications, such as ethanol production.

A decrease in ozone production is one of ethanol's most serious environmental warnings. As a result, it reduces the need for foreign-produced oil by shifting the

52   Biowaste and Biomass in Biofuel Applications

demand for indigenously power sources. It takes longer for ethanol to burn and is less pronounced (complete combustion). The amount of high-octane additives can be reduced by using ethanol. Biodegradation or diluting ethanol spills to safe levels is a more straightforward solution. Ethanol production necessitates a significant amount of energy and a large area of land. Non-E85-ready fuel systems may not be able to handle fuels with a little more than 10% ethanol content, which may lead to the corrosion of ferrous components [26]. It may cause electric gasoline pumps to wear out and create sparks that aren't necessary. It doesn't work well with capacitance fuel gauges. It's possible that automobiles in the system will display the wrong amount of fuel because of this. As a food crop, soybeans are expensive, but they are nevertheless a vital ingredient in the manufacture of biofuel. For biodiesel production, soybeans are utilized instead of ethanol. To make biofuels, soybean is almost certainly the worst feedstock.

As a result of their high costs and stringent growth requirements, these feedstocks competed directly with food supplies and farming land allocations. They raised sustainable and ethical development challenges, such as the unavoidably rising staple-food costs in poor and developing countries [27,28]. They also caused adverse effects on the environment, including soil and water contamination, increased greenhouse gases (when planted outside of traditional agricultural settings), a decrease in biodiversity, the spread of insects and pathogens in crops [29], and sustainability issues, such as low energy and/or cultivation yields (i.e., for corn, sugar cane, soybeans), also arose [30]. Even soybeans, which had an overall negative energy balance, could only be justified by mismanaged incentive structures [31] for a short time. Food crops, including cane sugar, rapeseed, and peanuts, have all functioned as a source for first-generation biofuels in the past because of their food value. Fermentation was the primary method used to produce the first generation of biofuels, with mechanical and occasionally thermal pre-treatment.

Second (and later third) generation fuels eventually supplanted all first-generation feedstocks due to comparable limitations. There will be better biofuel substitutes in the future, but for the time being, some of the first-generation feedstocks are still useful for biofuel production [32] due to their pros and disadvantages and how they stack up against each other.

4.2.2 Second Generation

In comparison to first-generation fuels, second-generation biofuels are much more industrially developed. While they aren't directly derived from crop production, they are made from sustainable feedstock like first-generation fuels. In general, these kinds of feedstocks aren't intended for human consumption in any way.

That is to say, human consumption does not benefit from second-generation feedstock. Despite the fact that it is a food crop, the plants have lost their nutritional value and cannot be consumed. Advanced biofuels are commonly referred to as such since the harvesting of fuels from this source is extremely challenging. Timber, agricultural leftovers, organic matter waste, household waste, and particular biomass crops, as well as cellulosic, hemicellulose, and lignin, are all potential non-food biomass sources for second-generation biofuels [5]. With this biofuel, existing IC engines can

Challenges and Future Prospects of Biofuel Generations

be altered to utilize it, or they can be used in slightly modified vehicles with internal combustion that can be pumped through existing facilities. In order to produce fuel, this species binds plants together. Two of the most common second-generation biofuels are lignocellulose ethanol and biomass-to-liquid diesel. Many pilot and demonstration facilities have been established in recent years, with most of the research taking place in North America, Europe, and a few newer nations. Second-generation biofuels have not yet been made commercially. There must be huge volumes of biomass available to manufacture the second generation, and this will necessitate an early investigation of both active and potential biomass sources.

Energy can be extracted from second-generation biofuels using a variety of technologies. One example is lignocellulose feedstock, which can sometimes necessitate several steps before ethanol can be produced. In the production of second-generation biofuels, several chemical and biochemical methods have been applied; thermochemical processes, like gasification, pyrolysis, and torrefaction, are also utilized [33,34]. Switchgrass, Indian grass, and other grasses (based on area and climatic condition) are the most widely used important raw materials of the second generation [35], followed by seed crops, like jatropha, Karanja, rapeseed, and camelina [36]; waste vegetable oil; and municipal solid waste [37]. There are numerous advantages to using grasses as a feedstock, including the fact that they are everlasting and rapidly growing on marginal terrain with minimum fertilizer use, allowing them to be cultivated frequently and with significant overall energy yields [38].

In second generation, besides crops, grass, and municipal waste, many other fuels are obtained from various sources. Bio-butanol is made using other microbes. However, bio-butanol can be utilized as a stand-alone alternative for gasoline without the need for any mixing. For biologically derived liquids for making gasoline, diesel, and jet fuel, the Fischer-Tropsch process begins with the preparation of a synthesis gas (syngas). Catalytic synthesis can also produce methanol, dimethyl ether, and mixed alcohols from syngas. Some specialized bacteria may also ferment syngas to produce alcohol [39]. It is possible to obtain biosynthetic natural gas (Bio-SNG) via gasification, followed by methanation and purification. Anaerobic digestion using microorganisms can produce biogas. Methane and carbon dioxide make up the majority of this gas's composition. Vehicles can run on compressed natural gas (CNG), liquefied natural gas (LNG), or even natural gas cylinders if it is injected into them.

Fuel qualities, including high cetane, non-aromatic, and sulfur-free, make hydrotreated vegetable oil a popular diesel replacement. Bio crude is a by-product of pyrolysis oil production. In this case, the ash is pyrolyzed at 1,000 °C and then cooled rapidly. Liquid fuels for transportation or stationary use (in boilers and turbines) can be produced by refinement and upgrading [40]. For a variety of reasons, second-generation biofuels are expected to be superior to first-generation biofuels: (a) They utilize lignocellulosic biomass material, such as ground agricultural wastes, sustainable forestry residues, or rapidly specialized energy crops. (b) The fuel is a call to substitute for existing petroleum-based fuel, meaning there are no constraints on combining, or they can also be used as is in current vehicles without mixing. (c) The second-generation biofuel is more eco-friendly and generates fewer greenhouse gases. (d) It's more cost-effective than first-generation technologies since they don't come from food crops like corn or soybean.

Commercial production of second-generation fuels has not yet begun. As the procedures are not conclusively demonstrated. Extraction, handling, and transportation infrastructure are not sufficiently accurate for big-scale production and handling of biomass. A concise and long-term regulatory framework is required to ensure that the corporate world and financiers can endow with affirmation. The agricultural/forestry sector actually changes the need to supply different biomass stock from residues and harvests, which appears to suggest a considerable conversion in the existing business. The second-generation fuels are environmentally friendly, and the costs should be kept to a minimum. These fuels are related to a lower risk of causing food shortages in underdeveloped countries or harming the pricing of consumers in rich countries. There are numerous advantages to using these feedstocks for biofuel production, including the wide variety of feedstocks available and the low cost of feedstocks (such as cellulose crops). Although real cost assessments are impossible, biofuels offer significant economic benefits over fossil fuels when seen as a whole. Fossil fuel-related costs, such as military spending and environmental health and safety costs, are often undervalued. However, the usage of biofuels can reduce greenhouse gas emissions, improve air quality, and create jobs. On the other hand, biofuels reduce our reliance on foreign crude oil. Figure 4.2 shows the biofuel production for different generations.

As an outcome, biofuels are better for the environment, economy, and society. Direct costs are often overlooked when it comes to liquid fuel. Consequently, biofuels are typically seen as non—competitive, despite the fact that, when evaluating environmental externalities, a biofuel market may actually provide long-term economic benefits [41].

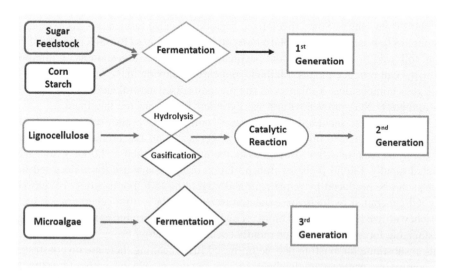

FIGURE 4.2 Biofuel production – schematic image for various generations.

Challenges and Future Prospects of Biofuel Generations 55

4.2.3 THIRD GENERATION

The widely accepted definition of third-generation biofuels includes fuels made from microalgae biomass, which grows at a higher rate than lignocellulosic (wood) biomass. In the third generation of biofuels, algae are the primary feedstock [5]. More energy is produced per hectare than land commodities like soybeans. A typical alga is a mixture of eukaryotic and prokaryotic species. Autotrophic and heterotrophic algae are the two main types of algae. Algae biomass can be converted into sources of energy in three ways: biochemical, chemical, and thermochemical [42]. Inorganic chemicals such as CO_2, salts, and a light energy source are necessary for autotrophic algae's growth. Because they are not phototrophs, heterotrophs must obtain their energy from other sources, such as organic substances like nutrition [43].

Microalgae are microscopic organisms that are usually measured on a micrometer scale. These species develop more quickly in water bodies or ponds than macroalgae and contain more lipids. Algae have a harvesting period of just a few weeks, whereas most crops have a harvesting cycle of a few months or more. For this reason, algal biomass has received the most interest as a biofuel source. In addition to biodiesel, butanol, gasoline, and methane gas, algae may produce ethanol, vegetable oil, and jet fuel.

A variety of techniques exist for cultivating algae. Algae grow in open-air ponds in a straightforward manner using this method. Although algae can be easily cultivated and have cheap asset costs, they are less effective than other systems. Other creatures have the ability to poison the pond, making them a major source of concern, even if just because of the algae-killing anxiety they inspire.

In contrast to open ponds, which are exposed to the atmosphere, closed-loop systems employ a sterilized source of CO_2. It has enormous potential since every time it is used, a small amount of carbon dioxide is released into the air. A photo-bioreactor is a complex and expensive technology to build since it requires a large amount of capital investment. Photobioreactors with high levels of efficiency are essential for developing algae's full potential. Photobioreactors have been proposed in substantial numbers, but only a few of them can actually be utilized to mass-produce algae. Mass transfer is a critical stumbling block to the practical implementation of algae mass cultures [44]. Photobioreactors must accept mass transfer rates methodically if large-scale algal cultures are to operate smoothly. Despite this, their benefits in terms of yield and control remain unmatched.

Algae can be cultivated practically anyplace (provided the ambient temperature is warm enough), and no farmland would need to be converted according to these methods. Algae can also be cultivated in wastewater, which has the added benefit of performing tertiary municipal wastewater treatment without using extra land [45]. Algae may be easier to grow than any conventional biofuels crop because of all these qualities [46]. Simultaneously, they represent the single significant drawback of algal technology, namely their high water and nutrient consumption requirements [47]. To produce one kilogram of biodiesel from microalgae, it is estimated that 0.33 kilogram of nitrogen, 0.71 kilogram of phosphorus, and 3726 kilograms of water are required. Using wastewater as a growth condition would reduce the water requirement by 90% and provide all of the nutrients microalgae require [47].

4.3 SUSTAINABILITY CONSIDERATIONS AND ECONOMIC FACTORS

The fact that biofuels can't be generated indefinitely, despite popular belief, is due to a simple fact: land availability. Producing renewable fuel obviously conflicts with food production operations, which is contrary to popular belief [48]. The availability of water is a secondary consideration, as alluded to earlier. In order to keep the relatively straightforward process of cultivating feedstock and generating biofuels becoming much less expensive than fossil fuel, the equilibrium among food and biofuel demand must be maintained. As a result of this, the industrial value of fossil fuels remains lower than that of biofuels. Feedstock costs and availability are the most important factors in determining the economic viability of a fuel.

Researchers have spent the last two decades developing microorganisms that can ferment pentose carbohydrates. To be cost-effective, these must be able to co-ferment glucose and xylose sources [49]. C5 pentoses are hard to ferment; however, new microbes are being produced that are capable of doing so [50]. There is currently no evidence that natural organisms can convert mixed C6 and C5 sugars at excellent yield; however, genetically altered microbes have made some claims toward this goal [51]. Employing non-commercial biomass, such as forest leftovers, as feedstock and selling co-products generated during the production process could improve the economic sustainability of greener energy production [52].

Extraction from algae has also produced high-value co-products, such as colorants, enzymes, fatty acids, carbs, vitamin supplements, and antioxidants, with application areas in the beauty, health and nutrition, and drug development [53–55]. Improved microalgae biorefinery plans are being developed to help ensure the long-term viability of these processes; cutting-edge technology can utilize supercritical fluid extraction technologies to increase productivity and simplicity of handling [56]. Increased production efficiency and improved energy and material recovery are already benefits of multi-product cogeneration. However, the economic analysis of algal biomass still needs to be significantly improved to compete with fossil fuels. If all by-products were utilized effectively, several conversion processes that are still in use could become financially viable despite their complexity and cost [36].

4.4 FUTURE PROSPECT AND CONCLUSION

The published literature on the future of biofuels can be used to identify a variety of complicated models, detailed narrative approaches, trends, argumentative discussions, and protracted plans. If you think about it, it's easy to wonder if research done two decades ago is still relevant or if its conclusions differ significantly from those in the current publication. The development time might range from 20 to 50 years in forecasting and future studies. Despite the fact that the current study focused on more recent studies, research from earlier periods was not completely neglected. These future-oriented works were examined and critiqued from a variety of angles in this review. It is these assumptions and motivating factors that have been used in these studies to help shape the future of biofuels; limitations, obstacles, issues, and prospects that these studies have identified; and a variety of visions and roadmaps

Challenges and Future Prospects of Biofuel Generations

that these studies have developed and proposed that have all contributed to the lessons learned. An alternative to a collaborative thought method (or a participatory study) was produced by analyzing these significant findings and providing ideas for the biofuels researchers, practitioners, and policymakers.

Biohydrogen production can now employ microalgae as a feedstock [57]. It has been found that some algae species can accumulate carbohydrates up to half their dry mass [58]. It's not easy to find enzyme targets and metabolic pathways that can be modified or replaced when using metabolic engineering to transform microscopic organisms into epithelial cells [59,60]. The functioning of a new metabolic route is influenced by a wide range of parameters, some of which may be hard to pinpoint. Emerging developments in metabolic engineering may one day enable the synthesis of bio-based products not found naturally by microbes [61,62]. Biofuel parent organisms and industrial activities could benefit from all these metabolic modification techniques. In terms of high sequencing for decrypting genomes [63], extremely sensitive exome sequencing [64,65], and advances in fluxomics [66], several new techniques are evolving [67]. Metabolic engineering can affect biofuel production through the use of various computational methods. In the future, microalgae may be used as a possible feedstock for native apps. Methods like burning biomass and fermentation, which can be used in both home and industrial settings while still being environmentally friendly, should take precedence over other energy conversion techniques.

In order to increase the financial viability of algae biofuel and safeguard our human and environmental health from harmful impacts, professionals from a variety of sectors must create environmentally acceptable processing and extraction strategies for biofuel and bioproducts. Numerous businesses could benefit from the simultaneous production of valuable bioproducts, according to this analysis. Researchers must conduct more research into discovering commercially valuable potential goods and their role in the treatment or prevention of diseases. Novel algal strains must be used to investigate the intended chemicals. Researchers must investigate whether:

- Microalgae harvests to the land can enhance crop growth and seedling growth;
- Liquid fertilizers from microalgal species can improve nutrient retention;
- Microalgae can elicit the progress of beneficial microorganisms; and
- Microalgae can elicit the performance and productivity of fruits and vegetables.

REFERENCES

[1] Goss, R. M., "BP statistical review of world energy 1982," *bp.com*, 1983.

[2] Shafiee, S. and E. Topal, "When will fossil fuel reserves be diminished?," *Energy Policy*, vol. 37, no. 1, pp. 181–189, January 2009.

[3] Dincer, I., "Renewable energy and sustainable development: A crucial review," *Renew. Sustain. Energy Rev.*, vol. 4, no. 2, pp. 157–175, 2000.

[4] Jacobsson, S., B. A. Sandén, and L. Bångens, "Transforming the energy system-the evolution of the German technological system for solar cells," *Technol. Anal. Strateg. Manag.*, vol. 16, no. 1, pp. 3–30, 2004.

[5] Berla, B. M., R. Saha, C. M. Immethun, C. D. Maranas, T. S. Moon, and H. B. Pakrasi, "Synthetic biology of cyanobacteria: Unique challenges and opportunities," *Front. Microbiol.*, vol. 4, August 2013.

[6] Bender, M. H., "Potential conservation of biomass in the production of synthetic organics," *Resour. Conserv. Recycl.*, vol. 30, no. 1, pp. 49–58, July 2000.

[7] Demirbas, A., "Biofuels sources, biofuel policy, biofuel economy and global biofuel projections," *Energy Convers. Manag.*, vol. 49, no. 8, pp. 2106–2116, August 2008.

[8] Ahlgren, E. O., M. Börjesson Hagberg, and M. Grahn, "Transport biofuels in global energy–economy modelling – a review of comprehensive energy systems assessment approaches," *GCB Bioenergy*, vol. 9, no. 7, pp. 1168–1180, July 2017.

[9] Awudu, I. and J. Zhang, "Uncertainties and sustainability concepts in biofuel supply chain management: A review," *Renew. Sustain. Energy Rev.*, vol. 16, no. 2, pp. 1359–1368, 2012.

[10] Ayoub, M. and A. Z. Abdullah, "Critical review on the current scenario and significance of crude glycerol resulting from biodiesel industry towards more sustainable renewable energy industry," *Renew. Sustain. Energy Rev.*, vol. 16, no. 5, pp. 2671–2686, 2012.

[11] Mahmudul, H. M., F. Y. Hagos, R. Mamat, A. A. Adam, W. F. W. Ishak, and R. Alenezi, "Production, characterization and performance of biodiesel as an alternative fuel in diesel engines – A review," *Renew. Sustain. Energy Rev.*, vol. 72, pp. 497–509, 2017.

[12] Othman, M. F., A. Adam, G. Najafi, and R. Mamat, "Green fuel as alternative fuel for diesel engine: A review," *Renew. Sustain. Energy Rev.*, vol. 80, pp. 694–709, 2017.

[13] Hill, J., "Environmental costs and benefits of transportation biofuel production from food-and lignocellulose-based energy crops: A review," *Sustain. Agric.*, pp. 125–139, 2009.

[14] Grahn, M., C. Azar, and K. Lindgren, "The role of biofuels for transportation in CO_2 emission reduction scenarios with global versus regional carbon caps," *Biomass and Bioenergy*, vol. 33, no. 3, pp. 360–371, March 2009.

[15] Gustavsson, L., P. Börjesson, B. Johansson, and P. Svenningsson, "Reducing CO_2 emissions by substituting biomass for fossil fuels," *Energy*, vol. 20, no. 11, pp. 1097–1113, 1995.

[16] Kopetz, H., "Renewable resources: Build a biomass energy market," *Nature*, vol. 494, no. 7435, pp. 29–31, February 2013.

[17] Balat, M. and M. Balat, "Political, economic and environmental impacts of biomass-based hydrogen," *Int. J. Hydrogen Energy*, vol. 34, no. 9, pp. 3589–3603, 2009.

[18] Tyndall, J. C., E. J. Berg, and J. P. Colletti, "Corn stover as a biofuel feedstock in Iowa's bio-economy: An Iowa farmer survey," *Biomass and Bioenergy*, vol. 35, no. 4, pp. 1485–1495, April 2011.

[19] Bentsen, N. S. and C. Felby, "Biomass for energy in the European Union—A review of bioenergy resource assessments," *Biotechnol. Biofuels*, vol. 5, 2012.

[20] Guo, M., W. Song, and J. Buhain, "Bioenergy and biofuels: History, status, and perspective," *Renew. Sustain. Energy Rev.*, vol. 42, pp. 712–725, 2015.

[21] Berndes, G., M. Hoogwijk, and R. Van Den Broek, "The contribution of biomass in the future global energy supply: A review of 17 studies," *Biomass and Bioenergy*, vol. 25, no. 1, pp. 1–28, 2003.

[22] Datta, A., A. Hossain, and S. Roy, "An overview on biofuels and their advantages and disadvantages," *Asian J. Chem.*, vol. 31, no. 8, pp. 1851–1858, 2019.

[23] Foster, E., M. Contestabile, J. Blazquez, B. Manzano, M. Workman, and N. Shah, "The unstudied barriers to widespread renewable energy deployment: Fossil fuel price responses," *Energy Policy*, vol. 103, pp. 258–264, 2017.

[24] Callegari, A., S. Bolognesi, D. Cecconet, and A. G. Capodaglio, "Production technologies, current role, and future prospects of biofuels feedstocks: A state-of-the-art review," *Crit. Rev. Environ. Sci. Technol.*, vol. 50, no. 4, pp. 384–436, 2020.

[25] Azad, A. K., M. G. Rasul, M. M. K. Khan, S. C. Sharma, and M. A. Hazrat, "Prospect of biofuels as an alternative transport fuel in Australia," *Renew. Sustain. Energy Rev.*, vol. 43, pp. 331–351, 2015.

[26] Delavarrafiee, M. and H. C. Frey, "Real-world fuel use and gaseous emission rates for flex fuel vehicles operated on E85 versus gasoline," *J. Air Waste Manag. Assoc.*, vol. 68, no. 3, pp. 235–254, March 2018.

[27] Gerbens-Leenes, P. W., "Bioenergy water footprints, comparing first, second and third generation feedstocks for bioenergy supply in 2040," *Eur. Water*, vol. 59, pp. 373–380, 2017.

[28] Renzaho, A. M. N., J. K. Kamara, and M. Toole, "Biofuel production and its impact on food security in low and middle income countries: Implications for the post-2015 sustainable development goals," *Renew. Sustain. Energy Rev.*, vol. 78, pp. 503–516, 2017.

[29] Embury, O., C. J. Merchant, and M. J. Filipiak, "A reprocessing for climate of sea surface temperature from the along-track scanning radiometers: Basis in radiative transfer," *Remote Sens. Environ.*, vol. 116, pp. 32–46, 2012.

[30] Kumar, A., A. Rashmi, A. Agarwal, T. Gupta Bhola, and R. Gurjar. *Biofuels.* Springer, 2017.

[31] Pimentel, D., "Ethanol fuels: Energy balance, economics, and environmental impacts are negative," *Nat. Resour. Res.*, vol. 12, no. 2, pp. 127–134, 2003.

[32] Hirani, A. H., N. Javed, M. Asif, S. K. Basu, and A. Kumar, "A review on first- and second- generation biofuel productions," *Biofuels Greenh. Gas Mitig. Glob. Warm. Next Gener. Biofuels Role Biotechnol.*, pp. 141–154, February 2018.

[33] Manara, P. and A. Zabaniotou, "Towards sewage sludge based biofuels via thermochemical conversion—A review," *Renew. Sustain. Energy Rev.*, vol. 16, no. 5, pp. 2566–2582, June 2012.

[34] Peterson, A. A., F. Vogel, R. P. Lachance, M. Fröling, M. J. Antal, and J. W. Tester, "Thermochemical biofuel production in hydrothermal media: A review of sub- and supercritical water technologies," *Energy Environ. Sci.*, vol. 1, no. 1, pp. 32–65, 2008.

[35] Ho, D. P., H. H. Ngo, and W. Guo, "A mini review on renewable sources for biofuel," *Bioresour. Technol.*, vol. 169, pp. 742–749, October 2014.

[36] Mekhilef, S., R. Saidur, and M. Kamalisarvestani, "Effect of dust, humidity and air velocity on efficiency of photovoltaic cells," *Renew. Sustain. Energy Rev.*, vol. 16, no. 5, pp. 2920–2925, 2012.

[37] Shi, A. Z., L. P. Koh, and H. T. W. Tan, "The biofuel potential of municipal solid waste," *GCB Bioenergy*, vol. 1, no. 5, pp. 317–320, September 2009.

[38] Cheng, J. J. and G. R. Timilsina, "Status and barriers of advanced biofuel technologies: A review," *Renew. Energy*, vol. 36, no. 12, pp. 3541–3549, December 2011.

[39] Rival, T. et al., "Fenton chemistry and oxidative stress mediate the toxicity of the -amyloid peptide in a Drosophila model of Alzheimer's disease," *Eur. J. Neurosci.*, vol. 29, no. 7, pp. 1335–1347, April 2009.

[40] Wongkhorsub, C. and N. Chindaprasert, "A comparison of the use of pyrolysis oils in diesel engine," *Energy Power Eng.*, vol. 05, no. 04, pp. 350–355, 2013.

[41] Naik, S. N., V. V. Goud, P. K. Rout, and A. K. Dalai, "Production of first and second generation biofuels: A comprehensive review," *Renew. Sustain. Energy Rev.*, vol. 14, no. 2, pp. 578–597, February 2010.

[42] Behera, S., R. Singh, R. Arora, N. K. Sharma, M. Shukla, and S. Kumar, "Scope of algae as third generation biofuels," *Front. Bioeng. Biotechnol.*, vol. 2, February 2015.

[43] Brennan, L. and P. Owende, "Biofuels from microalgae-A review of technologies for production, processing, and extractions of biofuels and co-products," *Renew. Sustain. Energy Rev.*, vol. 14, no. 2, pp. 557–577, February 2010.

[44] Ugwu, C. U., H. Aoyagi, and H. Uchiyama, "Photobioreactors for mass cultivation of algae," *Bioresour. Technol.*, vol. 99, no. 10, pp. 4021–4028, July 2008.

[45] Wang, L. et al., "Cultivation of green algae Chlorella sp. in different wastewaters from municipal wastewater treatment plant," *Appl. Biochem. Biotechnol.*, vol. 162, no. 4, pp. 1174–1186, October 2010.

[46] Milledge, J. J., B. V. Nielsen, and D. Bailey, "High-value products from macroalgae: The potential uses of the invasive brown seaweed, Sargassum muticum," *Rev. Environ. Sci. Biotechnol.*, vol. 15, no. 1, pp. 67–88, March 2016.

[47] Yang, J., M. Xu, X. Zhang, Q. Hu, M. Sommerfeld, and Y. Chen, "Life-cycle analysis on biodiesel production from microalgae: Water footprint and nutrients balance," *Bioresour. Technol.*, vol. 102, no. 1, pp. 159–165, January 2011.

[48] Rathmann, R., A. Szklo, and R. Schaeffer, "Land use competition for production of food and liquid biofuels: An analysis of the arguments in the current debate," *Renew. Energy*, vol. 35, no. 1, pp. 14–22, January 2010.

[49] You, Y., P. Li, F. Lei, Y. Xing, and J. Jiang, "Enhancement of ethanol production from green liquor-ethanol-pretreated sugarcane bagasse by glucose-xylose cofermentation at high solid loadings with mixed Saccharomyces cerevisiae strains," *Biotechnol. Biofuels*, vol. 10, no. 1, April 2017.

[50] Yusuf, F. and N. A. Gaur, "Engineering Saccharomyces cerevisiae for C5 fermentation: A step towards second-generation biofuel production," *Metab. Eng. Bioact. Compd. Strateg. Process.*, pp. 157–172, October 2017.

[51] Konsta-Gdoutos, M. S., Z. S. Metaxa, and S. P. Shah, "Highly dispersed carbon nanotube reinforced cement based materials," *Cem. Concr. Res.*, vol. 40, no. 7, pp. 1052–1059, 2010.

[52] Dalvand, K., J. Rubin, S. Gunukula, M. Clayton Wheeler, and G. Hunt, "Economics of biofuels: Market potential of furfural and its derivatives," *Biomass and Bioenergy*, vol. 115, pp. 56–63, August 2018.

[53] Chew, K. W. et al., "Microalgae biorefinery: High value products perspectives," *Bioresour. Technol.*, vol. 229, pp. 53–62, 2017.

[54] Steinman, A. D., G. A. Lamberti, P. R. Leavitt, and D. G. Uzarski, "Biomass and pigments of benthic algae," *Methods Stream Ecol. Third Ed.*, vol. 1, pp. 223–241, February 2017.

[55] Li, W. et al., "Characteristics of self-alkalization in high-rate denitrifying automatic circulation (DAC) reactor fed with methanol and sodium acetate," *Bioresour. Technol.*, vol. 154, pp. 44–50, 2014.

[56] De Melo, M. M. R., A. J. D. Silvestre, and C. M. Silva, "Supercritical fluid extraction of vegetable matrices: Applications, trends and future perspectives of a convincing green technology," *J. Supercrit. Fluids*, vol. 92, pp. 115–176, 2014.

[57] Kumar, G. et al., "Biomass based hydrogen production by dark fermentation—Recent trends and opportunities for greener processes," *Curr. Opin. Biotechnol.*, vol. 50, pp. 136–145, 2018.

[58] Markou, G., I. Angelidaki, and D. Georgakakis, "Microalgal carbohydrates: An overview of the factors influencing carbohydrates production, and of main bioconversion technologies for production of biofuels," *Appl. Microbiol. Biotechnol.*, vol. 96, no. 3, pp. 631–645, November 2012.

[59] Majidian, P., M. Tabatabaei, M. Zeinolabedini, M. P. Naghshbandi, and Y. Chisti, "Metabolic engineering of microorganisms for biofuel production," *Renew. Sustain. Energy Rev.*, vol. 82, pp. 3863–3885, February 2018.

[60] Nakanishi, A. et al., "Effect of pretreatment of hydrothermally processed rice straw with laccase-displaying yeast on ethanol fermentation," *Appl. Microbiol. Biotechnol.*, vol. 94, no. 4, pp. 939–948, May 2012.

[61] Chubukov, V., A. Mukhopadhyay, C. J. Petzold, J. D. Keasling, and H. G. Martín, "Synthetic and systems biology for microbial production of commodity chemicals," *npj Syst. Biol. Appl.*, vol. 2, April 2018.

[62] Koppolu, V. and V. K. Vasigala, "Role of Escherichia coli in Biofuel Production," *Microbiol. Insights*, vol. 9, p. MBI.S10878, January 2016.

[63] Medema, M. H., P. Cimermancic, A. Sali, E. Takano, and M. A. Fischbach, "A systematic computational analysis of biosynthetic gene cluster evolution: Lessons for engineering biosynthesis," *PLoS Comput. Biol.*, vol. 10, no. 12, p. e1004016, December 2014.

[64] Alonso-Gutierrez, J. et al., "Principal component analysis of proteomics (PCAP) as a tool to direct metabolic engineering," *Metab. Eng.*, vol. 28, pp. 123–133, 2015.

[65] Tang, X., H. Feng, J. Zhang, and W. N. Chen, "Comparative proteomics analysis of engineered Saccharomyces cerevisiae with enhanced biofuel precursor production," *PLoS One*, vol. 8, no. 12, December 2013.

[66] George, K. W. et al., "Correlation analysis of targeted proteins and metabolites to assess and engineer microbial isopentenol production," *Biotechnol. Bioeng.*, vol. 111, no. 8, pp. 1648–1658, 2014.

[67] Melchiorre, M. G. et al., "Social support, socio-economic status, health and abuse among older people in seven European countries," *PLoS One*, vol. 8, no. 1, January 2013.

5 A Comparative Study of Physicochemical Properties and Performance Characteristics of Various Biodiesel Feedstock

An Overview

Harish Chandra Joshi[1], Waseem Ahmad[2], Neetu Sharma[1], Vinod Kumar[3], Sanjeev Kimothi[4], and Bhawana[1]

1 Department of Chemistry, Graphic Era deemed to be University, Dehradun, Uttarakhand

2 Department of Chemistry, Uttaranchal University, Dehradun, Uttarakhand, India

3 Department of Life Science, Graphic Era deemed to be University, Dehradun, Uttarakhand

4 Research & Development Division, Uttaranchal University, Dehradun, Uttarakhand, India

CONTENTS

5.1 Introduction 64
    5.1.1 Feedstock 64
    5.1.2 Chemical Compositions of Fatty Esters 66
5.2 Physicochemical Properties of Biodiesel 69
    5.2.1 Density 69
    5.2.2 Specific Gravity 69
    5.2.3 Kinematic Viscosity (KV) 69
        5.2.3.1 Acid Number 69

DOI: 10.1201/9781003265597-5

5.2.4	Saponification Value	69
5.2.5	Iodine Value	73
	5.2.5.1 Flash Point	73
5.2.6	Cloud and Pour Point	73
5.2.7	Diesel Index	73
5.2.8	Moisture Content	73
5.2.9	Aniline Point	73
5.3	Characteristics of Emission and Performance	73
5.4	Conclusion and Summary of Result	78
References		84

5.1 INTRODUCTION

Consumption of fossil fuels is increasing daily, so researchers are focusing on alternative renewable fuels. Since innovation in biodiesel, a lot of innovative work has also been done on the diesel engine and finding an appropriate fuel (Canakci, 2019). Biodiesel has become an interesting alternative renewable fuel to be used in an engine due to biodegradability, unadulterated, physicochemical performance, and emission characteristics of conventional fossil fuel (Islam et al., 2014; Belaid et al., 2011). This renewable fuel is environmentally friendly without or with fewer oxides of sulfur relative to fossil fuel (Zagonel et al., 2004; Knothe & Steidley, 2005; Pimentel et al., 2006).

5.1.1 FEEDSTOCK

The production of biodiesel depends upon the different feedstocks, and the Biodiesel production costs are usually 70–80% depending on the percentage of oil within the feedstock (Joshi et al., 2019; Foglia et al., 2005). There are heterogeneous sources of biodiesel production. There are three-type generation feedstocks of fuel. The first generation is edible seed oil, like sunflower seed oil; the second-generation feedstock is non-edible seed oil (Mahua, neem seed oil); and the third-generation feedstock is microalgae. However, the first and second-generation feedstocks are high in cost and limited in quantity. Of them, some seed oils are unfeasible for the production of biodiesel (Leung & Leung, 2010; Sanchez et al., 2015; Pinzi et al., 2014; Balat, 2011; Hossain et al., 2018; Brennan & Owende, 2010; Jain et al., 2017). Table 5.1 shows the vegetable feedstock details with oil content percentage. Generally, biodiesel feedstock is divided into four categories (Knothe & Steidley, 2009; Ghazali et al., 2015):

1) Different types of vegetable oil
2) Animal Fats
3) Waste cooking oil (WCO)
4) Microalgae

The oil percentage in waste cooking oil does not depend on any substances and can be obtained from commercially available sources. The percentage of bio-oil in algae or microalgae is 2–20% (Kumar et al., 2019; Schenk et al., 2008). The

A Comparative Study of Various Biodiesel Feedstock

TABLE 5.1
Vegetable Seed Oil Feedstock.

Vegetable oil (non-edible seed oil)	Oil content (wt%)
Karanja	25–40 (Azam et al., 2005; Bryan & Chadha, 2005)
Polanga	65–75 (Azam et al., 2005;
Mahua	30–50 (Joshi & Negi, 2017; Kumar & Sharma, 2011; Jeena et al., 2010)
Neem	20–50 ((Azam et al., 2005; Pinzi et al., 2009; Joshi & Negi, 2017; Sanfor et al., 2009)
Rubber Seed oil	50–60 (Gill et al., 2011)
Sugar apple	15–20 (Borugadda & Goud, 2012)
Cotton Seed oil	17–25 (Fontaras et al., 2007; Nabi et al., 2009; Ilkilic & Yucesu, 2008)
Silkweed	20 (Borugadda & Goud, 2012)
Ethiopian Mustard	42 (Borugadda & Goud, 2012)
Semal	18–26 (Borugadda & Goud, 2012)
Undi	65 (Borugadda & Goud, 2012)
Jojoba	40–50 (Al-Widyan & Al-Widyan, 2010)
Hathichuk or Cardoon	25–26 (Borugadda & Goud, 2012)
Abyssinian mustard	30–38 (Borugadda & Goud, 2012)
Tobacco	35–49 (Usta et al., 2011; Giannelos et al., 2009)
White silk cotton	24–40 (Borugadda & Goud, 2012)
Suicide tree	54 (Borugadda & Goud, 2012)
Sea mango	50 (Gui et al., 2008)
Kapok	24–40 (Ghazali et al., 2015)
Croton tiglium	30 (Muliyansh & Atikash, 2014)
Linseed	35–45 (Puhan et al., 2010; Dixit & Rehman, 2012)
Jatropha	20–60 (Openshaw, 2000)
Cuphea (Cigar Plant)	20–38 Knothe et al., 2009)
Crotalaria retusa (Ghunghunia)	15 (Umerie et al., 2010)
Schlichera oleosa (Kusum)	30–45 (Joshi et al., 2020; Babu et al., 2018; Yadav, 2017)
Michelia champaca (Champa)	45 (Joshi et al., 2020; Hosamani et al., 2009)
Putranjiva roxburghii	42 (Joshi et al., 2020; Tripathi & Kumar, 2017)
Mesua ferrea (Indian Rose)	35–50 (Borugadda & Goud, 2012; Aslam et al., 2014)
Blackseed	50–60 (Yerranguntla et al., 2013)
Tung	30–40 (Park et al., 2008)
Sour Garcinia	45 (Tan et al., 2020)
Raphanus sativus	40–45 (Faria et al., 2018)
Sterculia foetida	40 (Akhtar et al., 2019)

(*Continued*)

TABLE 5.1 *(Continued)*

Vegetable oil (non-edible seed oil)	Oil content (wt%)
Flax	35–45 (Xie et al., 2020; Bacenetti et al., 2017)
Melia azedarach	37 (Bachheti et al., 2012)
Ricinus communis	50 (Figueroa et al., 2020)
Salvadora oleoides	45–50 (Borugadda & Goud, 2012; Tripathi & Kumar, 2020)
Sterculia foetida	50–60 (Borugadda & Goud, 2012; Kale et al., 2011)
Thlaspi arvense L.	36 (Borugadda & Goud, 2012; Bryan et al., 2016)
Citrus maxima	30–40 (Joshi et al., 2019)
Tomato seed	33.6–37.4 (Fahim, 2013; Lazos and Kalathenos (1998)
Moringa oleifera	70 (Benzard et al., 1971)

TABLE 5.2
Edible Vegetable Seed Oil Feedstock.

Edible vegetable seed oil	Oil content (wt%)
Coconut	30–50 (Borugadda & Goud, 2012; Tupufia, 2012)
Palm	20 (Kumar et al., 2016)
Rape seed	37–50 (Kumar et al., 2016)
Soyabean	20 (Kumar et al., 2016; Sanchez & Vasudevan, 2006)
Olive	45 (Kumar et al., 2016; Al-Jasass & Al-Jasass, 2012)
Mustard	28–32 (Kumar et al., 2016; Afif & Biradar, 200)
Hemp	26–42 (Schumann et al., 2004; Mirza & Ahmad, 2008)

auspicious prospective alternate renewable sources for biodiesel production is due to a high content of lipid in algae 30% or microalgae 30–40% by dry weight and high rates of growth, while edible oil have not more than 5% lipids content by dry weight (Amaro et al., 2011; Lam & Lee, 2011; Lam & Lee, 2012; Kligerman & Bouwer, 2015; Tredici, 2010). The advantages of algae or microalgae in the production of biodiesel is possible to expand on a wide scale and alter the cultivation conditions for the biochemical compositions such as high lipids and carbohydrate (Pittman et al., 2011; Mutlu & Meier, 2010). Table 5.2 shows the feedstock for edible oils.

5.1.2 CHEMICAL COMPOSITIONS OF FATTY ESTERS

The fuel properties of biodiesel may vary due to origination, saturation or unsaturation, and length of the fatty acid alkyl chain. There is main compositional contrast between fossil fuels, and biodiesel is oxygen content. There are various constituents of fatty acids present in fatty ester Figure 5.1.

Most feedstocks are used for medicinal purposes, cosmetics, chemicals, etc. Nowadays, biodiesel is produced due to its physicochemical properties.

A Comparative Study of Various Biodiesel Feedstock

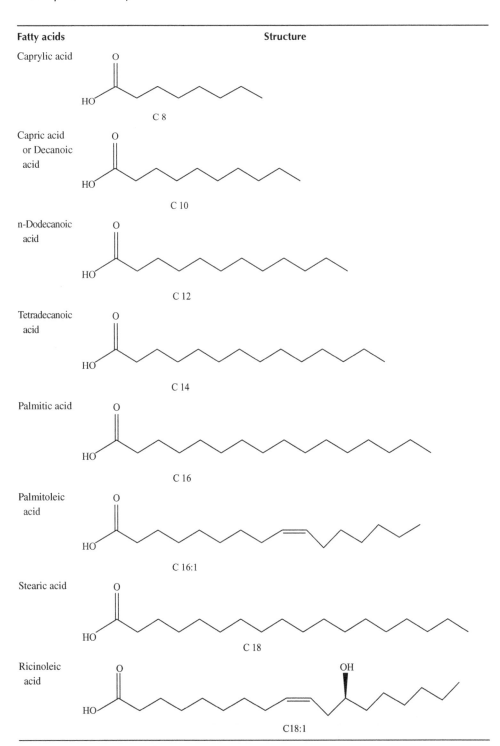

FIGURE 5.1 Chemical structure of fatty acids present in methyl ester.

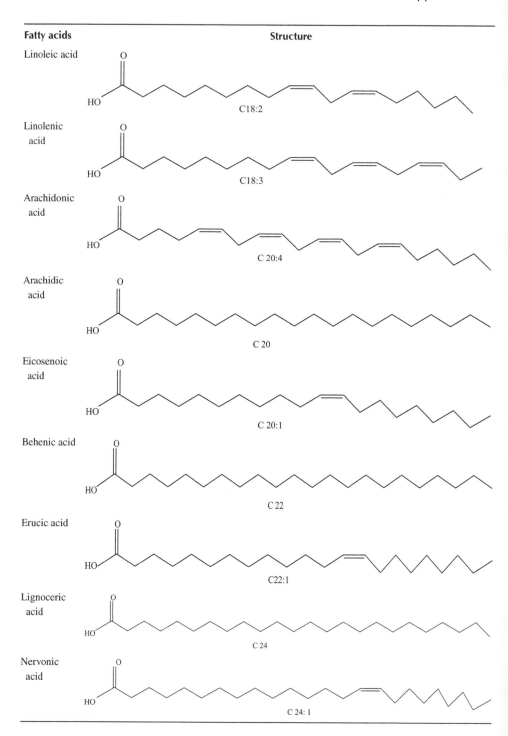

FIGURE 5.1 *(Continued)*

A Comparative Study of Various Biodiesel Feedstock

5.2 PHYSICOCHEMICAL PROPERTIES OF BIODIESEL

The major fuel properties appraise in the implementation of biodiesel, which may be originated from, non-edible, edible, animal fat or microalgae. The above properties of biodiesel depend on their constituent of chemical compositions and fatty acids (Nabi et al., 2009; Giannelos et al., 2002; Abebayo et al., 2011). The physicochemical properties of biodiesel are given in Table 5.3. In this section, fuel properties of biodiesel are discussed.

5.2.1 DENSITY

Generally, density is measured at 15 °C or 40 °C. The average density of the diesel has been reported in the range of 816–840 kg/m³ (Hoekmana et al., 2016). Table 5.3 represents the density of biodiesel. Neem biodiesel has the highest density, while coconut has the lowest density.

5.2.2 SPECIFIC GRAVITY

Diesel fuel has a specific gravity of 0.825 (Bobade & Khyade, 2012); however, the specific gravity of all methyl esters is higher than that of diesel oil.

5.2.3 KINEMATIC VISCOSITY (KV)

A high kinematic viscosity value leads to the delayed combustion of fuel due low flow of liquid fuel into combustion chamber of engine, taking too much time to mix with air. KV of biodiesel can be improved by decreasing with increasing temperature. The KV can determine by ASTM D445 standards (Kumar et al., 2009). Table 5.3 shows that the value of KV of Neem, Karanja, Mahua is 155.72, 40.2, and 37.86 mm²/s, respectively, is much higher than the standard value of biodiesel >1.9–6.0 mm²/s while all other feedstock methyl esters are close to standard biodiesel ≤1.9–6.0 mm²/s. Therefore, these feedstock methyl esters give better engine performance than the Neem, Karanja, and Mahua biodiesel.

5.2.3.1 Acid Number

Acid value measures the amount of fatty acid. Higher activation values allow faster appearing but less stable suds creation or vice versa. The acid value is determined by ASTM D 664 (ASTM 1998). The acid value of Neem and *Michalis Champaca* is >0.5 standard biodiesel.

5.2.4 SAPONIFICATION VALUE

ASTM D 5558 measures saponification value (SV or SN) (Nahak et al., 2010; Reda, 2014). SV measures the average molecular weight (Amw), or chain length of all fatty acids present in fat (Leal et al., 2008). Higher the SV, lower the fatty acid chain length. SV of *Salvadora oleoides* (SV = 228.9 mg KOH/g) is much higher than the reported work.

TABLE 5.3
The Physicochemical Properties of Different Feedstocks of Methyl Ester.

Feedstock/ Properties	Density	Specific gravity	Kinematic viscosity	Acid number	Saponification value	Iodine value	Flash Point (°C)	Cloud point (°C)	Pour point (°C)	Diesel index	Moisture content	Aniline point (°F)
Karanja	0.924	-	40.2	0.620	-	-	223	3.5	-3	-	0.03	**87**
Polanga	0.888	-	4.37	-	-	-	187	13	-3	-	-	-
Mahua	0.88	0.88684	37.86	8	1.12	7.03	167	-2	-6	24.6325	77	**87.8**
Neem	1.002	1.00636	155.72	74	92.4	14.72	110	-3	-5	7.83124	68	**86**
Rubber Seed oil	0.881	0.874	5.3	0.118	-	-	140	5	-8	-	-	-
Sugar apple	0.865	-	5.90	0.34	-	-	161	2	5	-	-	-
Cotton seed oil	0.848	-	6.1	-	-	-	200	-2	-5	-	-	-
Silkweed	-	-	5.2	-	-	-	-	-0.8	-6.7	-	-	-
Semal	0.875	-	4.78	-	-	-	155	3	-4	-	-	-
Ethiopian mustard	0.810	-	4.88	0.06	-	109.4	-	-	-	-	0.03	-
Undi	0.869	-	4	1.62	-	-	140	13.2	4.3	-	0.005	-
Jojoba	0.886	-	25	-	-	-	75	16	-6	-	0.026	-
Hathichuk or cardoon	0.880	-	3.56	-	-	-	175	-1	-	-	-	-
Tobacco	0.888	-	4.2	0.3	-	136	165	-	-12	-	-	-
White silk cotton	0.883	-	4.69	0.18	-	-	158.5	-3	-2	-	-	-
Sea mango	0.885	-	2.89	0.37	-	-	133	-	-	-	-	-
Kapok	0.860	-	4.2	0.38	-	-	148	4	-4.4	-	-	-
Croton tiglium	0.867	-	4.5	-	-	-	-	-	-	-	-	**109.83**
Tomato seed	0.922	-	38	1.68	-	118.4	-	-	-	-	-	-
Citrus maxima	0.892	0.8964	13	0.5	10	8.3	110	14	4.9	-	10	**87.8**

A Comparative Study of Various Biodiesel Feedstock

Thlaspi arvense L	-	-	5.24	0.04	-	-	-	-10	-18	-	-	-
Sterculia foetida	0.897	-	3.96	.14	-	-	160.5	-3	-3	-	-	-
Salvadora oleoides	0.875	-	3.25	0.45	228.9	11.97	130	-	3	-	-	-
Ricinus communis	0.9	0.95	25	0.9	170.73	83.5	-	-	-	-	-	-
Melia azedarach	0.9	0.89	3.2	-	48.9	119	131	-10	-28	-	-	-
Flax	0.886	-	4.24	0.5	-	120	170	-3	-8	-	-	-
Raphanus sativus	0.879	0.82	2.6	0.65	-	119	65	-15	-5	-	-	-
Tung	0.9030	-	7.53	0.001	-	-	160	-	-10	-	0.067	-
Blackseed	0.890	-	4.1	-	-	-	128	3	5	-	-	-
Mesua ferrea (Indian Rose)	0.898	-	6.2	0.01	-	-	112	-	3	-	-	-
Putranjiva roxburghii	0.8694	0.8820	9	2.8	0.56	8.88	110	-2	-12	-	0.6	-
Schlichera oleosa (Kusum)	0.8779	0.8804	8	3	0.56	7	130	-2	-6	-	0.6	-
Michelia champaca (Champa)	0.8873	0.8899	15	10	6	12	110	-5	-15	-	1.4	-
Cuphea (Cigar plant)	-	-	2.38	-	-	-	-	-9.1	-21.5	-	-	-
Jatropha	0.876	-	4.75	0.15	-	-	109.5	5	9	-	0.05	-
Moringa Olefera	0.8770	0.87830	4.008	0.185	-	9.89	160	NA	13.3	-9	0.065	-
Linseed	0.8925	-	3.7	-	-	-	108	1.7	-4	-	0.042	-

(Continued)

TABLE 5.3 (Continued)

Feedstock/Properties	Density	Specific gravity	Kinematic viscosity	Acid number	Saponification value	Iodine value	Flash Point (°C)	Cloud point (°C)	Pour point (°C)	Diesel index	Moisture content	Aniline point (°F)
Coconut	0.8073	-	2.7	0.106	-	-	115	-	0	-	0.034	-
Hemp	0.8885	-	3.87	0.097	177	-	160	-	-1.3	-	0.017	-
Mustard	0.88	0.672	4.10	1.5	-	54	156	-	-4	-	0.039	-
Olive	0.860	-	4.18	-	-	-	174	-	-	-	-	-
Soyabeen	0.8840	0.8814	4.039	0.8	-	62.6	118	-	0.9	-	0.409	-
Rape seed	0.844	0.882	4.5	-	-	-	170	-4	-12	-	-	-
Palm	0.8925	0.860	4.5	0.46	-	-	160	-	13	-	0.083	-
Waste cooking oil (WCO)	0.8555	-	4.3	0.332	-	-	170	-	2.4	-	0.242	-
Algae or microalgae	0.8780	-	4.5	0.22	-	-	95	16.1	-5.2	-	0.021	-

Canakci, 2005; Joshi et al., 2019, 2020; Hossain et al., 2018; Karmee & Chadha, 2005; Pinzi et al., 2009; Usta et al., 2011; GUi et al., 2008; Muliyansh & Atikash, 2014; Puhan et al., 2010; Schumann et al., 2004; Hotii & Hebbal, 2015; Agarwal & Kumar, 2017; An et al., 2013; Ahmad et al., 2014; Ikwuagu et al., 2000; Huzayyin et al., 2004; Shehata & Razek, 2011; Velikovic et al., 2006; Lin & Lin, 2012; Omprakash et al., 2015; Holser & Harry O Kuru, 2006; Bouaid et al., 2005; Harsha et al., 2018; Ong et al., 2011, 2019; Encinar et al., 1999; Silitonga et al., 2013, 2019; Lie et al., 2018; Giuffre et al., 2015; Moser et al., 2009; Kaul et al., 2007; Budhwani et al., 2019; Iiaz et al., 2016; Awais et al., 2020; Ciubta et al., 2013; Silveria et al., 2019; Kumar & Kumar, 2013; Kumar, 2006; Tulip & Radha, 2012; Shahid & Jamal, 2011.

A Comparative Study of Various Biodiesel Feedstock

5.2.5 Iodine Value

Iodine value (IV) is determined according to ASTM D 5558 (ASTM 1998). IV gives the amount of unsaturation contained in fatty acid and gives the efficient viscosity characteristics in cold conditions (Boog et al., 2011). Most of the methyl ester feedstock have IV ≤ 112.69 g I_2/100mL.

5.2.5.1 Flash Point

ASTM D93 standard is used to determine the flash point of biodiesel. Each biodiesel has its own flash point, and this point estimates the flammability hazard of substances. Many aspects affect the flash point, including residual alcohol and the number of double bonds and chemical compositions (Carareto et al., 2012; Ferando et al., 2007). *Citrus maxima*, *Raphanus sativus*, *Putranjiva Roxburghii*, Linseed, and microalgae have flash points less than 130 °C and it is the minimum flash point for the biodiesel according to the standards followed.

5.2.6 Cloud and Pour Point

This test is measured the ASTM D 2500 and ASTM D97 (Fernando et al., 2007; Haile et al., 2013). In Table 5.3, *Melia azedarach* and *Raphanus sativus* have the lowest cloud point −10 °C and −15 °C, respectively. On the other hand, *Melia azedarach* has the lowest pour point, that is, −28 °C.

5.2.7 Diesel Index

ASTM D4737 is used for the calculation of the diesel index. DI indicates the combustion and ignition quality of biodiesel. The typical value is between 35 and 60. Most of the methyl ester in Table 5.3 does not meet the standards.

5.2.8 Moisture Content

The moisture content of biodiesel is determined by Mebrahtu (2013) method (Kumar et al., 2009). The moisture content is in the range of 0.05 biodiesel. Moreover, the entire methyl ester meets the standards.

5.2.9 Aniline Point

The aniline point (AP) correspondence is the type and amount of aromatic hydrocarbons in biodiesel. A higher AP is indicative of lower aromatic hydrocarbon content or vice versa. AP of oil gives an indication of deterioration of oil when it is exposed to packing rubber sealing etc. In literature, most of the methyl esters do not have AP, but some methyl esters, such as *Croton tiglium*, Karanja and Mahua, have 109.83 F, 87 F, and 87.8 F AP, respectively.

5.3 CHARACTERISTICS OF EMISSION AND PERFORMANCE

The performance and emission generation of blended edible, non-edible, and microalgae biodiesel with conventional biodiesel on an engine can be evaluated by BTE and BSFC properties. The performance of biodiesel or blend biodiesel is given in Table 5.4.

TABLE 5.4

Performance Characteristics of Engine Using Different Biodiesels.

Feedstock/Properties	Engine type and characteristics	Result	
		Brake thermal efficiency	**BSFC**
Karanja	Four stroke, single cylinder, 1500 rpm constant speed with CI engine, blended fuel is 20% with various load	Greater under all load conditions	Decreases as the load increases
Polanga	Four stroke, single cylinder, DI, WC, CI, 1500 rpm constant speed with various mixes	Increases when mixed biodiesel and additives	Decreases with use of higher blended biodiesel and additives
Mahua	Single Cylinder, four Stroke, WC, DI, CR: 16.5:1, RP: 3.7 kw 1500 rpm constant speed	Compared to ordinary diesel fuel, it is much greater	Higher than the conventional diesel fuel
Neem	Four stroke, single cylinder, DI, WC, RS: 1500 rpm, RP:3.7 kw, CR: 16.5:1, Variable loads and constant speed	Low at high load	High at low load
Rubber	Single cylinder, four stroke, AC, CR: 17.5:1, DI, CI engine, RP: 4.4 kw, RS: 1500 rpm, leasing net RSO and Different diethyl ether with RSO (50 g/h, 100 g/h, 150 g/h, 200 g/h, and 250 g/h) and full stack condition	Lower than diesel fuel when utilizing net RSO and better with DEE injection when using RSO	
Sugar apple	3.6kW, Dual ignition diesel engine, computerized, vertical, one cylinder, four stroke, water-cooled, naturally aspirated. The engine is loaded using an eddy current dynamometer	Higher with the increase of blend percentage in biodiesel due to the presence of excess oxygen in the blend	Increase with the load
Cotton Seed	Four stroke, single cylinder, diesel engine with constant speed and water cooling, HP: 5.2 KW @ 1500 rpm/7.2 HP; Bore × Stroke: 87.5 × 110 mm; Compression ratio: 17.5:1	Fuel performance increases with increased engine torque until it reaches its optimum value, at which point it reduces	Engine performance reduces as engine torque rises, reaches a low, and then rises again
Jojoba	Four stroke, single cylinder, AC, DI, NA, CR: 17:1, different injection rates and timings of 24 CAD	Increase with EGR operation, full load, and high speed engine	Decrease with EGR operation and high speed engine
Hathichuk or Cardoon	The fuel injection system is of the rail type, with an injector feeding five holes with a diameter of 170 m. A charge amplifier is built inside a piezoelectric sensor (AVL QC33C) (AVL 3066A01)	For all of the fuels evaluated, the % load was raised	Increased by increasing in the engine load

Tobacco	Four stroke, single cylinder, NA, DI, RP: 14.7:1, RS: 2500 rpm, different speeds and a full load (1200, 1400, 1600, 1800, 2000, 2200, and 2400 rpm)		Slightly increased compared with conventional fuel at lower engine speed
White Silk cotton	Variable compression ratio engine, single cylinder, fuel injection timing BTDC (Degree) 0–25, RS: 1500 rpm, compression ratio: 12:1–19:1, water cooling	As the engine's injection timing order is improved, the brake thermal efficiency is doubled for all of the fuel types tested	
Kapok	TF 120 M Yanmar, single cylinder, cylinder bore × stroke volume: 92 mm × 96 mm, compression ratio: 17.7:1, 7.7 kW maximum power, 2400 rpm maximum engine speed, water cooling	For all biodiesel blends, the B20, B30, and B50 have the lowest performance due to the presence of oxygen in biodiesel mixes	The friction heat is lost at high speeds, resulting in poor combustion
Tomato seed	Kirloskar TAF-1, single cylinder, rated speed: 1500 rpm, bore 87.5 mm, stroke 110 mm, air cooling	The BTE of an engine rises with load and with blend concentration.	
Sterculia foetida	Single cylinder, four stroke, diesel engine, direct injection, bore × stroke: 87.5 × 110 mm, 17.5:1 compression ratio, 1500 rpm speed, 5.2 kW rated power, water cooling	Because of its lower viscosity, spray qualities, and calorific value, it has a higher viscosity, spray characteristics, and calorific value than the reference fuel	
Ricinus communis	Kirlosakar AVI; bore ×stroke: 80 mm × 110 mm; compression ratio: 12:1–20:1; Fuel used: diesel, CME, and their blends; Rated speed: 1500 rpm	BTE decreases in composites as the proportion of biodiesel component increases	For all composite ratios, BSFC decreases when BP rises and vice versa
Flax	Mitsubishi center, 4D34–2A, Inline 4, bore 104 mm, torque 295 Nm at 1800 rpm	When utilizing bogus flax biodiesel instead of diesel fuel, as well as adding butanol to both diesel and biodiesel, engine power, performance, and torque reduced	
Tung	Six cylinder, Four stroke turbocharged, intercooled, common rail direct injection compression ratio 17.5:1, maximum torque 1080 Nm@1400–1600 rpm, bore ×stroke: 112 mm × 132 mm	Due to the addition of ethanol to diesel-tung oil, the BTE increased	Due to the reduced calorific values, the combination of tung oil and ethanol resulted in a higher BSFC

(Continued)

TABLE 5.4 *(Continued)*

Feedstock/Properties	Engine type and characteristics	Result	
		Brake thermal efficiency	**BSFC**
Blackseed	Kirloskar TV1, direct injection system, fourstroke, water-cooled diesel engine, fuel injection pressure to 900 bar, RS:1500 rpm	In comparison to the NSME25, BTE climbed by 18.37% (blend)	Due to complete fuel combustion, the BSFC values for all nanofuel mixes with n-butanol declined.
Mesua ferrea (Indian Rose)	Kirloskar TV1 VCR diesel engine, single cylinder, four stroke, rated power at 1500 rpm, hp 5.20, bore ×stroke: 87.5 × 110, water cooled	Due to incomplete combustion and increased blend viscosity, BTE is lowest with diesel in all loads. Increases when the load and compression ratio rise	The BSFC decreases with load, which is consistent across all tested fuels
Putranjiva roxburghii	Ricardo diesel engine, fourstroke, single cylinder, speed: 1000–300 rpm, different blends used, range of compression ratio: 4.5:1–20:1	30% blend of Putranjiva oil with diesel gives quite a satisfactory performance	The performance of a 30% Putranjiva oil/diesel combination is quite acceptable
Schlichera oleosa (Kusum)	Kirloskar oil TV1 engine, single cylinder, four stroke, bore ×stroke: 87.50 × 110, compression ratio: 17.5, rated speed: 1500 rpm	Increases with the rise in the load	Consumption is decreased due to an increase in the brake power
Jatropha	Four stroke, single cylinder, the test engine is attached to an eddy current type dynamometer for load fluctuations, and it is water-cooled, electric start direct-injection diesel engine. RP: 3.5kW, RS: 1500 rpm	Blended biodiesel have a greater fuel efficiency than standard diesel. This is because of improved atomization, combustion, and ignition delay characteristics	Efficiency is decreases with increase in load
Moringa Olefera	Mitsubishi Pajero (4D56T), four cylinder inline, compression ratio: 21:1, bore × stroke (mm): 92 × 96, radiator cooling, maximum engine speed (rpm): 4200, maximum power (kW): 55		BSFC values are higher (5.42–8.39%) than conventional fuel and give a lower calorific value
Linseed	Four stroke, single cylinder, Di, WC, variable blends (B5, B10, B15, and B20), constant speed 1500 rpm, and different loads, RP: 3.5 kw, CR: 17.5:1, RS:1500 rpm	High percentage of biodiesel in fuel blend, high injection pressure and high load increases the thermal efficiency	The BSFC is reduced by a high % biodiesel in the fuel blend, high injection pressure, and a high load
Coconut	Motorsazan Model MT4.244, bore ×stroke (mm): 100 × 127, four cylinders, four stroke, compression ratio: 17.25:1, water-cooled		BSFC of all fuels increased with increasing percentage of biodiesel in blend fuel

Hemp	Kirloskar TV1, single cylinder, four stroke, DI engine, 87.50 mm × 110.00 mm bore × stroke, 18:01 compression ratio, 1500 rpm rated speed	Increases with increasing load up to 80%, then falls at maximum load due to incomplete combustion	All test fuels first decline with an increase in load, up to 80%, and then begin to increase with an increase in load
Mustard	AVL 5402, four stroke, single cylinder, rated speed: 1300 rpm, bore diameter (D): 87.5 mm, stroke (L): 110 mm, compression ratio 17:1	Increase with brake power and also increase with blended fuels	Increase with the 100% of blended biofuel
Soyabeen	Four-cylinder, fourstroke, variable speed, turbocharged DI diesel engine, compression ratio: 16.8:1		Due to a higher amount of biodiesel in the fuel blend and a higher heating value (HHV), reduction in efficiency was attained
Rape seed	Kirloskar, single cylinder, four stroke water cooled VCRDE, speed 1500 rpm @ compression ratio of 16:1, 110 mm × 80 mm bore × stroke	The maximum BTE was attained at 80% engine load. Following that, with all of the observed fuels, the engine's BTE drops slightly	As the engine's load grows, it decreases. The similar pattern was seen up to an engine load of 80%, after which the succeeding loading condition showed a modest rise
Palm	Single cylinder, four stroke, direct injection, naturally aspirated, air cooled, 78 mm bore, 6 mm in length, 3600 rpm rated speed, 17.5:1 compression ratio	In comparison to diesel, the blend sample has a minor improvement in brake power of 4.65% on average	When compared to diesel fuel, the average decrease in blend sample is 0.91%
Waste cooking oil (WCO)	Euro IV, in-line four cylinder, turbocharged, DI 18.5:1, compression ratio 21 with 75 kW at 3600 rpm is the rated power, denso common rail fuel injection system, operate in a variety of mixes and load conditions	Higher at 50% and 100% engine loads due to the improved combustion caused by biodiesel's fuel borne oxygen	When the biodiesel blend ratio was improved to 50% and 100%, a significant improvement in BSFC was found at 800 rpm
Algae or microalgae	Single-cylinder, fourstroke diesel engine, Lombardini 3LD 510, compression ratio: 17.5:1, cooling: forced-air cooling		Increased because biodiesel has a lower calorific value and a higher oxygen content than conventional fuel

Kavitha et al., 2019; Baijju et al., 2009; Sharma et al., 2009; Hegde & Rao, 2012; Puhan et al., 2005; Geo et al., 2010; Shehata & Razek, 2011; Parlak et al., 2013; Jindal & Salvi, 2012; Haldar et al., 2009; Canakci, 2005; Suldhal & Shrigiri, 2016; Kumar et al., 2018, 2019; Jaliliantabar et al., 2018; Tamilselvan et al., 2018; Ong et al., 2014; Nalgundwar et al., 2016; Sivasubramanian et al., 2017; Kavitha & Murugavelh, 2019; Rashed et al., 2016; Akar, 2016; Qi et al., 2017; Khan et al., 2020; Singh et al., 2015; Gugulothu, 2020; Afif & Biradar, 2019; Devarajan et al., 2018; Zareh et al., 2017; Saravanan et al., 2019; Velikovic et al., 2006; Sahoo et al., 2007.

78   Biowaste and Biomass in Biofuel Applications

Brake thermal efficiency (BTE) demonstrates the conversion or transfer of energy similarly to conventional biodiesel. At first, it was seen that warm productivity diminishes with an increment in the biodiesel rate in the fuel. Nevertheless, as the mixing level of biodiesel was expanded past 50% by volume, the warm productivity keeps on expanding. This might be because biodiesel's high oxygen substance brings about great fuel burning.

According to the literature, BSFC was lowered as a result of lower viscosity, density, and calorific value. However, due to poor biodiesel blend mixing, decreased atomization, and greater engine load, the BSFC of certain mixed fuels increases.

The emission characteristics are given in Table 5.5. Researchers found that utilizing oxygenated fuels lowered CO emissions by up to 30% depending on engine type, age, RS, and other factors (Alptekin & Canakci, 2008). In blended fuel, CO emission is reduced due to the higher content of oxygen, the combustion is complete, leading to the lower formation of CO than the fossil fuel. However, CO emission is increased in Polanga (Bajju et al., 2009), Putranjiva Roxburghii (Rashed et al., 2016), and Cardoon (Jindal & Salvi, 2012) due to higher biodiesel blends, resulting in higher viscosity and poor air mixing of fuel. Smoke was observed with blended fuel

5.4 CONCLUSION AND SUMMARY OF RESULT

This review concluded that non-edible oils and microalgae are promising sustainable renewable energy sources for biodiesel. These biodiesel provide the energy required for transportation and other purposes. Most of the investigators focused on the physicochemical properties, performance, and emission characteristics of different engines with different loads of biodiesel.

The fatty acid compositions influence the physicochemical properties of produced biodiesel and blended biodiesel. The physicochemical properties of edible, nonedible, and microalgae are measured according to ASTM and EN standards. Previous studies show that most of the physicochemical properties are close to the standards.

The inclusion of mono-, di-, and tri-saturated fatty acids in blends at low temperatures improved the fuel properties, stability, safety, and ignition efficiency. Study shows that low heating, high density, and high viscosity value of biodiesel lead to reduced engine power and increased fuel exhaustion. Engine power and fuel exhaustion properties can be enhanced through the blending process by adding a low percentage of biodiesel in the blended fuel, such as ethanol, butanol, or diesel.

Break specific fuel consumption (BSFC) of the blended fuel increases the efficiency of the engine on increases the load and percentage of biodiesel in the fuel blend. Some fuel blends decrease the BSFC of the engine due to a higher content of oxygen in blend fuel and high heating value.

Studies of literature agreed that the emission of CO will be reduced with the increased engine load. The emission of NOx increases due to a higher content of oxygen in biodiesel. HC emission will also be reduced, increasing load and fueled

TABLE 5.5
Emission Characteristics of Diesel Engine Using Different Biodiesel.

Feedstock/ Properties	Emission characteristics				
	CO	NO_x	HCs	PM	Smoke
Karanja	Decreases with increased high load	Increases when the load is high and the proportion of biodiesel in the fuel is high	With a heavy load and a low proportion of biodiesel in the mix fuel, the efficiency drops	Decreases with increases in biodiesel content	Smoke is reduced with high load
Polanga	Higher CO emission with higher blended biodiesel ratio	Increases when the percentage ratio of mixed gasoline increases	Decreases with higher blended biodiesel ratio	Decreases with higher blended biodiesel ratio	Decreases with higher blended biodiesel ratio and engine speed
Mahua	Emissions drop as the percentage of biodiesel in the blended fuel increases	Increased engine load as well as mixed biodiesel ratio	Increase in biodiesel percentage in blended fuel and heavy load cause a decrease	–	With a high proportion of biodiesel in blended fuel, the overall load reduced
Neem	Decreases with increases engine load and ethanol content in biodiesel	Decreases with the increases of half load and full load	Reduces as load rises, and increases when ethanol is added to the blend fuel	–	All load circumstances resulted in a reduction
Rubber Seed	With a high load and a low biodiesel content in mixed fuel, emissions are reduced	With a high proportion of biodiesel in the fuel blend and a high load, the percentage of biodiesel increases	Low proportion of biodiesel in blended fuel decreases with heavy load, additives, and low percentage of biodiesel in mixed fuel	–	Low load and a high proportion of biodiesel in the fuel cause a reduction
Sugar apple	Decreases with the increasing load for all the test fuels	Increases with increasing loads	Decreases slightly with the increase in loads	–	–
Cotton Seed	CO emission is lower than the conventional fuel due to biodiesel contain some extra oxygen in their molecules	At the same engine torque, NOx levels were greater for biodiesel blends than for regular diesel fuel. The inclusion of additional oxygen in the molecules of biodiesel blends causes this	–	Biodiesel mixtures reduced PM by 24%	Biodiesel mixtures reduced the smoke emission by 14%

(Continued)

TABLE 5.5 *(Continued)*

Feedstock/ Properties	Emission characteristics				
	CO	NOx	HCs	PM	Smoke
Jojoba	EGR operation and a high amount of biodiesel in blended fuel lead to an increase. High engine speed, on the other hand, might cause a drop in performance	High engine speed causes an increase, but EGR activation causes a drop	Decrease with low engine speed but increase with EGR operation	-	-
Hathichuk or Cardoon	CO emission increased with increasing engine speed and low load	At lower engine loads (15% and 30%) and engine speeds (1200–1700), as well as at 45% engine load, NOx emissions were decreased (at all engine speeds)	-	-	-
Tobacco	CO emissions drop as engine load and biodiesel concentration in the fuel blend rise. However, if the injection pressure is excessive, it should be increased	Increase when the load is full and the injection pressure is high	Reduction in emissions by increasing engine load and biodiesel percentage in the fuel blend. However, if the injection pressure is excessive, increase it	-	With a full load and a high-speed engine, the reduction is smaller
White silk cotton	The CO emission of the blend B10 is comparable to that of high-quality gasoline, with a minor increase at injection timing 18°bTDC	With a reduction in the injection timing relationship, emissions for diesel and B10 and B20 mixes drop	For blends B10 and B20, organic compound emission is lower with greater injection time order	-	-
Kapok	CO emissions significantly decreased due to reduction in biodiesel blend ratio	With a lower amount of biodiesel in the fuel blend, emissions are reduced	At full load, biodiesel blends produce more HC emissions	-	Reduced as the biodiesel blending percentage was increased, owing to a reduction in carbon residual

Tomato seed	As the blend percentage rises, CO decreases	Increase as the blend percentage increases	Decrease with the increase in blend percentage	-	Decrease with load and blend percentage
Sterculia foetida	With the higher biodiesel blends, CO emissions decreased during maximum load	At 0% load, the emission of NOx for STB and the reference fuel was found to be almost identical. At higher loads, NOx is emitted by all biodiesel blends	Reduced emissions by increasing engine load and increasing biodiesel percentage in the fuel blend	-	-
Ricinus communis	Reduction in 8.2% of CO exhalation level	Increase with optimization of load	If the load increases, the HC exhalation also increases for the diesel. This is due to the shortage of oxygen	-	Smoke level decreases with slow combustion. It can be increased by increase in the composite ratio
Flax	Emission decreases with blended biodiesel-butanol-diesel	Emission decreases with blended biodiesel-butanol-diesel	-	-	
Tung	CO emission was high at low load	Minimal engine load resulted in low emissions; however, high engine load resulted in somewhat higher emissions	CO emission was high at low load	-	Due to the increased oxygen concentration in ethanol, it was reduced at higher engine loads
Black seed	Emission decreases at maximum load	Due to an excess of oxygen molecules in the combustion chamber and a high temperature, emissions increased	At maximum load, emission decreases	-	At maximum load, emission decreases
Mesua ferrea (Indian rose)	With an increase in CR, emissions decrease in sequence	Emission increases with increasing load and CR	Emission decreasing with the increase in load	-	-
Putranjiva roxburghii	Emissions decrease with increase load due to uses of blend and higher ignition temperature	Fuel blends emit much less pollution than diesel fuel at greater loads	-	Reduced the emission with 30% use of blends	Higher NO_x was observed at 30% blend of biodiesel

(Continued)

TABLE 5.5 *(Continued)*

Feedstock/ Properties	Emission characteristics				
	CO	NOₓ	HCs	PM	Smoke
Schlichera oleosa (Kusum)	Higher CO emission is produced at low loads due to low in-cylinder temperature	Emission increases due to full load	Due to a longer ignition delay interval, HC emissions increase	-	Due to the sufficient amount of oxygen atoms present in biodiesel blends, smoke production was reduced
Jatropha	When the amount of biodiesel in a blend fuel is reduced, emissions fall	At the same engine torque, biodiesel and biodiesel blends emit more NOx than standard diesel fuel. The availability of oxygen in methyl esters is higher than in diesel, which might be the cause for this	At all power outputs, increasing biodiesel proportion lowered HC emissions	-	-
Moringa olefera	Blended biodiesel fuels reduced emission (22.93–32.65%) more efficiently than diesel fuel	Emission slightly reduced about 6.91–18.56% than diesel fuel	Blended biodiesel fuels reduced emissions (11.84–30.26%) more efficiently than diesel fuel	-	-
Linseed	Increases with percentages of biodiesel in the fuel blend, but decreases with increasing engine load	Slightly increases	Emissions are reduced by increasing engine load and increasing biodiesel content in the fuel blend		
Coconut	As the amount of biodiesel in the fuel blend rises, CO emissions fall	Increased NOx exhausting the engine. Increased load caused NOx levels to rise in comparison to diesel decreases	-	Decrease in PM in the engine exhaust gases and increase with load	-
Hemp	CO emission level is increased for all test fuel on increased the load due to incomplete combustion of fuel	NOx emissions are greater in all biodiesel blends than those in conventional diesel fuel. NOx emissions of B10 increase by 2%	Because of the increased oxygen content, HC emissions are higher for basic diesel and lowest for all blends	-	At greater load conditions, B10's smoke cloudiness was reduced by 10%

Feedstock	CO emission	NOx emission	HC emission	Smoke
Mustard	Increases with increases percentage of biodiesel in blended fuel	Increases with increase in the percentage of blend fuel when compared to diesel at rated load, while NOx emissions of B100 increase by 20%. The amount of biodiesel in a mix affects NOx emissions significantly	Emission decreases with increase in the percentage of blend fuel	–
Soyabean	Emission reduced on blending of fuel	Decreases with increase in percentage of blends in biodiesel	Decrease with increase in percentage of blends in biodiesel	The smoke levels were significantly low
Rape seed	More efficient reduction in the CO emission for all tested biodiesel and blend fuel than the conventional fuel	The emissions of biodiesel and blends tested were greater than diesel fuel, with the B20 mix emitting 3.77% more NOx than diesel	All of the biodiesel and blends tested had lower HC emissions than diesel fuel. The B 20 blend has 8.56% fewer HC emissions than diesel	All of the biodiesel and blends that were evaluated had lower smoke cloudiness than diesel
Palm	Emission reduced on lower percentage of blending in blended fuel	Lower blends of biodiesel increase the emission	–	–
Waste cooking oil (WCO)	Increases at 25% load due to high viscosity	Emission is optimum at engine operating conditions	HCs emission is low	–
Algae or microalgae	Reduced emission compared to the conventional diesel fuel because biodiesel contains more oxygen and this oxygen enhances the complete combustion of fuel	In comparison to diesel fuel, the amount of butanol added to the blends reduced	–	–

Kavitha et al., 2019; Baijiu et al., 2009; Sharma et al., 2009; Hegde & Rao, 2012; Puhan et al., 2005; Geo et al., 2010; Shehata & Razek, 2011; Parlak et al., 2013; Jindal & Salvi, 2012; Haldar et al., 2009; Canakci, 2005; Suldhal & Shrigiri, 2016; Kumar et al., 2018, 2019; Jaliliantabar et al., 2018; Tamilselvan et al., 2018; Ong et al., 2014; Nalgundwar et al., 2016; Sivasubramanian et al., 2017; Kavitha & Murugavelh, 2019; Rashed et al., 2016; Akar, 2016; Qi et al., 2017; Khan et al., 2020; Singh et al., 2015; Gugulothu, 2020; Afif & Biradar, 2019; Devarajan et al., 2018; Zareh et al., 2017; Saravanan et al., 2019; Velikovic et al., 2006; Sahoo et al., 2007.

with biodiesel. PM and smoke of blend fuel are reduced instead of conventional fossil fuel due to a higher content of oxygen in biodiesel.

Furthermore, there are more prominent factors affecting the different engine types, to be considered while assessing the physicochemical properties, engine performance and emission characteristics.

REFERENCES

Adebayo, G. B., Ameen, O. M.& Abass, L. T., 2011. Physico-chemical properties of biodiesel produced from Jatropha Curcas oil and fossil diesel. *Journal of Microbiology and Biotechnology Research.* 1(1), 12–16.

Afif, Mohammed Kinan & Biradar, C. H., 2019. Production of biodiesel from *Cannabis Sativa* (Hemp) seed oil and its performance and emission characteristics on DI engine fuelled with biodiesel blends. *IRJET.* 6(8), 246–253.

Agarwal, A. K., 2007. Biofuels (alcohols and biodiesel) applications as fuels for internal combustion engines. *Prog Energy Combust Sci.* 33(3), 233–2371.

Agarwal, Deepak & Agarwal, Avinash Kumar, 2007. Performance and emissions characteristics of Jatropha oil (preheated and blends) in a direct injection compression ignition engine. *Applied Thermal Engineering.* 27, 2314–2323 doi:10.1016/j. applthermaleng.2007.01.009

Ahmad, A., Yasin, N., Derek, C. & Lim, J.K., 2011. Microalgae as a sustainable energy source for biodiesel production: a review. *Renewable and Sustainable Energy Reviews.* 15, 584–593. Doi: 10.1016/j.rser.2010.09.018

Ahmad, J., Yusup, S., Bokhari, A. & Kamil, R.N.M., 2014. Study of fuel properties of rubber seed oil based biodiesel. *Energy Convers Manage.* 78, 266–275.

Aitani, Abdullah M., 2004. Book oil refining and products. *Encyclopedia of Energy.* 4, 715–729.

Akar, M. A., 2016. Performance and emission characteristics of compression ignition engine operating with false flax biodiesel and butanol blends. *Advances in Mechanical Engineering.* 8(2), 1–7. Doi: 10.1177/1687814016632677.

Akhtar, M. T., Ahmad, M., Shaheen, A., Zafar, M., Ullah, R., Asma, M. & Waseem, Amir, 2019. Comparative study of liquid biodiesel from Sterculia foetida (bottle tree) using CuO-CeO$_2$ and Fe$_2$O$_3$ nano catalysts. *Frontiers in Energy Research.* 7, 4. Doi: 10.3389/ fenrg.2019.00004

Al-Jasass, F. M. & Al-Jasser, M. S., 2012. Chemical composition and fatty acid content of some spices and herbs under Saudi Arabia conditions. *The Scientific World Journal.* 1–5. Doi: 10.1100/2012/859892

Alptekin, E. & Canakci, M., 2008. Determination of the density and the viscosities of biodiesel–diesel fuel blend. *Renew Energy.* 33, 2623–2630.

Al-Widyan, M. I. & Al-Muhtaseb, M. T. A., 2010. Experimental investigation of jojoba as a renewable energy source. *Energy Convers Manage.* 51, 1702–1707.

Amaro, H. M., Guedes, A. C. & Malcata, F. X., 2011. Advances and perspectives in using microalgae to produce biodiesel. *Applied Energy.* 88(10), 3402–3410.

American Society for Testing and Materials (ASTM). 1998. *Standard Specification For Biodiesel Fuel (B100) Blend Stock For Distillate Fuels.* Designation ASTM D 6751. ASTM International, West Conshohocken, PA.

An, H., Yang, W. M., Maghbouli, A., Li, J., Chou, S. K. & Chua, K. J. 2013. Performance, combustion and emission characteristics of biodiesel derived from waste cooking oils. *Applied Energy.* 112, 493–499. Doi: 10.1016/j.apenergy.2012.12.044

Arun Kumar, M., Kannan, M. & Murali, G., 2019. Experimental studies on engine performance and emission characteristics using castor biodiesel as fuel in CI engine. *Renewable Energy.* 131, 737–744. Doi: 10.1016/j.renene.2018.07.096

A Comparative Study of Various Biodiesel Feedstock 85

Aslam, Mohammad, Saxena, Prashant & Sharma, Anil K., 2014. Green technology for biodiesel production from Mesua Ferrea L. seed oil. *Energy and Environment Research.* 4(2), 11–21. Doi: 10.5539/eer.v4n2p11.

Avramovic, J. M., Stamenkovic, O. S., Todorovic, Z. B., Lazic, M. L. & Veljkovic, V. B., 2010. The optimization of the ultrasound-assisted base-catalyzed sunflower oil methanolysis by a full factorial design. *Fuel Process. Technol.* 91, 1551–1557.

Awais, M., Musmar, S. A., Kabir, F., Batool, I., Rasheed, M. A., Jamil, F. & Tlili, I., 2020. Biodiesel production from *Melia azedarach* and *Ricinus communis* oil by transesterification process. *Catalysts.* 10(4). 427.10.3390/catal10040427

Bacenetti, J., Restuccia, A., Schillaci, G. & Failla, S., 2017. Biodiesel production from unconventional oilseed crops (*Linum usitatissimum* L. and *Camelina sativa* L.) in Mediterranean conditions: environmental sustainability assessment. *Renewable Energy.* 112, 444–456. Doi: 10.1016/j.renene.2017.05.044

Bachheti, R. K., Dwivedi, Himanshu, Rana, Vikas, Rai, Indra & Joshi, Archana 2012. Characterization of fatty acids in *Melia Azedarach* L. seed oil. *International Journal of Current Research and Review.* 4(3), 108–111.

Baiju, B., Naik, M. K. & Das, L. M. A. 2009. Comparative evaluation of compression ignition engine characteristics using methyl and ethyl esters of Karanja oil. *Renew. Energy.* 34, 1616–1621.

Balat, M., 2011. Potential alternatives to edible oils for biodiesel production e a review of current work. *Energy Conversion and Management.* 52(2), 1479–1492. Doi: 10.1016/j. enconman.2010.10.011

Balat, M. & Balat, H., 2010. Progress in biodiesel processing. *Applied Energy.* 87, 1815–1835.

Batista, A. C. F., Vieira, A. T., Rodrigues, H. S., Silva, T. A., Assunção, R. M. N., Beluomini, M. A., Rezende, H. P. & Hernandez-Terrones, M. G., 2014. Production and physico-chemical characterization of methylic and ethylic biodiesel from canola oil/obtenção e caracterização do biodiesel de canola pelas rotas metílica e etílica. *Rev. Bras. Eng. Biossistemas.* 8, 289–298. Doi: 10.18011/bioeng2014v8n4p289–298

Belaid, M., Muzenda, E., Mitilene, G. & Mollagee, M., 2011. Feasibility study for a castor oil extraction plant in South Africa. *World Academy of Science, Engineering and Technology.* 52, 740–744.

Benzard, J., Bugaut, M. & Clement, G., 1971. Triglycerides composition of coconut oil. *Journal of American Oil Chem Society.* 3, 134–139.

Bobade, S. N. & Khyade, V. B., 2012. Detail study on the properties of Pongamia Pinnata (Karanja) for the production of biofuel. *Research Journal of Chemical Sciences.* 2(7), 16–20.

Boog, J. H. F., Silveira, E. L. C., De Caland, L. B. & Tubino. M. 2011. Determining the residual alcohol in biodiesel through its flash point. *Fuel.* 90, 905–907.

Borugadda, V. B. & Goud, V. V., 2012. Biodiesel production from renewable feedstocks: status and opportunities. *Renew Sustain Energy Rev.* 16, 4763–4784.

Bouaid, A., Diaz, Y., Martinez, M. & Aracil, J., 2005. Pilot plant studies of biodiesel production using Brassica carinata as raw material. *Catalysis Today.* 106(1–4), 193–196. Doi: 10.1016/j.cattod.2005.07.163

Brennan, L. & Owende, P., 2010. Biofuels from microalgae; a review of technologies for production, processing, and extractions of biofuels and co-products. *Renewable Sustainable Energy Rev.* 14, 557–577.

Bryan, R. M., 2009 Biodiesel production, properties and feedstocks. *Vitro Cell Dev Biol—Plant.* 45, 229–66.

Budhwani, A. A. A., Maqbool, A., Hussain, T. & Syed, M. N., 2019. Production of biodiesel by enzymatic transesterification of non-edible *Salvadora persica* (Pilu) oil and crude coconut oil in a solvent-free system. *Bioresources and Bioprocessing.* 6, 41. Doi: 10.1186/s40643-019-0275-3

Canakci, M., 2005. Performance and emissions characteristics of biodiesel from soybean oil. *Proceedings of the Institution of Mechanical Engineers, Part D: Journal of Automobile Engineering.* 219(7), 915–922. Doi: 10.1243/095440705X28736.

Carareto, N. D. D., Kimura, C. Y. C. S., Oliveira, E. C., Costa, M. C. & Meirelles, A. J. A., 2012. Flash points of mixtures containing ethyl esters or ethylic biodiesel and ethanol. *Fuel.* 96, 319–326.

Ciubota-Rosie, C., Ruiz, J. R., Ramos, M. J. & Perez, A., 2013. Biodiesel from *Camelina sativa*: a comprehensive characterisation. *Fuel.* 105, 572–577. Doi: 10.1016/j.fuel.2012.09.062

Da Rós, P. C. M., Freitas, L., Perez, V. H. & De Castro, H. F., 2013. Enzymatic synthesis of biodiesel from palm oil assisted by microwave irradiation. *Bioprocess Biosyst. Eng.* 36, 443–451.

Devarajan, Y., Munuswamy, D. B., Nagappan, B. & Pandian, A. K., 2018. Performance, combustion and emission analysis of mustard oil biodiesel and octanol blends in diesel engine. *Heat and Mass Transfer.* 54(6), 1803–1811. Doi: 10.1007/s00231-018-2274-x

Dixit, S. & Rehman, A., 2012. Linseed oil as a potential resource for bio-diesel: a review. *Renew Sustain Energy Rev.* 16, 4415–4421.

Du, Z., Hu, B., Ma, X., Cheng, Y., Liu, Y., Lin, X., Wan, Y., Lei, H., Chen P. & Ruan R., 2013. Catalytic pyrolysis of microalgae and their three major components: carbohydrates, proteins, and lipids. *Bioresour. Technol.* 130, 777–782.

Encinar, J. M., Gonzalez, J. F., Sabio, E. & Ramiro, M. J., 1999. Preparation and properties of biodiesel from *Cynara cardunculus* L. oil. *Industrial & Engineering Chemistry Research.* 38(8), 2927–2931. Doi: 10.1021/ie990012x

Fahim, Danesh M. & Bahrami, M. E., 2013. Evaluation of physicochemical properties of Iranian tomato seed oil. *J Nutr Food Sci.* 3, 206. Doi: 10.4172/2155–9600

Faria, Douglas, Santos, Fernando, Machado, Grazielle, Lourega, Rogério, Eichler, Paulo, De Souza, Guilherme & Lima, Jeane, 2018. Extraction of radish seed oil (*Raphanus sativus* L.) and evaluation of its potential in biodiesel production. *AIMS Energy.* 6(4), 551–565.

Fernando, S, Karra, P., Hernandez, R., Jha, S. K. 2007. Effect of incompletely converted soybean oil on biodiesel quality. *Energy.* 32, 844–851.

Foglia, T. A., Jones, K. C. & Phillips, J. G., 2005. Determination of biodiesel and triacylglycerol in diesel fuel by LC. *Chromatographia.* 66, 115.

Fontaras, G., Tzamkiozis, T., Hatziemmanouil, E. & Samaras, Z., 2007. Experimental study on the potential application of cottonseed oil–diesel blends as fuels for automotive diesel engines. *Process Safety Environ. Protect.* 85, 396–403.

Geo, V. E., Nagarajan, G. & Nagalingam, B., 2010. Studies on improving the performance of rubber seed oil fuel for diesel engine with DEE port injection. *Fuel.* 89, 3559–3567.

Ghazali, W. N. M. W., Mamat, R., Masjuki, H. H. & Najafi, Gholamhassan, 2015. Effects of biodiesel from different feedstock on engine performance and emissions: a review. *Renew Sust Energy Rev.* 51, 585–602.

Giannelos, P., Zannikos, F., Stournas, S. & Lois, E., 2002. Anastopoulos. Tobacco seed oil as an alternative diesel fuel: physical and chemical properties. *Ind. Crops Prod.* 16, 1–9.

Gill, P., Soni, S. K., Kundu, K. & Srivastava, S., 2011. Effect of blends of rubber seed oil on engine performance and emissions. *Fuel.* 88, 738–743.

Giuffre, A. M., Capocasale, M., Zappia, C., Sicari, V., Pellicano, T. M., Poiana, M. & Panzera, G., 2015. Tomato seed oil for biodiesel production. *European Journal of Lipid Science and Technology.* 118(4), 640–650. Doi: 10.1002/ejlt.201500002

Gugulothu, S. K., 2020. Performance and emission analysis of SOME (Schleichera oleosa oil methyl ester) on DI diesel engine. *SN Applied Sciences.* 2(4). Doi: 10.1007/s42452-020-2494-9

Gui, M. M., Lee, K. T. & Bhatia, S., 2008. Feasibility of edible oil vs. non-edible oil vs. waste edible oil as biodiesel feedstock. *Energy.* 33(11), 1646–1653. Doi: 10.1016/j.energy.2008.06.002.

A Comparative Study of Various Biodiesel Feedstock 87

Haile, Mebrahtu, Asfaw Araya & Asfaw, Nigist, 2013. Investigation of waste coffee ground as a potential raw material for biodiesel production. *International Journal of Renewable Energy Research*. 3, 855–860.

Haldar, S. K., Ghosh, B. B. & Nag, A., 2009. Utilization of unattended Putranjiva Roxburghii non edible oil as fuel in diesel engine. *Renewable Energy*. 34(1), 343–347.

Harsha, Hebbar, Math, H. R., M. C. & Yatish, K. V., 2018. Optimization and kinetic study of CaO nano-particles catalyzed biodiesel production from *Bombax Ceiba* oil. *Energy*. 143, 25–34. Doi: 10.1016/j.energy.2017.10.118

Hegde, A. K. & Rao, K. S., 2012. Performance and emission study of 4S CI engine using calophyllum inophyllum biodiesel with additives. *Int J Theor Appl Res Mech. Eng. (IJTARME)*. 1, 2319–3182.

Hoekmana, S., Broch, A., Robbins, C., Ceniceros, E. & Natarajan, M., 2016. Review of biodiesel composition, properties, and specifications. *Renewable and Sustainable Energy Reviews*. 16, 143–169. Doi: 10.1016/j.rser.2011.07.143.

Holser, R. A. & Harry-O'Kuru, R., 2006. Transesterified milkweed (Asclepias) seed oil as a biodiesel fuel. *Fuel*. 85(14–15), 2106–2110. Doi: 10.1016/j.fuel.2006.04.001

Hosamani, K. M., Hiremath, V. B. & Keri, R. S., 2009. Renewable energy sources from Michelia champaca and Garcinia indica seed oils: a rich source of oil. *Biomass Bioenergy*. 33, 267–270.

Hossain, F. M., Rainey, T. J., Ristovski, Z. & Brown, R. J., 2018. Performance and exhaust emissions of diesel engines using microalgae FAME and the prospects for microalgae HTL bio crude. *Renewable and Sustainable Energy Reviews*. 82, 4269–4278. Doi: 10.1016/j.rser.2017.06.026.

Hotti, Siddalingappa R. & Hebbal, Omprakash D., 2015. Biodiesel production process optimization from sugar apple seed oil *(Annona squamosa)* and its characterization. *Journal of Renewable Energy*. 1–6. Doi: 10.1155/2015/148587.

Huzayyin, A., Bawady, A., Rady, M. & Dawood, A., 2004. Experimental evaluation of diesel engine performance and emission using blends of jojoba oil and diesel fuel. *Energy Convers Manage*. 45, 2093–2112.

Ijaz, M., Bahtti, K. H., Anwar, Z., Dogar, U. F. & Irshad, M., 2016. Production, optimization and quality assessment of biodiesel from Ricinus communis L. oil. *Journal of Radiation Research and Applied Sciences*. 9(2), 180–184. Doi: 10.1016/j.jrras.2015.12.005.

Ikwuagwu, O., Ononogbu, I. & Njoku, O., 2000. Production of biodiesel using rubber [*Hevea brasiliensis* (Kunth. Muell.)] seed oil. *Ind Crops Prod*. 12, 57–62.

Ilkilic, C. & Yücesu, H., 2008. The use of cottonseed oil methyl ester on a diesel engine. *Energy Sources, Part A: Recovery, Utilization, and Environmental Effects*. 30, 742–753.

Islam, Md. Saiful, Ahmed, Abu Saleh, Islam, Aminul, Aziz, Sidek Abdul, Xian, Low Chyi & Mridha, Moniruzzaman, 2014. Study on emission and performance of diesel engine using castor biodiesel. *Journal of Chemistry*. 1–8. Doi: 10.1155/2014/451526.

Jain, P., Arora, N., Mehtani, J., Pruthi, V. & Majumder, C. B., 2017. Pretreated algal bloom as a substantial nutrient source for microalgae cultivation for biodiesel production. *Bioresource Technology*. 242, 152–160.

Jaliliantabar, F., Ghobadian, B., Carlucci, A. P., Najafi, G., Ficarella, A., Strafella, L. & De Domenico, S., 2018. Comparative evaluation of physical and chemical properties, emission and combustion characteristics of brassica, cardoon and coffee based biodiesels as fuel in a compression-ignition engine. *Fuel*. 222, 156–174. Doi: 10.1016/j.fuel.2018.02.145.

Jena, P. C., Raheman, H., Kumar, G. Prasanna & Machavaram, R., 2010. Biodiesel production from mixture of mahua and simarouba oils with high free fatty acids. *Biomass Bioenergy*. 34, 1108–1116.

Jindal, S. & Salvi, B., 2012. Sustainability aspects and optimization of linseed biodiesel blends for compression ignition engine. *J Renew Sustain. Energy*. 4, 043111.

Joshi H. C., Grag, Nitika, Kumar, Sanjay & Ahmad, Waseem, 2021. Influence of the catalytic activity of MgO catalyst on the comparative studies of Schlichera oleosa, Michelia champaca and Putranjiva based biodiesel and its blend with ethanol-diesel. *Materials Today: Proceedings*. 38, 18–23. Doi: 10.1016/j.matpr.2020.05.432

Joshi, H. C. & Negi, Mahesh, 2017. Study the production and characterization of Neem and Mahua based biodiesel and its blends with diesel fuel: an optimum blended fuel for Asia. *Energy Sources, Part A: Recovery, Utilization, and Environmental Effects*. 39(17), 1894–1900.

Joshi, H. C., Singh, Jitendra & Aggarwal, Aishwarya, 2019. Thermochemical conversion of non-food feedstock of Moringa oleifera seed bio-oil to the biodiesel and its blends with n-butanol-diesel and utilization of glycerol obtained as by-product. *Clay Research*. 38(2), 75–82.

Kale, S. S., Darade, Vijaya & Thakur, H. A., 2011. Analysis of fixed oil from *Sterculia Foetida Linn*. *Ijpsr*. 2(11), 2908–2914.

Karmee, S. K. & Chadha, A., 2005. Preparation of biodiesel from crude oil of Pongamia pinnata. *Bioresour Technol*. 96, 1425–1429.

Kaul, S., Saxena, R. C., Kumar, A., Negi, M. S., Bhatnagar, A. K., Goyal, H. B. & Gupta, A. K., 2007. Corrosion behaviour of biodiesel from seed oils of Indian origin on diesel engine parts. *Fuel Processing Technology*. 88(3), 303–307. Doi: 10.1016/j.fuproc.2006.10.011

Kavitha, K. R., Kumar, N. Beem & Rajasekar, R. 2019. Experimental investigation of diesel engine performance fuelled with the blends of *Jatropha curcas*, ethanol, and diesel. *Environmental Science and Pollution Research*. 26(9), 8633–8639. Doi: 10.1007/s11356–019–04288-x

Kavitha, M. S. & Murugavelh, S. 2019. Optimization and transesterification of sterculia oil: Assessment of engine performance, emission and combustion analysis. *Journal of Cleaner Production*. 234, 1192–1209. Doi: 10.1016/j.jclepro.2019.06.240

Khan, H., Soudagar, M. E. M., Kumar, R. H., Safaei, M. R., Farooq, M., Khidmatgar, A. & Taqui, S. N., 2020. Effect of Nano-graphene oxide and n-butanol fuel additives blended with diesel—Nigella sativa biodiesel fuel emulsion on diesel engine characteristics. *Symmetry*. 12(6), 961. Doi: 10.3390/sym12060961

Kligerman, D. C. & Bouwer, E. J., 2015. Prospects for biodiesel production from algae based wastewater treatment in Brazil: a review. *Renewable and Sustainable Energy Reviews*. 52, 1834–1846.

Knothe, G. & Steidley, K. R., 2005. Kinematic viscosity of biodiesel fuel components and related compounds. Influence of compound structure and comparison to petro diesel fuel components. *Fuel*. 84, 1059–1065. Doi: 10.1016/j.fuel.2005.01.016

Knothe, G. & Steidley, K. R., 2009. A comparison of used cooking oils: a very heterogeneous feedstock for biodiesel. *Bioresource Technol*. 100, 5796–5801.

Knothe, G., Steven, C., Cermak & Evangelista, Roque L., 2009. Cuphea oil as source of biodiesel with improved fuel properties caused by high content of methyl decanoate. *Energy & Fuels*. 23, 1743–1747.10.1021/ef800958t

Kumar, A. & Sharma, S., 2011. Potential non-edible oil resources as biodiesel feedstock: an Indian perspective. *Renew Sustain Energy Rev*.15, 1791–800.

Kumar, A. S., Maheswar, D. & Reddy, K. Vijaya Kumar, 2009. Comparison of diesel engine performance and emissions from neat and transesterified cotton seed oil. *Jordan Journal of Mechanical and Industrial Engineering*. 3(3), 190–197.

Kumar, Bhabesh & Joshi, Harish Chandra, 2016. Characteristics and composition of soyabean oil seed from India by Alkali—catalysed transesterification and its potential as biodiesel feedstock. *Asian Journal of Chemistry*. 29(3), 525–528.

Kumar, Sanjay, Kaur, Gurpreet, Joshi, Anjali & Joshi, Harish Chandra, 2019. Production of biodiesel from citrus maxima (Chakotara) seed oil, a potential of non-food feedstock and its blends with n butanol-diesel and purification, utilization of glycerol obtained as byproduct from biodiesel. *Energy Sources, Part A: Recovery, Utilization, and Environmental Effects*. 41(12), 1508–1517. Doi: 10.1080/15567036.2018.1549125

Kumar, V. & Kant, P., 2013. Study of physical and chemical properties of biodiesel from sorghum oil. *Research Journal of Chemical Sciences*. 3(9), 64–68.

Kumar, V., Kumar, Sanjay, Chauhan, P. K., Verma, Monu, Bahuguna, Vivekanand, Joshi, Harish Chandra, Ahmad, Waseem, Negi, Poonam, Sharma, Nishesh, Ramola, Bharti, Rautela, Indra, Nanda, Manisha & Vlaskin, Mikhail S., 2019. Low-temperature catalyst based hydrothermal liquefaction of harmful Macroalgal blooms, and aqueous phase nutrient recycling by microalgae. *Scientific Reports*. 9, 11384. Doi: 10.1038/s41598-019-47664-w

Kumar, V., Nanda, M. Joshi, H. C., Singh, A., Sharma, S. & Verma, M., 2018. Production of biodiesel and bioethanol using algal biomass harvested from fresh water river. *Renewable Energy*. 116, 606–612. Doi: 10.1016/j.renene.2017.10.016

Lam, M. K. & Lee, K. T., 2011. Renewable and sustainable bioenergies production from palm oil mill effluent (POME): wine win strategies toward better environmental protection. *Biotechnology Advances*. 29(1), 124–141.

Lam, M. K. & Lee, K. T., 2012. Microalgae biofuels: a critical review of issues, problems and the way forward. *Biotechnology Advances*. 30(3), 673–690.

Lazos, E. S. & Kalathenos, P., 1988. Technical note: composition of tomato processing wastes. *Int J Food Sci Technol*. 23, 649–652.

Leal, R. V. P., Borges, P. P. & Seid, P. R., 2008. Metrological evaluation of titration technique for the determination of the iodine value in biodiesel. In *International Conference on Metrology of Environmental, Food and Nutritional Measurements*, Budapest, Hungary. 10–12.

Leung, D. Y., Wu, X. and Leung, M., 2010. A review on biodiesel production using catalysed transesterification. *Applied Energy*. 87, 1083–1095.

Lie, J., Rizkiana, M. B., Soetaredjo, F. E., Ju Yi-Hsu & Ismadji, Suryadi, 2018. Production of biodiesel from sea mango (*Cerbera odollam*) seed using in situ subcritical methanol–water under a non-catalytic process. *Int J. Ind. Chem*. 9, 53–59. Doi: 10.1007/s40090-018-0138-3

Lin, Cherng-Yuan & Lin, Yi-Wei, 2012. Fuel characteristics of biodiesel produced from a high-acid oil from soybean soapstock by supercritical-methanol transesterification. *Energies*. 5, 2370–2380. Doi: 10.3390/en5072370.

Mahajan, S., Konar, S. K. & Boocock, D. G. B., 2006. Determining the acid number of biodiesel. *Journal of the American Oil Chemists Society*. 83(6), 567–570. Doi:10.1007/s11746-006-1241-8

Mahesh, Babu T. N. V., Srinivasa P. Rao, Sudheer B. & Kumar, Prem, 2018 Parametric optimization of kusum oil biodiesel production using Taguchi-PCA method. *IJCRT National Conference Proceeding NTSET*. 234–240.

Mirza, U. K., Ahmad, N. & Majeed, T., 2008. An overview of biomass energy utilization in Pakistan. *Renewable and Sustainable Energy Reviews*. 12(7), 1988–1996.

Mohibbe, Azam M., Waris, A. & Nahar, N. M., 2005. Prospects and potential of fatty acid methyl esters of some non-traditional seed oils for use as biodiesel in India. *Biomass Bioenergy*. 29, 293–302.

Moser, B. R., Knothe, G., Vaughn, S. F. & Isbell, T. A., 2009. Production and evaluation of biodiesel from field pennycress (*Thlaspi arvense* L.). oil. *Energy & Fuels*. 23(8), 4149–4155. Doi: 10.1021/ef900337g

Moser, B. R., Roque, L., Evangelista & Isbell, Terry A., 2016. Preparation and fuel properties of field pennycress *(Thlaspi arvense)* seed oil ethyl esters and blends with ultralow-sulfur diesel fuel. *Energy Fuels*. 30(1), 473–479.

Muliyansah, Saputera & Tintin Apung Atikah, 2014. Extraction & transesterification of croton tiglium oil seeds from central Kalimantan, Indonesia as an alternatives biodiesel raw materials. *Asian Journal of Applied Sciences*. 7(3), 140–149.

Mutlu, H. & Meier, M. A. R., 2010. Castor oil as a renewable resource for the chemical industry. *Eur. J. Lipid Sci. Technol*. 112, 10–30.

Nabi, M. N., Rahman, M. M. & Akhter, M. S., 2009. Biodiesel from cotton seed oil and its effect on engine performance and exhaust emissions. *Appl Therm. Eng.* 29, 2265–2270.

Nahak, G., Samantray, D., Mohapatra, N. K. & Sahu, R. K., 2010. Comparative study of enzymatic transesterification of Jatropha oil using lipase from *Jatropha curcas* and *Jatropha gossipyfolia*. *Continental Journal of Biological Sciences*. 3, 33–45.

Nalgundwar, A., Paul, B. & Sharma, S. K., 2016. Comparison of performance and emissions characteristics of DI CI engine fueled with dual biodiesel blends of palm and jatropha. *Fuel*. 173, 172–179. Doi: 10.1016/j.fuel.2016.01.022.

Omkaresh, B. R., Suresh, R., Arun, S. B., Yathish, K. V., 2015. Biodiesel production from custard apple seed (*Annona squamosa*) oil and its performance test on CI engine. *International Journal of Applied Engineering Research*. 10(2), 1938–1942.

Ong, H. C., Mahlia, T. M. I., Masjuki, H. H. & Norhasyima, R. S., 2011. Comparison of palm oil, Jatropha curcas and Calophyllum inophyllum for biodiesel: a review. *Renewable and Sustainable Energy Reviews*. 15(8), 3501–3515. Doi: 10.1016/j.rser.2011.05.005

Ong, H. C., Masjuki, H. H., Mahlia, T. M. I., Silitonga, A. S., Chong, W. T. & Yusaf, T., 2014. Engine performance and emissions using *Jatropha curcas*, *Ceiba pentandra* and *Calophyllum inophyllum* biodiesel in a CI diesel engine. *Energy*. 69, 427–445. Doi: 10.1016/j.energy.2014.03.035

Ong, H. C., Milano, Jassinnee, Silitonga, Arridina Susan, Hassan, Masjuki Haji, Shamsuddin, Abd Halim, Wang, Chin-Tsan, Mahlia, Teuku Meurah Indra, Siswantoro, Joko, Kusumo, Fitranto & Sutrisno, Joko, 2019. Biodiesel production from *Calophyllum inophyllum-Ceiba pentandra* oil mixture: optimization and characterization. *Journal of Cleaner Production*. 219, 183–198.

Openshaw, K., 2000. A review of Jatropha curcas: an oil plant of unfulfilled promise. *Biomass Bioenergy*. 19, 1–15.

Palash, S., Masjuki, H., Kalam, M., Masum, B., Sanjid, A. & Abedin, M., 2013. State of the art of NOx mitigation technologies and their effect on the performance and emission characteristics of biodiesel-fueled compression ignition engines. *Energy Convers Manage*. 76, 400–420.

Park, Ji-Yeon, Kim, Deog-Keun, Wang, Zhong-Ming, Lu, Pengmei, Park, Soon-Chul & Lee, Jin-Suk, 2008. Production and characterization of biodiesel from tung oil. *Appl Biochem Biotechnol*. 148, 109–117.

Parlak, A., Ayhan, V., Cesur, I. & Kokkulunk, G., 2013. Investigation of the effects of steam injection on performance and emissions of a diesel engine fuelled with tobacco seed oil methyl ester. *Fuel Process Technol*. 116, 101–109.

Pimentel, Maria Fernanda, Ribeiro, Grece M. G. S., Cruz, Rosenira S. Da., Stragevitch, Luiz, Filho, Jose Geraldo A. Pacheco & Teixeira, Leonardo S. G., 2006. Determination of biodiesel content when blended with mineral diesel fuel using infrared spectroscopy and multivariate calibration. *Microchemical Journal*. 82, 201–206. Doi: 10.1016/j.microc.2006.01.019

Pinzi, S., Garcia, I. L., Gimenez, F. J. L., Castro, M. D. L., Dorado, G. & Dorado, M. P., 2009. The ideal vegetable oil-based biodiesel composition: a review of social. *Econ Tech Implic Energy Fuels*. 23, 2325–2341.

Pinzi, S., Leiva, D., Lopez-Garcia, Isabel, Redel-Macías, M. Dolores & Dorado, M. Pilar, 2014. Latest trends in feedstocks for biodiesel production. *Biofpr*. 8, 126–143. Doi: 10.1002/bbb.1435.

Pittman, J. K., Dean, A. P. & Osundeko, O., 2011. The potential of sustainable algal biofuel production using wastewater resources. *Bioresour Technol*. 102(1), 17–25.

Puhan, S., Saravanan, N., Nagarajan, G. & Vedaraman, N., 2010. Effect of biodiesel unsaturated fatty acid on combustion characteristics of a DI compression ignition engine. *Biomass Bioenergy*. 34, 1079–1088.

Puhan, S., Vedaraman, N., Rambrahamam, B. & Nagarajan, G., 2005. Mahua (Madhuca indica) seed oil: a source of renewable energy in India. *J Sci Ind Res*. 64, 890.

Qi, D. H., Yang, K., Zhang, D. & Chen, B., 2017. Combustion and emission characteristics of diesel-tung oil-ethanol blended fuels used in a CRDI diesel engine with different injection strategies. *Applied Thermal Engineering*. 111, 927–935. Doi: 10.1016/j.applthermaleng.2016.09.157

Rajkumari, K. & Rokhum, L., 2020. A sustainable protocol for production of biodiesel by transesterification of soybean oil using banana trunk ash as a heterogeneous catalyst. *Biomass Convers. Biorefinery*. 10(4), 839–848. Doi: 10.1007/s13399-020-00647-8

Rao, Rajeshwer, Yerranguntla, Zubaidha, Pudukulathan Kader, Reddy, Jakku Narender, Kondhare, Dasharath, Deshmukh, Sushma, Saiprakash & Santoshi Pondicherry, 2013. Production of Biodiesel from Guizotia abyssinica seed oil using crystalline Manganese carbonate ($MnCO_3$) a green catalyst. *Catalysis for Sustainable Energy*. 22–27.

Rashed, M. M., Kalam, M. A., Masjuki, H. H., Mofijur, M., Rasul, M. G. & Zulkifli, N. W. M., 2016. Performance and emission characteristics of a diesel engine fueled with Palm, Jatropha, and Moringa oil methyl ester. *Industrial Crops and Products*. 79, 70–76. Doi: 10.1016/j.indcrop.2015.10.046

Rashid, U., Anwar, F., Moser, B. R. & Knothe, G., 2008. *Moringa oleifera* oil: a possible source of biodiesel. *Bioresour Technol*. 99, 8175–8179.

Ravi Kumar, V. & Senthilkumar, D., 2013. Reduction of NOx emission on NiCrAl-titanium oxide coated direct injection diesel engine fuelled with radish (Raphanus sativus) biodiesel. *Journal of Renewable and Sustainable Energy*. 5(6), doi: 063121.10.1063/1.4843915

Reda, Abebe. 2014. Production and characterization of biodiesel from the traditional tannery fleshing wastes. *Ethiop. J. Sci. & Technol*. 7(1), 1–13.

Rial, R. C., De Freitas, O. N., Nazario, C. E. D. & Viana L. H., 2020. Biodiesel from soybean oil using porcine pancreas lipase immobilized on a new support: P-nitrobenzyl cellulose xanthate. *Renew. Energy*. 149, 970–979.

Roman-Figueroa, Celian, Cea, Mara, Paneque, Manuel & Gonzalez, Maria Eugenia, 2020. Oil content and fatty acid composition in castor bean naturalized accessions under Mediterranean conditions in Chile. *Agronomy*. 10(8), 1145 doi: 10.3390/agronomy10081145

Sahoo, P., Das, L., Babu, M. & Naik. S., 2007. Biodiesel development from high acid value polanga seed oil and performance evaluation in a CI engine. *Fuel*. 86, 448–454.

Sanchez, F. & Vasudevan, P. T., 2006. Enzyme catalysed production of biodiesel from olive oil. *Applied Biochemistry and Biotechnology*. 135(1), 1–14. Doi: 10.1385/abab:135:1:1

Sanchez-Arreola, E., Martin-Torres, G., Lozada-Ramirez, J. D., Hernandez, Luis R., Bandala-Gonzalez, Erick R. & Bach, Horacio, 2015. Biodiesel production and de-oiled seed cake nutritional values of a Mexican edible Jatropha curcas. *Renew. Energy*. 76, 143–147. Doi: 10.1016/j.renene.2014.11.017

Sanford, S. D., White, J. M., Shah, P. S., Wee, C., Valverde, M. A. & Meier, G. R., 2009. Feedstock and biodiesel characteristics report. *Renew Energy Group*. 416.

Saravanan, A., Murugan, M., Reddy, Sreenivasa & Parida, Satyajeet, 2020. Performance and emission characteristics of variable compression ratio CI engine fueled with dual biodiesel blends of Rapeseed and Mahua. *Fuel*. 263, 116751. Doi: 10.1016/j.fuel.2019.116751

Schenk, Peer M., Thomas-Hall, Skye R., Stephens, Evan, Marx, Ute C., Mussgnug, Jan H., Posten, Clemens, Kruse, Olaf & Hankamer, Ben, 2008. Second generation biofuels: high-efficiency microalgae for biodiesel production. *Bioenergy Research*. 1, 20–43. Doi: 10.1007/s12155-008-9008-8

Schumann, E., Weber, W. E., Matthaus, B., Brühl, L., Kriese, U. & Beyer, M., 2004. Oil content, tocopherol composition and fatty acid patterns of the seeds of 51 Cannabis sativa L. genotypes. *Euphytica*. 137, 339–351. Doi: 10.1023/b:euph.0000040473.23941.76.

Shahabuddin, M., Kalam, M., Masjuki, H., Bhuiya, M. & Mofijur, M., 2012. An experimental investigation into biodiesel stability by means of oxidation and property determination. *Energy.* 44, 616–622.

Shahid, E. M. & Jamal, Y., 2011. Production of biodiesel: a technical review. *Renewable and Sustainable Energy Reviews.* 15(9), 4732–4745. Doi: 10.1016/j.rser.2011.07.079.

Sharma, Anil Kumar. 2006. *Thesis, Biodiesel Production from Mesua ferrea Lnahar and Pongamia glabra Vent Koroch Seed Oil.* Lambert Academic Publishing.

Sharma, D., Soni, S. & Mathur, J., 2009. Emission reduction in a direct injection diesel engine fueled by neem–diesel blend. *Energy Sources, Part A: Recovery, Utilization, and Environmental Effects.* 31, 500–508.

Shehata, M. & Razek, S., 2011. Experimental investigation of diesel engine performance and emission characteristics using jojoba/diesel blend and sunflower oil. *Fuel.* 90, 886–897.

Silitonga, A. S., Ong, H. C., Masjuki, H. H., Mahlia, T. M. I., Chong, W. T. & Yusaf, T. F., 2013. Production of biodiesel from *Sterculia foetida* and its process optimization. *Fuel.* 111, 478–484. Doi: 10.1016/j.fuel.2013.03.051

Silitonga, A. S., Shamsuddin, A. H., Mahlia, T. M. I., Milano, J., Kusumo, F., Siswantoro, J. & Ong, H. C., 2020. Biodiesel synthesis from *Ceiba pentandra* oil by microwave irradiation-assisted transesterification: ELM modelling and optimization. *Renewable Energy.* 146, 1278–1291. doi: 10.1016/j.renene.2019.07.065.

Silveira, E. G., Barcelos, L. F. T., Perez, V. H., Justo, O. R., Ramirez, L. C., Rego Filho, L. de M. & de Castro, M. P. P., 2019. Biodiesel production from non-edible *Forage turnip* oil by extruded catalyst. *Industrial Crops and Products.* 139, 111503. Doi: 10.1016/j.indcrop.2019.111503

Singh, N., Kumar, H., Jha, M. K. & Sharma, A. K., 2015. Complete heat balance, performance, and emission evaluation of a CI engine fueled with *Mesua ferrea* methyl and ethyl ester's blends with petrodiesel. *Journal of Thermal Analysis and Calorimetry.* 122(2), 907–916. Doi: 10.1007/s10973-015-4777-8

Sivasubramanian, H., Sundaresan, V., Ramasubramaniam, S. K., Shanmugaiah, S. R. & Nagarajan, S. K., 2017. Investigation of biodiesel obtained from tomato seed as a potential fuel alternative in a CI engine. *Biofuels.* 1–9. Doi: 10.1080/17597269.2017.1338124

Suldhal, Arun, A. & Shrigiri, Basavaraj M., 2016. Performance and emission characteristics of diesel engine using custard apple seed oil methyl ester and blends. *IRJET.* 3(6), 2068–2072.

Tamilselvan, R., Rameshbabu, R., Thirunavukkarasu, R. & Periyasamy. 2018. Effect of fuel injection timing on performance and emission characteristics of *Ceiba Pentandra* Biodiesel. *Materials Today: Proceedings.* 5(2), 6770–6779. Doi: 10.1016/j.matpr.2017.11.336

Tan, Wen-Nee, Tong, Woei-Yenn, Leong, Chean-Ring, Syazni, Nik Nur, Kamal, Mohamed, Muhamad, Musthahimah, Lim, Jun-Wei, Khairuddean Melati & Man, Maizatul Balqis Her, 2020. Chemical composition of essential oil of Garcinia gummi-gutta and its antimicrobial and cytotoxic activities. *Journal of Essential Oil Bearing Plants.* 1–11. Doi: 10.1080/0972060X.2020.1828179.

Tredici, M. R., 2010. Photobiology of microalgae mass cultures: understanding the tools for the next green revolution. *Biofuels.* 1(1), 143–162.

Tripathi, N. N. & Narendra, Kumar, 2017. Putranjiva roxburghii oil—a potential herbal preservative for peanuts during storage. *J. Stored Products Res.* 43, 435–442.

Tripathi, Y. C. & Kumar, Hemant, 2020. Biochemical and physicochemical changes in seeds and fatty oil of Salvadora oleoides and Salvadora persica by soil borne fungi. *J Chem. Sci. Chem Engg.* 1(2), 1–6.

Tulip, D. & Radha, K. V., 2013. Production of biodiesel from mustard oil its performance and emission characterization on internal combustion engine. *Advanced Engineering and Applied Sciences: An International Journal.* 3(3), 37–42.

A Comparative Study of Various Biodiesel Feedstock   93

Tupufia, Samani Carel, 2012. Thesis, biodiesel production from coconut oil. School of Biotechnology and Biomolecular Science University of New South Wales.

Umerie, S. C., Okonlkwo, I. F., Nwadialor, N. A. & Okonlkwo, J. C., 2010. Studies on the oil and nutritive value of seeds of Crotalaria retusa L. (Fabaceae). *Pakistan Journal of Nutrition.* 9(9), 912–914.

Usta, N., Aydogan, B., Çon, A., Uguzdogan, E. & Ozkal, S., 2011. Properties and quality verification of biodiesel produced from tobacco seed oil. *Energy Convers Manage.* 52, 2031–2039.

Veljkovic, V., Lakicevic, S., Stamenkovic, O., Todorovic, Z. & Lazic, M., 2006. Biodiesel production from tobacco (Nicotiana tabacum L.) seed oil with a high content of free fatty acids. *Fuel.* 85, 2671–2675.

Xie, Y., Yan, Z., Niu, Z., Coulter, J. A., Niu, J., Zhang, J. & Wang, L., 2020. Yield, oil content, and fatty acid profile of flax (*Linum usitatissimum* L.) as affected by phosphorus rate and seeding rate. *Industrial Crops and Products.* 145, 112087. Doi: 10.1016/j.indcrop.2020.112087

Yadav, A. K., 2017. Optimum production of biodiesel from an under-utilized and potential feedstock, Kusum seed oil. *Iranica J. Energy Environ.* 8(1), 6–10. Doi: 10.5829/idosi.ijee.2017.08.01.02.

Yathish, K. V., Omkaresh, B. R. & Suresh, R. 2013. Biodiesel production from custard apple seed *(Annona Squamosa)* oil and its characteristics study. *International Journal of Engineering.* 2(5), 31–36.

Zagonel, G. F., Peralta-Zamora, P. & Ramos, L. P., 2004. Multvariate monitoring of soybean oil ethanolysis by FTIR. *Talanta.* 63, 1021. Doi: 10.1016/j.talanta.2004.01.008

Zareh, P., Zare, A. A. & Ghobadian, B., 2017. Comparative assessment of performance and emission characteristics of castor, coconut and waste cooking based biodiesel as fuel in a diesel engine. *Energy.* 139, 883–894. Doi: 10.1016/j.energy.2017.08.040

6 Chemical Processing Techniques Related to Bio-Waste for Their Conversion to Biofuel

Harish Chandra Joshi[1], Nitika Grag[2], and Waseem Ahmad[3]

1 Department of Chemistry, Graphic Era deemed to be University, Dehradun, Uttarakhand

2 Department of Chemistry, RKGIT, Ghaziabad, Uttar Pradesh, India

3 Department of Chemistry Uttaranchal University, Dehradun, Uttarakhand, India

CONTENTS

6.1 Introduction 96
6.2 Techniques of Conversion of Waste into Bioenergy 96
    6.2.1 Thermochemical Process 96
        6.2.1.1 Gasification 97
            6.2.1.1.1 Chemistry of Gasification 97
            6.2.1.1.2 Downdraft Gasifier 98
            6.2.1.1.3 Updraft Gasifier 98
        6.2.1.2 Hydrothermal Liquefaction 99
        6.2.1.3 Pyrolysis 99
    6.2.2 Biochemical Process 100
        6.2.2.1 Anaerobic Digestion 100
        6.2.2.2 Alcoholic Fermentation 101
        6.2.2.3 Photobiological Hydrogen Production 102
        6.2.2.4 Supercritical Fluid Method 103
    6.2.3 Transesterification 104
6.3 Conclusion 105
References 105

DOI: 10.1201/9781003265597-6

6.1 INTRODUCTION

Biofuels are inexhaustible transportation fuels developed from biomass-based sustainable assets like plants, animals or microorganisms. Years ago, peanut oil was used as diesel fuel (Roberts & Patterson 2014). Biomass has been considered the major source of sustainable energy throughout the world (Alam & Tanveer 2020; Kumar et al. 2018). Uses of biofuel in existing engines, there is no need for modification in an engine. Thus based on performance requirements, there is a significant similarity allying the characteristics and properties of fossil fuel and renewable biofuel.

Various feedstocks are available for biofuel generation, such as agricultural waste, forest crops, agricultural crops, waste from foods, and animal fats. Based on the feedstock, the biofuel can be classified into the following categories: (i) first generation: biomass produced from edible oils (Bhuiya et al. 2016; Lee & Lavoie 2013); (ii) second generation: biofuel can be produced from a variety of feedstock like municipal solid waste, lignocellulose; and (iii) third generation: biofuel produced from algae and microalgae (Figure 6.1)

6.2 TECHNIQUES OF CONVERSION OF WASTE INTO BIOENERGY

Generally, there are three techniques for the conversion of biomass and waste into bioenergy, that is, thermochemical, biochemical, and transesterification processes.

6.2.1 Thermochemical Process

The thermochemical (TCC) processes involve the gasification, pyrolysis, and liquefaction processes. The selection of the process depends on the types of feedstock and

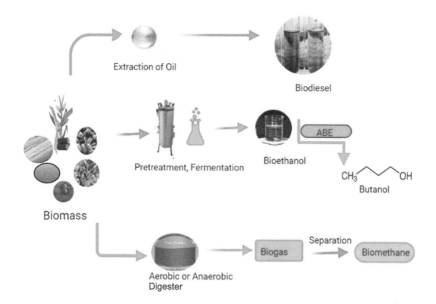

FIGURE 6.1 Conversion of biomass into biofuels.

Chemical Processing Techniques Related to Bio-Waste

preferred type of energy. TCC is involved in high-temperature chemical processes that require breaking bonds and converting organic matter into bio-char, synthesis gas, and bio-oil (Lee et al. 2019; Joshi et al. 2019).

6.2.1.1 Gasification

During the last few years, there has been a growing awareness among scientists to develop new methods for the production of biofuel. Biomass is considered one of the most important sources of biofuels (Pragya et al. 2013). Biomass is considered one of the most important renewable sources of energy. Biomass contains a significant amount of carbon, hydrogen, oxygen, and nitrogen (Damartzis et al. 2011). Biomass is considered a more significant renewable energy source than solar energy, wind energy, and other available energy sources due to their non-dependency on climatic conditions (Alonso et al. 2010). In the context of India, biomass has become more important because India is considered a rich country with tremendous biomass reserves (DeLasa et al. 2011). In India, biomass is easily available, making it one of the most suitable sources to generate biofuels (Wang et al. 2008). Biofuels are further classified based on the biomass that is used in their production. Bio-ethanol, bio-methanol, and bio-butanol are considered first-generation biofuels produced by biomass having sugar starch and vegetable oils. Ethanol is generally popular as a second-generation biofuel, and its production involves biomass having lignocelluloses. The third- and fourth-generation biofuels are produced by using algal biomass (Stoholm et al. 2010). The production of biofuel by using biomass is considered one of the latest and hot topics among researchers in this field. Many researchers are going on to develop new methods for producing biofuel by using biomass (Nacken et al. 2007). There are many methods available in the production of biofuel by using biomass like gasification, hydrothermal, liquefaction, and pyrolysis (Lv et al. 2004).

Gasification is basically a conversion process in which the organic or carbon-containing compound is converted into carbon mono oxide, carbon dioxide, and hydrogen by heating it at a temperature higher than 700 °C. Biomass is considered one of the most important alternative sources of energy (Lucas et al. 2004). Biomass is used to generate energy using different methods; the gasification of biomass is one of the most important ways to generate energy (Gupta et al. 2007). Gasification involves different steps, like oxidation, drying, pyrolysis, and reduction. Gasification is one of the oldest techniques to generate energy. The first time, it was used in Sweden to generate energy using wood biomass (Hanping et al. 2008).

6.2.1.1.1 Chemistry of Gasification

Gasification is generally considered a thermal transformation of solid or liquid biomass into a mixture of gasses. Gasification is a complicated process involving different processes, like oxidation-reduction and pyrolysis (Buragohain et al. 2010).

In the next step of the gasification, there is a drying process in which the feedstock is heated to remove the moisture present in the biomass (Karellas et al. 2007). The drying process is achieved at a temperature of 150 °C.

In the next step, the biomass undergo thermal decomposition, commonly known as pyrolysis. Pyrolysis was carried out at 250–700 °C. In this step, the biomass is converted into H_2, CO, CO_2, methane, and tar. The energy required for this process is derived from the oxidation process (Kirubakaran et al. 2009).

In the last step, the products formed in the pyrolysis step react with each other and give the ultimate gaseous mixture. The processes, which occur in this step, involve reduction reactions (Radwan et al. 2015).

The gasification process is operated in an apparatus called a gasifier. Different types of gasifier are generally used in the gasification process (Hamad et al. 2016).

6.2.1.1.2 Downdraft Gasifier

Downdraft gasifier is generally a counter-current reactor in which the biomasses enter from the top of the reactor, and the gaseous products are released from the bottom. In this gasifier, four regions generally occur in which the four processes are oxidation, drying, pyrolysis, and reduction process, as shown in Figure 6.2 (Asadullah et al. 2014).

6.2.1.1.3 Updraft Gasifier

In this type of gasifier, the air is injected from the bottom of the gasifier, and the gas mixture is finally released from the top of the gasifier. It is called an upward gasifier or updraft gasifier. In this gasifier too, there are four regions, and in these four regions, four different processes take place (Begum et al. 2014).

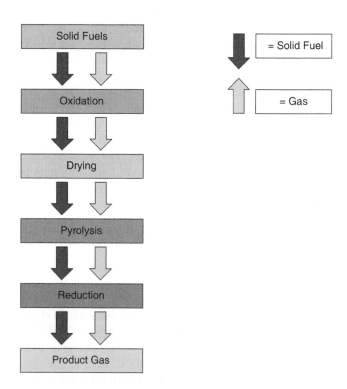

FIGURE 6.2 Process of conversion of solid fuels to gaseous fuels.

6.2.1.2 Hydrothermal Liquefaction

Hydrothermal liquefaction is generally considered a thermomechanical conversion of solid biomass into liquid biofuel (Adams et al. 2011). In hydrothermal liquefaction, we use solid mass without drying, which is one of the significant advantages of this process. Other processes, which are used to generate biofuel from biomass, require proper drying of the solid biomass. Due to this, all these are time-consuming processes, but hydrothermal liquefaction is a rapid process (Barbier et al. 2012). In the hydrothermal liquefaction process, the solid biomass is converted into liquid fuel in the presence of a hot and pressurized solvent medium. This method's liquid fuel is considered a high-energy condensed liquid fuel (Biller et al. 2013; Kumar et al. 2021).

The hydrothermal liquefaction process is generally classified into different categories depending upon the reaction condition (Biller et al.2012). The process, carried out at the temperature range of 180–250 °C and at pressure 2–10 MPa, is called hydrothermal carbonization. The processes performed at 250–374 °C and a pressure of 2–25 MPa is called hydrothermal liquefaction (Cherad et al. 2013). The processes, carried out at a temperature of more than 374 °C and pressure of more than 25 MPa, are called hydrothermal gasification (Elliott et al. 2011). In all processes, different products are obtained in the first process, which is known as hydrothermal carbonization hydrochar or bio char (Elliott et al. 2012). In the hydrothermal liquefaction process, bio-oil is obtained; in the hydrothermal gasification process, gaseous products are obtained, like methane, ethane, and hydrogen gases (Faeth et al. 2013).

In hydrothermal liquefaction, cellulose reacts with water at a higher temperature. Due to this reaction, the hydrogen bond in the cellulose molecule is broken down and the cellulose crystallinity is lost (Garcia Alba et al. 2013). The cellulose breaks down to give glucose and fructose, which on further degradation, give simple hydrocarbons (Goudriaan et al. 2008). The Hydrothermal liquefaction process is of two one is called a Batch Process and another one is called a continuous process. Most of the hydrothermal liquefaction process is carried out in a batch reactor (Jazrawi et al. 2013). The commonly used batch reactors are autoclaved reactors made from stainless steel.

In the batch reactor, the final temperature is reached after a long time; hence, the process takes a long time in this reactor. In order to reduce the time of the hydrothermal liquefaction process, the reaction was carried out in a continuous process.

6.2.1.3 Pyrolysis

Pyrolysis is a thermomechanical process producing biofuel by heating biomass from 400 °C to 500 °C without oxygen. Pyrolysis is a chemical conversation process used to bring changes in the chemical composition of biomass (Wang et al. 2008). Pyrolysis is considered a thermal treatment process but does not involve any kind of oxygen during the process (Abbasi et al. 2010). This oxygen-free thermal treatment of the biomass is known as pyrolysis. Due to the absence of oxygen, pyrolysis is considered an endothermic process, and the product obtained at the end of the pyrolysis process is energy-rich. Pyrolysis product contains a mixture of solid components, such as biochar charcoal and non-condensable gases (Howarth et al. 2010).

100   Biowaste and Biomass in Biofuel Applications

In pyrolysis, temperature plays a crucial role, and it is reported that as the temperature varies, the composition of the gaseous product varies. The temperature at which the pyrolysis is completed is called the pyrolysis temperature (Sdrula et al. 2010). If the pyrolysis is performed at a low temperature, then in the composition of the product, the concentration of char is increased. The product's composition also depends upon the composition of the biomass which undergo pyrolysis (Nanda et al. 2014). If pyrolysis is performed at a low temperature, then the solid product is obtained at a greater concentration, whereas pyrolysis is performed at a higher concentration than the gaseous product obtained at a higher concentration (Kamal et al. 2011).

Pyrolysis is considered an economical process, and it is also considered an eco-friendly process, but some toxic gases are also produced, like hydrogen sulfide and ammonia, etc. So, proper treatment of exhaust gases is necessary for the protection of the environment (Zhang et al. 2007). The solid, liquid, and gaseous products obtained in the pyrolysis process are generally known as biochar, bio-oil, and syngas, respectively. They all are considered valuable fuels (Muradov et al.2008).

Depending on the temperature at which the pyrolysis performed, it is classified into three classes: fast pyrolysis, slow pyrolysis, and flash pyrolysis (Thornley et al. 2009). If the pyrolysis is performed at a temperature range of 300–700 °C, it is called slow pyrolysis. If the pyrolysis is performed at a temperature range of 550–1250 °C, then it is called fast pyrolysis. If the pyrolysis is performed at the temperature range of800–1300 °C, it is called flash pyrolysis. The Qualitative and quantitative identification of pyrolysis products is carried out by using GC-MS Spectroscopy (Venderbosch et al. 2010).

6.2.2 Biochemical Process

In this technique, biomass or waste is converted into useful bioenergy by using yeast, microorganisms, or specialized bacteria. There are various biochemical processes, such as anaerobic digestion, photobiological hydrogen production, and alcoholic fermentation, to convert the different biofuels (Lee et al. 2019).

6.2.2.1 Anaerobic Digestion

Anaerobic digestion is a chemical digestion process that converts a complex organic feedstock into a series of simpler water-soluble organic molecules, which are then transformed into biogas containing methane. The process is anaerobic, which means it takes place without oxygen. This means it does not require oxygen or any other external electron acceptors like nitrate or sulfate to occur. Anaerobic digestion happens naturally in complete surroundings rich in organic carbon and limited by the input of electron acceptors or energy sources such as light. For example, natural environments include marshland, rice paddies, and the rumen of animals and insects. One of the main conceptual advantages of anaerobic digestion as biofuels producing bioprocess is the gaseous end product that evidently implies direct *in-situ* product separation. The biogas generated typically consists of 50–70 vol.% methane 442 biochemical conversion, anaerobic digestion, and 30–50% carbon dioxide, with tiny amounts of water, molecular hydrogen, and hydrogen sulfide. The anaerobic

Chemical Processing Techniques Related to Bio-Waste

digestion process is applied for the treatment of heterogeneous organic residues with a relatively high water content (>70 vol.%) and a high fraction of biodegradable matter, such as a portion of municipal solid trash that is organic (OFMSW), excreta, and numerous agro-industrial residues. Technologies applied for anaerobic wastewater treatment differ from those implemented for treating streams with a high solid content (Kleerebezem et al., 2014).

Anaerobic digestion is a type of biological fragmentation that occurs in the absence of oxygen. It entails microorganisms converting organic matter into a gaseous product known as biogas, leaving a stable solid product known as a digester.

Anaerobic digestion of organic waste has gotten a lot of press because it has many environmental and financial advantages. It can reduce local waste through reprocessing, saving resources, lowering greenhouse gas emissions, and increasing financial resilience in the face of an uncertain future for energy production and garbage disposal. By minimizing landfill area, the whole-of-life consequences of landfilling, and post-closure dump maintenance, the productive use of local garbage through reprocessing conserves resources. By minimizing harmful emissions and pollutants, converting garbage into a renewable energy source will aid in the economy's de-carbonization. Anaerobic digestion is breaking down organic waste to produce biogas and bio-fertilizers. Anaerobic digestion is a collection of mechanisms in which microorganisms break down biodegradable material without oxygen. This can be utilized for waste management in commercial, agricultural, or residential settings, as well as the creation of clean fuels. Anaerobic digestion is one of the most successful and dependable waste management strategies for dealing with the trash that has a lot of moisture. In the absence of oxygen, microbes break down biodegradable materials in a sequence of biological processes known as AD. Biological processes include hydrolysis, acidogenesis, acetogenesis, and biomethanation. (Uddin et al. 2021).

6.2.2.2 Alcoholic Fermentation

Food waste is widely recognized as a significant economic, social, and environmental issue. As previously stated, the food waste arrangement is not stable. It shows significant differences depending on the season, location, and population dietary practices. Despite the unavoidable variations in food waste composition, it is unquestionably rich in carbohydrates, proteins, lipids, and minerals, making it a perfect raw material for microbial conversion to produce biofuels. The use of food waste to make biofuels is also in keeping with the United Nations' 2030 Agenda for Sustainable Development, which was adopted in 2015. It is, to be more precise, intimately linked to the Sustainable Development Goals: Bioethanol production from lignocellulosic materials is a technology that has recently been explored from a technological standpoint. This process includes prearrangement, enzymatic hydrolysis, fermentation, and ethanol recovery. In terms of cost, the most expensive step is enzymatic hydrolysis, which clearly raises the total cost of bioethanol production and has been noted as a barrier to future ethanol production deployment. Instead of utilizing commercially available enzymes, on-site manufacture of the required enzymes is a desirable solution to this problem (Prasolulas et al. 2020).

Ethanol is one of the most auspicious products derived from renewable resources fermentation. Apart from its use as a fuel, it is widely employed as a feedstock for the production of various industrial products, such as ethene, which has an annual market demand of over 140 million tons. Ethene is also used to make polyethene and other types of polymers. Ethanol is widely manufactured via yeast and microbial-catalyzed fermentation. Amylum source materials such as sorghum corn, potato, and wheat serve as the main feedstock for ethanol fermentation. (Pietrzak & Kawa-Rygielska 2014). Food waste, such as wheat-rye bread, kitchen garbage, mixed food waste, and potato peel, has recently been accomplished and investigated as feedstocks for bio-ethanol production. However, due to the complicated lignocellulosic nature of food waste, it must be pretreated, which includes enzymatic and heating processes, as well as alkali and acid treatment, with the goal of improving cellulose and starch eat ability (Waqas et al. 2019). Bioenergy is defined as energy obtained from any biomass-derived fuel. Because biomass is a renewable natural resource, it has been proposed as an alternate fuel for generating long-term energy. Humans have traditionally relied on biomass in the form of firewood to provide direct combustion energy. In developed countries, a variety of feedstocks for biofuel production are abundant, including agricultural and forestry wastes, construction and industrial waste, and municipal solid waste (MSW). The renewable energy sources produced from these feedstocks are known as second-generation biofuels. Second-generation biofuels are made from lignocellulosic materials (such as cassava, switchgrass, wood, and straw) and biomass residues, as opposed to first-generation biofuels, which are made from palatable food crops (such as sugarcane, wheat, barley, corn, potato, soybean, sunflower, and coconut). The conversion of wastes that would otherwise decay into useful biofuels using biomass residues and trash as a key resource for biofuels is a potential concept to address environmental difficulties around waste disposal by converting wastes that would otherwise decay into valuable biofuels. Due to their tremendous potential for producing vast amounts of lipids suitable for biodiesel production, another biomass, algae, is presented as a feedstock for third-generation biofuels. Furthermore, this fast-growing biomass may be used directly to produce a variety of biofuels (Lee et al. 2019).

6.2.2.3 Photobiological Hydrogen Production

In terms of production, fossil fuels account for hydrogen production, providing the largest proportion, with 60 percent coming from dedicated primary hydrogen-producing plants. Natural gas (NG) produces roughly 71.27 percent of hydrogen, coal produces 27.27 percent, petroleum produces 0.7 percent, and water electrolysis produces the remaining 0.7 percent. Notably, the generation of hydrogen from fossil fuels is neither renewable nor carbon neutral, as the process generates many GHG emissions. Thermal decomposition, catalytic oxidation, steam gasification, and pyrolysis are some of the terms used to describe the water gas shift reaction, and auto thermal re-forming are all methods for producing hydrogen. The recent recognition of waste-to-energy programs has definitely influenced research into hydrogen synthesis from waste materials. Bio-hydrogen is created from a variety of organic wastes, and it simultaneously solves waste disposal and energy generation issues. Biodegradable waste products from plants or animals that can be broken down into CO_2, methane,

Chemical Processing Techniques Related to Bio-Waste

or simple organic molecules are referred to as organic waste. Among other organic wastes, industrial waste, municipal sewage sludge, solid waste, agricultural residues, and animal manure have the potential to be used in bioenergy production (Osman et al. 2020). In the presence of light, some biomasses, such as microalgae, have the natural potential to create hydrogen gas. Microalgae convert water molecules into O_2 and H^+ during photosynthesis. Under anaerobic conditions, hydrogenase enzymes convert H^+ to H_2 gas. The O_2 generated during photosynthesis quickly inhibits the hydrogenase enzymes, preventing the released H_2 gas. This means that anaerobic conditions are required for the cultivation of microalgae for the production of H_2 gas. (Cantrell et al. 2008). Microalgae can be used in two ways to collect photosynthetic H_2. The first method involves producing Oxygen and Hydrogen gas simultaneously in the presence of light. Hydrogenase enzymes utilize the created electrons by the water molecules' oxidation to produce hydrogen gas. Although this process has larger yields in theory than the second, the H_2 production is quickly hindered by the generation of O_2. The second method involves using a system with two phases, the first phase cultivating microalgae in natural settings and the second phase fostering continuous H_2 production under anaerobic conditions and Sulfur -displace conditions. Sulfur shortage causes the microalgae to enter a continuity mode, in which the cells obtain their energy from the production of H_2 The two-phase system's H_2 production would start to fail after 60 hours of operation, and the theoretical maximum H_2 yield may reach 198 kg H_2 ha 1 day 1 (Lee et al.2019).

6.2.2.4 Supercritical Fluid Method

The extraction process known as supercritical fluid extraction uses supercritical carbon dioxide as the solvent (SC-CO_2). The SC-CO_2 extraction procedure is a valuable tool for boosting yield and getting a range of profiles when extracting organic chemicals from plants (Azevedo et al.2008). Supercritical fluid extraction has a few advantages over typical extraction processes, including greater selectivity, faster processing time, and the use of non-toxic solvents. Other supercritical solvents that can be used include methanol, ethanol, propanol, acetone, methyl acetate, and dimethyl carbonate. When these solvents reach the supercritical state, their hydrogen bonds are considerably diminished, decreasing polarity and dielectric constant, allowing the solvent molecules to function as free monomers (Hoang et al.2013). For its moderate critical conditions (31.1°C and 74 bar), nonflammability, low toxicity, and wide availability, supercritical carbon dioxide (SC-CO_2) is one of the most often utilized compressed fluids for biomass processing. Because of its zero-dipole moment, SC-CO_2 is classified as a nonpolar molecule. Its maximum solvation power for non-polar or weakly polar compounds is inversely proportional to the solute's molar mass. CO_2, on the other hand, has a large quadrupole moment, and due to its microscopic solvent behavior, it may participate in hydrogen bond interactions and act as both a weak Lewis' acid and a weak Lewis' base. Its solvation power may also be affected by the addition of co-solvents, which can raise the polarity of the solvent system. SC-CO_2 also aids mass transfer by increasing diffusivity and lowering the solvent system's viscosity. Furthermore, the moisture in the biomass, when combined with CO_2, produces carbonic acid, which promotes hemicellulose hydrolysis. One of the most significant financial benefits of SC-CO_2 pretreatment is that no fermentation

104   Biowaste and Biomass in Biofuel Applications

inhibitors are formed; hence, after extraction, the biomass is ready to be hydrolyzed and then fermented without the need for detoxification or any other separation/purification step (Escobar et al. 2020).

6.2.3 TRANSESTERIFICATION

Transesterification is a kind of organic reaction in which an alcohol molecule reacts with an ester molecule and replaces the alkyl group in the alcohol with the alky group in the ester. Biodiesel, one of the most prominent biofuels, is produced by the transesterification of methanol with triglycerides (Mahlia et al. 2020; Joshi & Negi 2017). Transesterification has now become one the most popular tool for the production of biodiesel because in this process conversion rate is very high, and the conversation process is very rapid (Hendrawan et al.2020).

The name of esterification depends upon the product obtained at the end of the reaction. In this reaction, generally, an alcohol reacts with an acid to form an ester. Since ester is formed as a major product in this reaction, it is called esterification. The transesterification process is carried out in the presence of an acid or basic catalyst. Now, the process of transesterification is carried out in the presence of a biological catalyst (Goh et al. 2019; Kumar & Joshi 2016).

The transesterification reaction, which is frequently used in the production of biodiesel, is generally base-catalyzed (Romprasert et al. 2019). The major product obtained in the reaction of the production of biofuel by transesterification is fatty acid esters. One of the most important side products of this reaction is glycerine. As the reaction is completed, the two separate layers appear. One layer represents the fatty acid ester, and the second layer represents the glycerine. The fatty layer is separated out, but there are some impurities of glycerin which is must be removed; hence proper treatment is required (Chew et al. 2008; Joshi et al. 2020).

The Whole transesterification process is divided into different stages. In the first stage, raw materials are selected, and the free fatty acid content, water content, and the content of non-saponifiable substances are the major factors that play a crucial role in the selection of raw materials (Zhang et al. 2018).

In the next stage, the alcohol used in the production of biodiesels is first treated with the catalyst and generally a basic catalyst. In the transesterification process, an ahydrous alcohol is used (Rajaeifar et al. 2019). The molar ratio of alcohol and oil (triglycerides) is a very important parameter, and it is found that the ration of alcohol and oil is 3:1.

In this next stage, decide the different reaction conditions. Generally, the oil and alcohol are not mixed at room temperature, hence the transesterification is carried out at a higher temperature. The transesterification process is commonly performed at the temperature range of 50–60 °C (Silitonga et al. 2020).

After the reaction's completion, the two products are obtained, which the process of decantation (Sathiyamoorthi et al. 2019) separates. The final product obtained is a fatty acid methyl ester or fatty acid ethyl ester. These are properly washed with acidified water. After washing with acidified water, the products are also washed with normal distilled water. After washing with water, the traces water is removed by drying, and after drying, the products are suitable for the characterization process (Zhang et al. 2012).

6.3 CONCLUSION

Waste biomass can be converted into useful energy, such as bioelectricity, bio-fuel for transportation, etc., using the thermochemical conversion (TCC), trans-esterification process, and biochemical process, and the useful derivatives can be obtained from the glycerol. Bio-butanol and bioethanol can be obtained from biochemical pathways. In general, the transesterification process using an acid/base catalyst is a suitable pathway for converting waste into biofuel. Nowadays, researchers have modified the transesterification process by the use of nanoparticles and reached the maximum conversion. Now hydrothermal liquefaction (HTL) technology, with or without catalyst, is added to the extraction of bio- oil from waste, but cannot obtain a sufficient amount of bio-oil to be conversion. Yet, ongoing research investigations are focused on filling in the gaps in existing technologies and improving the efficiency and economics of the manufacturing processes.

REFERENCES

Abbasi, T., S.A. Abbasi. 2010. Biomass energy and the environmental impacts associated with its production and utilization. *Renew. Sustain. Energy Rev.* 14: 919–937.

Adams, J.M.M., A.B. Ross, K. Anastasakis, E.M. Hodgson, J.A. Gallagher, J.M. Jones, I.S. Donnison. 2011. Seasonal variation in the chemical composition of the bioenergy feedstock Laminaria digitata for thermo chemical conversion. *Bioresour. Technol.* 102 (1): 226–234.

Alam, Md. Saiful, Md. Sifat Tanveer, 2020. Conversion of biomass into biofuel: a cutting-edge technology. *Bioreactors.* 55–73. doi: 10.1016/B978-0-12-821264-6.00005-X

Alonso, D.M., J.Q. Bond, J.A. Dumesic. 2010. Catalytic conversion of biomass to biofuels. *Green Chem.* 12: 1493–1513.

Asadullah, M. 2014. Barriers of commercial power generation using biomass gasification gas: A review. *Renew. Sustainable Energy Rev.* 29: 201–215.

Azevedo A.B.A.d., P. Mazzafera, R.S. Mohamed, M.S.A.B.V. de, T.G. Kieckbusch. 2008. Extraction of caffeine, chlorogenic acids and lipids from green coffee beans using supercritical carbon dioxide and co-solvents. *Brazilian J. Chem. Eng.* 25: 543–552.

Barbier, J., N. Charon, N. Dupassieux, A. Loppinet-Serani, L. Mahe, J. Ponthus, M. Courtiade, A. Ducrozet, A. Quoineaud, F. Cansell. 2012. Hydro thermal conversion of lignin compounds. A detailed study of fragmentation and condensation reaction pathways. *Biomass Bioenergy* 46: 479–491.

Begum, S., M. Rasul, D. Cork, D. Akbar. 2014. An experimental investigation of solid waste gasification using a large pilot scale waste to energy plant. *Proc. Eng.* 90: 718–724.

Bensaid, Samir, Dung Hoang, Pierluig Bellantoni, Guido Saracco. 2013. Supercritical fluid technology in biodiesel production: pilot plant design and operation. *Green Processing and Synthesis* 2 (5): 397–406.

Bhuiya, M., M. Rasul, M. Khan, N. Ashwath, A. Azad. 2016. Prospects of 2nd generation biodiesel as a sustainable fuel—part: 1 selection of feedstocks, oil extraction techniques and conversion technologies. *Renew. Sustain. Energy Rev.* 55: 1109–1128.

Biller, P., C. Friedman, A.B. Ross. 2013. Hydrothermal microwave processing of microalgae as a pre-treatment and extraction technique for bio-fuels and bio products. *Bioresour. Technol.* 136: 188–195.

Biller, P., A.B. Ross. 2012. Hydrothermal processing of algal biomass for the production of biofuels and chemicals. *Biofuels* 3 (5): 603–623.

Buragohain, B., P. Mahanta, V.S. Moholkar. 2010. Biomass gasification for decentralized power generation: The Indian perspective. *Renew Sustainable Energy Rev.* 14: 73–92.

Cantrell, K.B., T. Ducey, K.S. Ro, P.G. Hunt. 2008. Livestock waste-to-bioenergy generation opportunities. *Bioresour Technol.* 99 (17): 7941–7953.

Cherad, R., J.A. Onwudili, U. Ekpo, P.T. Williams, A.R. Lea-Langton, M. Carmargo-Valero, A.B. Ross. 2013. Macro algae supercritical water gasification combined with nutrient recycling for microalgae cultivation. *Environ. Prog. Sustain. Energy* 32 (4): 902–909.

Damartzis, T., A. Zabaniotou. 2011. Thermochemical conversion of biomass to second-generation biofuels through integrated process. *Renew Sust. Energy Rev.* 15: 366–378.

DeLasa, H., Salaices E., J. Mazumder, R. Lucky. 2011. Catalytic steam gasification of biomass: catalysts, thermodynamics and kinetics. *Chem. Rev.* 111: 5404–5433.

Elliott, D.C. 2011. Hydrothermal processing. In: *Thermochemical Processing of Biomass.* John Wiley & Sons Ltd, Chichester, U.K., pp. 200–231.

Elliott, D.C., T.R. Hart, G.G. Neuenschwander, L.J. Rotness, M.V. Olarte, A.H. Zacher. 2012. Chemical processing in high-pressure aqueous environment. Process development for catalytic gasification of algae feed stocks. *Ind. Eng. Chem. Res.* 51: 10768–10777.

Escobar, E.L.N., T.A. da Silva, C.L. Pirich, M.L. Corazza, L. Pereira Ramos. 2020. Supercritical fluids: A promising technique for biomass pretreatment and fractionation. *Front. Bioeng. Biotechnol.* 23 (8): 252. doi: 10.3389/fbioe.2020.00252.

Faeth, J.L., P.J. Valdez, P.E. Savage. 2013. Fast hydrothermal liquefaction of Nano chloropsis sp. to produce bio crude. *Energy Fuels* 27 (3): 1391–1398.

Garcia Alba, L., C. Torri, D. Fabbri, S.R.A. Kersten, D.W.F. Brilman. 2013. Microalgae growth on the aqueous phase from hydrothermal liquefaction of the same microalgae. *Chem. Eng. J.* 228: 214–223.

Goh, B.H.H., H.C. Ong, M.Y. Cheah, W.H. Chen, K.L. Yu, T.M.I. Mahlia. 2019. Sustainability of direct biodiesel synthesis from microalgae biomass: A critical review. *Renew and Sustainable Energ. Rev.* 107: 59–74. doi: 10.1016/j.rser.2019.02.012.

Goudriaan, F., B. Van de Beld, F.R. Boerefijn, G.M. Bos, J.E. Naber, S. Van der Wal, J.A. Zeevalkink. 2008. Thermal efficiency of the HTU process for biomass liquefaction. In: *Progress in Thermo Chemical Biomass Conversion.* Black Well Science Ltd, Oxford, U.K., pp. 1312–1325.

Gupta, A.K., W. Cichonski. 2007. Ultrahigh temperature steam gasification of biomass and solid wastes. *Environ. Eng. Sci.* 24: 1179–1189.

Hamad, M.A., A.M. Radwan, D.A. Heggo, T. Moustafa. 2016. Hydrogen rich gas production from catalytic gasification of biomass. *Renew Energy* 85: 1290–1300.

Hanping, C.L. Bin, Y. Haiping, Y. Guolai, Z. Shihong, 2008. Experimental investigation of biomassgasification in a fluidized bed reactor. *Energy Fuels* 22: 3493–3498.

Hendrawan, Y., N.S. Maharani, B.D. Argo, Y. Wibisono. 2020. Modelling and optimization of palm oil moisture loss as biodiesel pretreatment. *E&ES* 456. doi: 10.1088/1755-1315/456/1/012035

Howarth, N.A.A., A. Foxall. 2010. The Veil of Kyoto and the politics of greenhouse gas mitigation in Australia. *Political Geogr.*29: 167–176.

Jazrawi, C., P. Biller, A.B. Ross, A. Montoya, T. Maschmeyer, B.S. Haynes. 2013. Pilot plant testing of continuous hydrothermal liquefaction of microalgae. *Algal Res.* 2 (3): 268–277.

Joshi, Harish Chandra, Nitika Garg, Sanjay Kumar, Waseem Ahmad. 2020. Influence of the catalytic activity of MgO catalyst on the comparative studies of Schlicheraoleosa, Michelia champaca and Putranjiva based biodiesel and its blend with ethanol-diesel. International Conference on FLAME 2020. *Materials Today: Proceedings* 38 (1): 18–23 2021. doi: 10.1016/j.matpr.2020.05.432

Joshi, Harish Chandra, Mahesh Negi. 2017. Study the production and characterization of Neem and Mahua based biodiesel and its blends with diesel fuel: An optimum blended fuel for Asia. *Energy Sources, Part A: Recovery, Utilization, and Environmental Effects* 39 (17): 1894–1900.

Joshi, Harish Chandra, Jitendra Singh, Aishwarya Aggarwal. 2019. Thermochemical conversion (TCC) of Moringa oleifera seed bio-oil to the production of biodiesel and its blends with n- butanol-diesel and utilization of glycerol obtained as by-product. *Clay Research* 38 (2): 75–82. doi: 10.5958/0974–4509.2019.00004.4

Kamal, G.M., F. Anwar, A.I. Hussain, N. Sarri, M.Y. Ashraf. 2011. Yield and chemical composition of citrus essential oils as affected by drying pretreatment of peels. *International Food Research Journal* 18 (4): 1275–1282.

Karellas, S., J. Karl. 2007. Analysis of the product gas from biomass gasification by means of Laser spectroscopy. *Opt. Las. Eng.* 45: 935–946.

Kirubakaran, V., V. Sivaramakrishnan, R. Nalini, T. Sekar, M. Premalatha, P. Subramanian. 2009. A review on gasification of biomass. *Renew Sustainable Energy Rev.* 13: 179–186.

Kleerebezem, R. 2014. Biochemical conversion. *Biomass as a Sustainable Energy Source for the Future* 441–468. doi: 10.1002/9781118916643.ch14

Kraus, T. 2007. Hydrogen fuel-an economically viable future for the transportation industry. *Duke J. Econ.* 19: 39.

Kumar, Bhabesh, Harish Chandra Joshi. 2016. Characteristics and composition of soyabean oil seed from India by Alkali-catalysed transesterification and its potential as biodiesel feedstock. *Asian Journal of Chemistry* 29 (3): 525–528.

Kumar, Sanjay, Gurpreet Kaur, Anjali Joshi, Harish Chandra Joshi. 2019. Production of biodiesel from citrus maxima (Chakotara) seed oil, a potential of non-food feedstock and its blends with n butanol-diesel and purification, utilization of glycerol obtained as by-product from biodiesel. *Energy Sources, Part A: Recovery, Utilization, and Environmental Effects* 41 (12): 1508–1517.

Kumar, Vinod, Krishna Kumar Jaiswal, Mikhail S. Vlaskin, Manisha Nanda, M.K. Tripathi, Prateek Gururani, Sanjay Kumar, Harish Chandra Joshi. 2021. Hydrothermal liquefaction of municipal wastewater sludge and nutrient recovery from the aqueous phase. *Biofuels* doi: 10.1080/17597269.2020.1863627

Kumar, Vinod, Manisha Nanda, Harish Chandra Joshi, Ajay Singh, Monu Verma. 2018. Production of biodiesel and bioethanol using algal biomass harvested from fresh water river. *Renewable Energy* 116: 606–612.

Lee, R.A., J.-M. Lavoie. 2013. From first-to third-generation biofuels: challenges of producing a commodity from a biomass of increasing complexity. *Anim. Front.* 3: 6–11.

Lucas, C., D. Szewczyk, W. Blasiak, S. Mochida. 2004. High-temperature air and steam gasification of densified biofuels. *Biomass Bioenergy* 27: 563–575.

Lv, P.M., Z.H. Xiong, J. Chang, C.Z. Wu, Y. Chen, J.X. Zhu. 2004. An experimental study on biomass air- steam gasification in a fluidized bed. *Bioresour. Technol.* 95: 95–101.

Mahlia, T.M.I., Z.A.H.S. Syazmi, M. Mofijur, A.P. Abas, M.R. Bilad, H.C. Ong, A.S. Silitonga. 2020. Patent landscape review on biodiesel production: Technology updates. *Renew and Sustainable Energ. Rev.* 118. doi: 10.1016/j.rser.2019.109526

Muradov, N.Z., T.N. Veziroglu. 2008. "Green" path from fossil-based to hydrogen economy: An overview of carbon-neutral technologies. *Int. J. Hydrog. Energy* 33: 6804–6839.

Nacken, M., L. Ma, K. Engelen, S. Heidenreich, G.V. Baron. 2007. Development of a tar reforming catalyst for integration in a ceramic filter element and use in hot gas cleaning. *Ind. Eng. Chem. Res.* 46: 1945–1951.

Nanda, M.R., Z. Yuan, W. Qin, M. Poirier, X. Chunbao. 2014. Purification of crude glycerol using acidification: Effects of acid types and product characterization. *Austin Chemical Engineering* 1 (1): 1–7.

Osman, A.I., T.J. Deka, D.C. Baruah. 2020. Critical challenges in biohydrogen production processes from the organic feedstocks. *Biomass Conv. Bioref.* doi: 10.1007/s13399–020–00965-x

Pragya, N., K.K. Pandey, P. Sahoo. 2013. A reviews on harvesting, oil extraction and bio fuels production technologies from microalgae. *Renew Sust. Energy Rev.* 24: 159–171.

Prasoulas, George, Gentikis Aggelos, Konti, Aikaterine, Kalantzi Styliani, Kekos Dimitris, Mamma Dioni. 2020. Bioethanol production from food waste applying the multienzyme system produced on-site by Fusarium oxysporum F3 and mixed microbial cultures. *MDPI Fermentation* 6: 39.

Radwan, A.M., M.A. Hamad, A.M. Singedy. 2015. Synthesis gas production from catalytic gasification of saw dust. *Life Sci. J.* 12: 104–118.

Rajaeifar, M.A., M. Tabatabaei, M. Aghbashlo, A.S. Nizami, O. Heidrich. 2019. Emissions from urban bus fleets running on biodiesel blends under real-world operating conditions: Implications for designing future case studies. *Renew. Sust. Energ. Rev.* 111: 276–292. doi: 10.1016/j.rser.2019.05.004.

Robert, Magda, Sandor Szlovak, Judit Toth. 2021. The role of using bioalcohol fuels in sustainable development. In *Book: Bio-Economy and Agri-Production*, Chapter 7. Academic Press, Elsevier, pp. 133–146.

Roberts, L.G., T.J. Patterson. 2014. *Book: Encyclopedia of Toxicology, Chapter: Biofuels*, Volume 1. pp. 469–475. doi: 10.1016/B978-0-12-386454-3.01054-X

Romprasert, S., K. Jermsittiparsert. 2019. Energy risk management and cost of economic production biodiesel project. *International J. Energ. Economics and Policy* 9: 349–357. doi: 10.32479/ijeep.8367.

Sathiyamoorthi, R., G. Sankaranarayanan, T. Chiranjeevi, D.D. Kumar. 2019. Experimental investigation on performance, combustion and emission characteristics of a single cylinder diesel engine fuelled by biodiesel derived from Cymbopogon Martinii. *Renew. Energ.* 132: 394–415. doi: 10.1016/j.renene.2018.08.001.

Sdrula, N. 2010. A study using classical or membrane separation in the biodiesel process. *Desalination* 250: 1070–1072.

Silitonga, A.S., A.H. Shamsuddin, T.M.I. Mahlia, J. Milano, F. Kusumo, J. Siswantoro, H.C. Ong. 2020. Biodiesel synthesis from Ceiba pentandra oil by microwave irradiation-assisted transesterification: ELM modelling and optimization. *Renew. Energ.* 146: 1278–1291. doi: 10.1016/j.renene.2019.07.065

Stoholm, P., J. Cramer, R.G. Nielsen, B. Sander, J. Ahrenfeldt, U.B. Henriksen. 2010. The low temperature CFB gasifier e 100 kWth tests on straw and new 6 MW the demonstration plant. In: *Proceedings of the 18th European Biomass Conference*, pp. 619–623. Lyon.

Sze Ying Lee, Revathy Sankaran, Kit Wayne Chew, Chung Hong Tan, Rambabu Krishnamoorthy, Dinh-Toi Chu, Pau-Loke Show. 2019. Waste to bioenergy: a review on the recent conversion technologies. *BMC Energy* 1: 4. doi: 10.1186/s42500-019-0004-7

Thornley, P., P. Upham, Y. Huang, S. Rezvani, J. Brammer, J. Rogers. 2009. Integrated assessment of bioelectricity technology options. *Energy Policy* 37: 890–903.

Uddin, M.N., S.Y. Arafat Siddiki, M. Mofijur, F. Djavanroodi, M.A. Hazrat, P. Loke Show, S.F. Ahmed, Y.M. Chu. 2021. Prospects of bioenergy production from organic waste using anaerobic digestion technology: a mini review. *Frontiers in Energy Research* 6270–6293.

Venderbosch, R.H., W. Prins. 2010. Review: fast pyrolysis technology development. *Biofuel* 4: 178–208.

Wang, G., W. Li, B. Li, H. Chen. 2008. study on pyrolysis of biomass and its three components under syngas. *Fuel* 87: 552–558.

Wang, L., C.L. Weller, D.D. Jones, M.A. Hanna. 2008. Contemporary issues in thermal gasification of biomass and its application to electricity and fuel production. *Biomass Bioenergy* 32: 573–581.

Waqas, M., M. Rehan, M.D. Khan, A.S. Nizami. 2018. Conversion of food waste to fermentation products. *Reference Module in Food Science*. doi: 10.1016/b978-0-08-100596-5.22294-4

Zhang, O., J. Chang, T. Wang, Y. Xu. 2007. Review of biomass pyrolysis oil properties and upgrading research. *Energy Convers Manag.* 48: 87–92.

Zhang, Y., A.E. Ghaly, B. Li. 2012. Availability and physical properties of residues from major agricultural crops for energy conversion through thermochemical processes. *Am. J. Agric. Biol. Sci.* 7: 312–321. doi: 10.3844/ajabssp.2012.312

Zhang, Y., A.E. Ghaly, B. Li. 2013. Determination of the exergy of four wheat straws. *Am. J. Biochem. Biotechnol.* 9: 338–347. doi: 10.3844/ajbbsp.2013.338.347

Zhang, Y., W. Zhao, B. Li, H. Li. 2018. Understanding the sustainability of fuel from the viewpoint of exergy. *Eur. J. Sustain. Dev. Res.*2. doi: 10.20897/ejosdr/76935.

7 The Effectiveness of *Balanites aegyptiaca* Oil Nanofluid Augmented with Nanoparticles as Cutting Fluids during the Turning Process

Nishant Kumar Singh[1], Yashvir Singh[2,3], Erween Abd Rahim[2], Abhishek Sharma[4], Amneesh Singla[5], and P.S. Ranjit[6]

1 Department of Mechanical Engineering, Harcourt Butler Technical University, Kanpur, Uttar Pradesh, India

2 Faculty of Mechanical and Manufacturing Engineering, Universiti Tun Hussein Onn Malaysia, Parit Raja, Batu Pahat, Johor, Malaysia

3 Department of Mechanical Engineering, Graphic Era Deemed to be University, Dehradun, Uttarakhand, India

4 Department of Mechanical Engineering, G L Bajaj Institute of Technology and Management, Greater Noida, Uttar Pradesh, India

5 Department of Mechanical Engineering, University of Petroleum and Energy Studies, Dehradun, Uttarakhand, India

6 Department of Mechanical Engineering, Engineering College, Surampalem, India

CONTENTS

7.1	Introduction	112
7.2	Experimental Procedure	113
	7.2.1 Bio-Based Nanofluid Lubricant Synthesis	113
	7.2.2 Physical and Chemical Characteristics	114
	7.2.3 Machining Performance	115

DOI: 10.1201/9781003265597-7

112 Biowaste and Biomass in Biofuel Applications

7.3 Results and Discussion 116
    7.3.1 Cutting Temperature 116
    7.3.2 Chip Thickness 117
    7.3.3 Surface Roughness of the Machined Sample 118
7.4 Conclusion 120
References 120

7.1 INTRODUCTION

Metalworking fluid (MWF) is a lubricant applied between two moveable surfaces to minimize the friction transfer heat, eliminate contaminants and improve efficiency. MWFs are essential production consumables. An MWF comprises more than 90% base oil and less than 10% additive package [1]. MWFs comprise crude oil, heavy oil, and vegetable oil. Despite the fact that it is renewable, vegetable oil is good for the environment. Furthermore, vegetable oil must be changed before use to enhance its limits in oxidation stability, high friction, high viscosity, thermal stability, and corrosion resistance [2].

Furthermore, the price of vegetable oil is lower than that of other MWFs. Due to the extremely growing focus on environmental sustainability, there has been an increase in the desire for environmentally acceptable MWFs. Vegetable oils are renewable ingredients that also function as short biodegradable fluids. Furthermore, it is an environmentally friendly alternative to base oils for lubrication [3].

Tribological aspects, such as friction, lubrication, and wear mechanism, are significant considerations for identifying a particular MWF [4] employed MWF in the cutting region to reduce friction and heat generation both outside and inside. Cutting efficiency is significantly improved. This study used minimum quality lubricant (MQL) as a metal-working fluid to improve manufacturing sustainability. Using bio-based oil obtained from vegetable oil gives potential ecological advantages, such as non-toxicity, stability, eco-friendliness, and high compost ability, for sustainable development in machining innovation [5]. With stringent environmental regulations, vegetable oil is making its way into lubricants for transport and power applications. Scientists, engineers, and innovators should be aware that green inventions and techniques are better for mother nature and can reduce energy bills while also providing cleaner and better products [6].

The use of vegetable oil as MWF, on the other hand, has drawbacks. Vegetable oil is considered a mediocre lubricant due to its weak thermal and oxidative endurance [7]. In its essential state, vegetable oil has various physical and chemical limitations [8]. Many experiments on enhancing vegetable oil have been conducted, encompassing chemical modifications and the inclusion of chemicals [9]. Many additives are compatible with vegetable oil, including molybdenum disulfide, hexagonal boron nitride, aluminum oxide, and copper oxide. Lubricant additives perform purposes such as antioxidants, anti-wear agents, rust and corrosion inhibitors, and viscosity index enhancers.

Moreover, nanofluids derived from the mixture of conventional oil and nanoparticles have shown significant promise as lubricants [10]. Nanofluids can enhance

The Effectiveness of *Balanites aegyptiaca* Oil Nanofluid

thermal conductivity between the fluid and the absorbers, increase density-specific heat capacity output, enabling the fluid to transfer more thermal energy, and improve thermal conductivity, leading to a greater heat transfer coefficient [11]. Nanofluids can also cut manufacturing costs, time, and energy in various machining techniques [12].

Few studies have been undertaken on the tribological efficacy features, and the machining behavior of Balanites Aegyptiaca oil as a lubricant has not been thoroughly examined. To the best of the evidence, no study has been documented that used a vegetable-based lubricant derived from Balanites Aegyptiaca oil and included two additives as an MWF. For this investigation, modified Balanites Aegyptiaca (desert date) oil (MBAO) was combined with two additives (silicon dioxide and activated carbon) to be employed as MWFs. The feasibility of modified Balanites Aegyptiaca nanofluids was determined using machinability in cutting temperature, chip thickness, and tool chip contact length.

7.2 EXPERIMENTAL PROCEDURE

7.2.1 BIO-BASED NANOFLUID LUBRICANT SYNTHESIS

Transesterification is required to modify the properties of Balanites Aegyptiaca oil in terms of making it appropriate for machining applications. The desert date oil was purchased locally in New Delhi, India, from a trader. Balanites Aegyptiaca oil provides a high concentration of unsaturated fatty acids, which are ideal for reducing friction and wear between the tool and the workpiece in interaction. The evaluation of unsaturated fatty acids is also becoming more significant since they can provide a reasonable preventative coating within a constrained capacity. The size of the nanoparticles evaluated in this study was 25 nm due to their beneficial role in reducing friction and wear of surfaces in contact. The SiO_2 and Activated Carbon nanoparticles were purchased from M/S Sigma Aldrich Chemicals in New Delhi, India, and the dealer specified the nanoparticles' size.

Modified Balanites Aegyptiaca (MBAO) production began with the chemical alteration of crude MBAO. MBAO is subjected to a two-step acid-based catalyst to yield Balanites Aegyptiaca methyl ester (BAME). The first stage is the esterification of MBAO and phosphoric acid, which reduces the fatty acid concentration (percent FFA) to less than 1%. The second step was to transesterify methanol with EBAO in a 6:1 ratio to generate BAME. Next, MBAO was synthesized by transesterifying trimethylolpropane ester (TMP) + Balanites Aegyptiaca methyl ester (BAME) in a 3.5:1 ratio with 1% (wt/wt) sodium methoxide ($NaOCH_3$) [12]. An ultrasonication process was used to add SiO_2 and Activated Carbon nanoparticles to the Balanites aegyptiaca oil to generate a consistent and persistent differential. SiO_2 nanoparticles were blended with *Balanites aegyptiaca* oil using an ultrasonicator. The MBAO was combined with SiO_2 and AC to create a nanofluid using vigorous stirring at 500 rpm and 50°C for 25 minutes. The provided electricity was 100 KW at a frequency of 50 KHz. SiO_2 has a thermal expansion coefficient of $5.1 \times 10^{-6}°C^{-1}$, and Activated Carbon has a thermal expansion coefficient of $3.6 \times 10^{-6}°C^{-1}$ [13]. Table 7.1 displays all of the lubricant samples made using nanoparticle additions. The methods

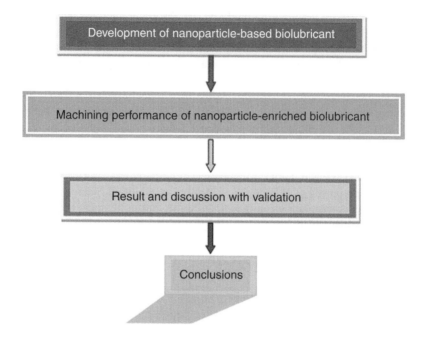

FIGURE 7.1 The techniques used to improve the machining performance of nanoparticle-enriched bio-lubricant are depicted schematically.

TABLE 7.1
MBAO Sample Specifications.

Name of sample	Concentration of additives (wt%)	Nanoparticle additives
MBAOs1	0.25	Silicon oxide
MBAOs2	0.50	
MBAOs3	0.75	
MBAOc1	0.25	Activated carbon
MBAOc2	0.50	
MBAOc3	0.75	

employed to increase nanoparticle-enriched bio-lubricant machining performance are schematically presented in Figure 7.1.

7.2.2 Physical and Chemical Characteristics

To determine the qualities of the oil, the feature had to be studied. Table 7.1 displays the MBAO sample specification. Table 7.2 shows the physicochemical properties of the samples used in the investigation. The density was determined using benchtop

TABLE 7.2
The Physical and Chemical Features of Unrefined *Balanites aegyptiaca* Oil and the Levels of SiO$_2$ Nanoparticles in the Oil.

Characteristics	Density @ 15 °C (g/cm³)	Kinematic viscosity @ 40 °C (mm²/s)	Kinematic @ 40 °C (mm²/s)	Viscosity	Kinematic (°C)	Viscosity (mg KOH/g)
Balanites aegyptiaca oil						
Balanites aegyptiaca oil + 0.25%	1.023	19.34	4.96	240	243.09	0.36
Balanites aegyptiaca oil +0.50%	1.024	19.62	5.08	248	243.72	0.34
Balanites aegyptiaca oil + 0.75%	1.036	19.70	5.16	253	243.82	0.38
Balanites aegyptiaca oil +0.7%	1.037	19.78	5.23	257	243.94	0.40
Balanites aegyptiaca oil +0.9%	1.039	19.86	5.28	261	244.04	0.41

density meters. The viscosity was measured using a Redwood viscometer. Using ASTM standards, the rheometer was leveraged to compute kinematic viscosity at 40°Cand 100°C. The viscosity index was calculated using kinematic viscosity measurements taken at different temperatures.

7.2.3 MACHINING PERFORMANCE

Table 7.3 shows the orthogonal cutting settings used on an NC lathe machine (MTAB-CNC Turn) for the turning operation. The workpiece in this exploration was made of EN19 steel. A triangular shape insert cutting tool with the model number TPMW-1.8–1.5-.5 HSS was employed. Feed rate and cutting speed are selected depending on exploratory experimentation and taking into account the material getting cut as well as the material the cutter is made of. During the cutting operation, the lubricant was supplied with an input pressure of 0.3 MPa using the minimum quantity lubrication (MQL) method. The lubricant flowed at a steady rate of 0.15 L/h from a nozzle with an inner diameter of 0.20 mm. The MQL nozzle was positioned at a 40° angle and roughly 7 mm from the cutting instruments' cutting edges.

During the machining process, a thermal imager camera HTI-19 was utilized to quantify the highest cutting temperature by putting the camera in the x-direction. Chip thickness was measured using a micrometer. Ten chips were collected to evaluate each machining factor, and the overall result of the chip thickness was elucidated. The tool chip contact length was measured using a toolmaker measuring microscope after the experimental process. The target area for analysis was rake surfaces.

TABLE 7.3
Orthogonal Cutting Factors.

Specification	Values
Cutting speed, V_c (m/min)	300
Feed rate, fr (mm/rev)	0.10
Width of cut, w (mm)	1.5
Axial cutting length (cm)	10
MQL input pressure (MPa)	0.3
Nozzle angle	40
Nozzle inner diameter (mm)	2
Oil flow rate (L/h)	0.15
Workpiece material	EN19

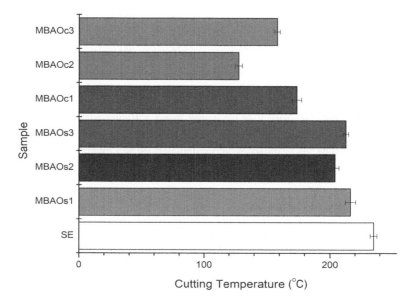

FIGURE 7.2 Cutting temperature.

7.3 RESULTS AND DISCUSSION

7.3.1 Cutting Temperature

Figure 7.2 depicts the result for the highest cutting temperature as a plot. According to the plot, SE had a greater cutting temperature than MBAO combined with additives. Because of the moderate Viscosity Index (VI) (139), the highest cutting temperature is SE, which is 244.1 °C [14]. The heat was created when the cutting tool made contact with the workpiece. Because of the large proportion of unsaturated

The Effectiveness of *Balanites aegyptiaca* Oil Nanofluid

fatty acid concentration in SE, low VI generated a thinner lubrication layer, allowing the carbon chains of SE to be easily broken and the lubricant film to evaporate at high temperatures [15]. Compared to SE, MBAO has a 3–15% lower cutting temperature. TMP trimester provides a solid lubricating coating as a direct outcome of vast, complicated branches and polarity molecular chains [16].

MBAOc2 has a reduced maximum cutting temperature of 135.5 °C. Adding Activated Carbon to MBAO helps to boost the lubricating capacity under high pressure. Still, too many additives can generate high stress and friction in the oil, resulting in fluid films that cannot shield the surface area and promote the temperature to rise. MBAO2 has the lowest temperature of 215.5 °C among the MBAOs, accompanied by MBAOs3 and MBAOs1. While assessing machining effectiveness, the maximum cutting temperature is significant since it can extend tool life [17]. Since the thermal expansion coefficient of Activated Carbon additions is lower than SiO_2, the maximum cutting temperature for MBAOc is lower than MBAOc [13]. The thermal expansion coefficient of additives has a significant impact on the cutting temperature. Due to the extreme material's high thermal expansion coefficient, the cutting temperature drops [16]. The thermal conductivity qualities of Activated Carbon and Silicon Oxide aid in enhancing the lubricating oil in MBAO, resulting in a robust lubricant layer compared to SE [18].

During machining, the thermal resistance can affect a piece's dimensional precision, surface polish, and tool life [8]. The formation of a lubricating layer from oil viscosity has the potential to minimize heat generation [9]. According to the findings of this investigation, the addition of 0.50 wt% nanoparticles in MBAO led to decreased maximum cutting temperature. At lower nanoparticle concentrations (at a level of 0.25wt%), fewer particles are entangled in the interface, resulting in a suboptimal lubrication film. At a level of 0.75wt%, a high concentration of SiO_2 and Activated Carbon created a high-stress concentration, aiding the abrasion characteristic of particles. This finding is consistent with recent research by Talib et al. [1]. The increasing the intensity of other particles, the greater the friction between the contact surface [19]. The lubrication film for MBAOs1, MBAOs3, MBAOc1, and MBAOc3 was entirely broken down, and the lubrication film was unable to preserve the contact surface between the tool and chips, causing the cutting temperature to rise. Finally, MBAOc2 has the lowest cutting temperature of all specimens due to the presence of fatty acids in the TMP trimester, which allow a high lubricating film formation between the contact surface of the tool and chips.

7.3.2 Chip Thickness

Figure 7.3 depicts a graph of chip thickness acquired following the machining operation. SE has the thickest chip of any specimen, measuring 0.223 mm. This is because the MBAO lubricating coating minimizes the contact area at the shear zone during machining. MBAO features a complex and challenging molecular chain that generates a durable lubricating coating, reducing friction at the tool-workpiece interface [20]. Although the lubricating layer between tool-chip surfaces is adequate, MBAOs2 has the thinnest chip [21]. MBAOs2 has a 15% reduction in chip thickness compared to SE.

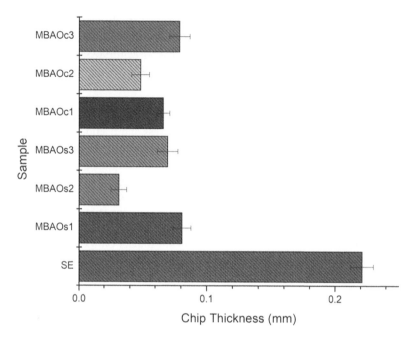

FIGURE 7.3 Chip thickness.

Furthermore, the creation of a lubricating film can aid in the movement of the chip over the tool, given the short contact length [16]. Furthermore, the MBAOs3 have an overabundance of fillers, leading to reduced shear angles and coarser chips. As a reason, the film layer cannot be created, leading to a large contact area. As a result, the creation of chips thickens. MBAOc2 has the most negligible chip thickness of 0.182mm, accompanied by MBAOc1 and MBAOc3. An enhancement induces friction between the tool and the contact surface [19]. Finally, MBAOs2 has better efficacy regarding chip thickness, which is 0.178mm, since it has a suitable lubricating film layer whenever the tool interfaces with the surface area [8]. The findings revealed that higher concentrations likely increase chip thickness. Overuse of additives enhanced friction during the machining operation, preventing the formation of a lubricating layer and resulting in thicker chips. Consequently, significant stress concentration resulted in a large quantity of force. As per Figure 2(b), high concentration induced dislocations as a result of large accumulation of particles, which caused severe friction on the tool-chip contact surface [12].

7.3.3 Surface Roughness of the Machined Sample

Figure 7.4 depicts the optical view of the surface roughness of the work sample following the orthogonal cutting procedure. The photos show how the varied compositions of Silicon Oxide and Activated Carbon have influenced the roughness of the

The Effectiveness of *Balanites aegyptiaca* Oil Nanofluid

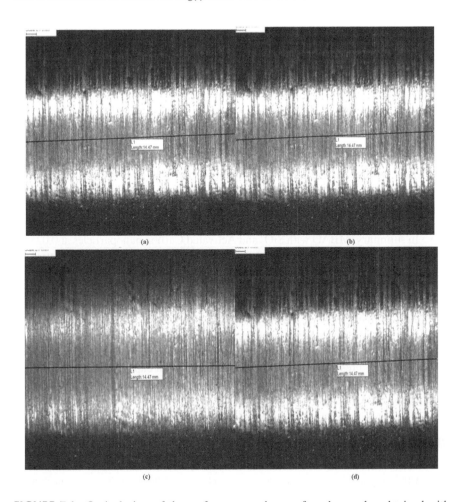

FIGURE 7.4 Optical view of the surfaces – roughness of work samples obtained with (a) MBAOc, (b) MBAOc2, (c) MBAOs, and (d) MBAOs2.

machined sample. It was consistent with the cutting temperature and chip thickness observed in this investigation. Different MWFs used in the cutting edge significantly impacted the surface roughness machined sample [22]. The MBAO has a better surface finish than the SE. It is due to the high creation of long and branching TMP triester, which resulted in less friction between the tool's contact area and the chips [9]. MBAOc2 and MBAOs2 have the better surface finish among MBAOs and MBAOc, measuring 0.32µm and 0.26µm, respectively. It was revealed that having adequate lubrication affects surface roughness decrease. Once lubricant seeped into the shearing zone, friction was reduced, resulting in a reduced surface roughness [12]. The considerable generation in MBAOs2 and MBAOc2 offer enough coverage to reduce tool chip contact length and friction between the tool and metal surface [23]. The MBAOc3 outcome was 10% more than the MBAOc2 result owing to the combination of extra additives, which resulted in inadequate lubrication and greater friction. As demonstrated in Table 7.3, adding additives in MBAOs1, MBAOs3, MBAOc1, and MBAOc3 resulted in poor surface finish behavior. The shielding coating of MBAO began to deteriorate due to the more significant content case. MBAOc2 has an outstanding surface finish due to adequate lubricant-produced defensive layers that can minimize friction and tool chip contact length [24].

7.4 CONCLUSION

This study compared the performance of modified Balanites Aegyptiaca (Desert date) oil with two additions (Silicon dioxide and Activated Carbon) to organic ester as MWFs. The following are the insights generated from the outcomes:

- In summary, MBAO with SiO_2 and Activated Carbon nanoparticles at 0.025 wt% displays improved turning process outcomes in the case of cutting temperature, chip thickness, and tool chip contact length compared to 0.01 and 0.05 wt% compositions.
- Furthermore, unlike organic ester, MBAO with additions inhibits superior cutting characteristics. MBAOs2 (MBAO plus 0.50 wt% Activated Carbon) has the highest effective machining performance.
- One of the significant cornerstones of sustainable manufacturing is environmental preservation. Furthermore, this has the capability to be present in the lubricants industry in the context of environmental consciousness and energy efficiency.

REFERENCES

[1] Talib, N., & Rahim, E. A. (2018). Performance of modified Jatropha oil in combination with hexagonal boron nitride particles as a bio-based lubricant for green machining. *Tribology International*, 118(March 2017), 89–104.

[2] Jamaluddin, N. A., Talib, N., Sahab, A., & Sani, A. (2020). Tribological assessment of modified Jatropha oil with hBN and graphene nanoparticles as a new preference for the metalworking fluid. *International Journal of Engineering and Advanced Technology*, 9(3), 3144–3149.

[3] Woma, T. Y., Lawal, S. A., Abdulrahman, A. S., Olutoye, M. A., & Ojapah, M. M. (2019). Vegetable oil based lubricants: Challenges and prospects. *Tribology Online*, 14(2), 60–70.

[4] Sayuti, M., Erh, O. M., Sarhan, A. A. D., & Hamdi, M. (2014). Investigation on the morphology of the machined surface in end milling of aerospace AL6061-T6 for novel uses of SiO_2 nanolubrication system. *Journal of Cleaner Production*, 66, 655–663.

[5] Lee, P. H., Nam, J. S., Li, C., & Lee, S. W. (2012). An experimental study on micro-grinding process with nanofluid minimum quantity lubrication (MQL). *International Journal of Precision Engineering and Manufacturing*, 13(3), 331–338.

[6] Srivastava, A., & Sahai, P. (2013). Vegetable oils as lube base stocks: A review. *African Journal of Biotechnology*, 12(9), 880–891.

[7] Yunus, R., Fakhru'l-Razi, A., Ooi, T. L., Iyuke, S. E., & Perez, J. M. (2004). Lubrication properties of trimethylolpropane esters based on palm oil and palm kernel oils. *European Journal of Lipid Science and Technology*, 106(1), 52–60.

[8] Talib, N., Sasahara, H., & Rahim, E. A. (2017). Evaluation of modified Jatropha-based oil with hexagonal boron nitride particle as a biolubricant in orthogonal cutting process. *International Journal of Advanced Manufacturing Technology*, 92(1–4), 371–391.

[9] Shashidhara, Y. M., & Jayaram, S. R. (2010). Vegetable oils as a potential cutting fluid-an evolution. *Tribology International*, 43(5–6), 1073–1081.

[10] Talib, N., Nasir, R. M., & Rahim, E. A. (2018). Investigation on the tribological behaviour of modified Jatropha oil with hexagonal boron nitride particles as a metalworking fluid for machining process. *International Journal of Integrated Engineering*, 10(3), 57–62.

[11] Hamdan, A., Fadzil, M., & Hamdi, M. (2012). Procitan rad—performance evaluation of different types of cutting fluid in the machining of Aisi 01 hardened steel using pulsed jet minimal quantity lubrication system. *Journal of Aerospace Engineering*, 11, 17–24.

[12] Osama, M., Singh, A., Walvekar, R., Khalid, M., Gupta, T. C. S. M., & Yin, W. W. (2017). Recent developments and performance review of metal working fluids. *Tribology International*, 114, 389–401.

[13] Chan, C. H., Tang, S. W., Mohd, N. K., Lim, W. H., Yeong, S. K., & Idris, Z. (2018). Tribological behavior of biolubricant base stocks and additives. *Renewable and Sustainable Energy Reviews*, 93(March 2017), 145–157.

[14] Talib, N., Sani, A. S. A., & Hamzah, N. A. (2019). Modified Jatropha nano-lubricant as metal working fluid for machining process. *Journal of Tribology*, 23(September), 90–96.

[15] Lawal, S. A. (2013). A review of application of vegetable oil-based cutting fluids in machining nonferrous metals. *Indian Journal of Science and Technology*, 6(1), 3951–3956.

[16] Atabani, A. E., Silitonga, A. S., Ong, H. C., Mahlia, T. M. I., Masjuki, H. H., Badruddin, I. A., & Fayaz, H. (2013). Non-edible vegetable oils: A critical evaluation of oil extraction, fatty acid compositions, biodiesel production, characteristics, engine performance and emissions production. *Renewable and Sustainable Energy Reviews*, 18, 211–245.

[17] Uysal, A., Demiren, F., & Altan, E. (2015). Applying minimum quantity lubrication (MQL) method on milling of martensitic stainless steel by using Nano MoS_2 reinforced vegetable cutting fluid. *Procedia—Social and Behavioral Sciences*, 195, 2742–2747.

[18] Katpatal, D. C., Andhare, A. B., Padole, P. M., & Khedkar, R. S. (2017). Study of dispersion stability and thermo-physical properties of CuO-Jatropha oil-based nanolubricants. *Journal of the Brazilian Society of Mechanical Sciences and Engineering*, 39(9), 3657–3668.

[19] Wan, Q., Jin, Y., Sun, P., & Ding, Y. (2015). Tribological behaviour of lubricant oil containing boron nitride nanoparticles. *Procedia Engineering*, 102, 1038–1045.

[20] Huang, S., Yao, W., Hu, J., & Xu, X. (2015). Tribological performance and lubrication mechanism of contact-charged electrostatic spray lubrication technique. *Tribology Letters*, 59(2).

[21] Dhar, N. R., & Kamruzzaman, M. (2005). A study of effects of MQL by vegetable oil on cutting temperature, chips and cutting forces in turning AISI-1060 steel. In: *Recent Advances in Manufacturing Technologies*. NIT Rourkela, Orissa, India.

[22] Abdul Sani, A. S., Rahim, E. A., Sharif, S., & Sasahara, H. (2019). Machining performance of vegetable oil with phosphonium- and ammonium-based ionic liquids via MQL technique. *Journal of Cleaner Production*, 209, 947–964.

[23] Ilhan, B., Kurt, M., & Ertürk, H. (2016). Experimental investigation of heat transfer enhancement and viscosity change of hBN nanofluids. *Experimental Thermal and Fluid Science*, 77, 272–283.

[24] Rahim, E. A., Talib, N., Amiril Sahab, A. S., Syahrullail, S., & Mohid, Z. (2017). Tribological evaluation on various formulation of modified RBD palm olein as sustainable metalworking fluids for machining process. *Materials Science Forum*, 882, 13–17.

8 Lignocellulose Biomass Pyrolysis for Bio-Oil Production

Biomass Pre-treatment Methods for Production of Drop-In Fuels

Kumar, R.[1], Strezov, V.[1], Weldekidan, H.[1], He, J.[1], Singh, S.[2], Kan, T.[1], and Dastjerdi, B.[1]

1 School of Natural Sciences, Faculty of Science & Engineering, Macquarie University, Sydney, NSW, Australia

2 Department of Organic and Petrochemical Technology, School of Chemical Engineering, Hanoi University of Science and Technology, 1 Dai Co Viet, Hanoi, Vietnam

CONTENTS

8.1 Introduction 124
8.2 Biomass Pyrolysis 128
8.3 Bio-Oil Properties 132
8.4 Pre-treatment of Biomass 136
    8.4.1 Physical and Thermal Methods 136
        8.4.1.1 Grinding 136
        8.4.1.2 Densification 139
        8.4.1.3 Dry Torrefaction 141
    8.4.2 Chemical Methods 148
        8.4.2.1 Acid Treatment of Biomass 148
        8.4.2.2 Alkali Treatment of Biomass 155
        8.4.2.3 Wet Torrefaction 157
        8.4.2.4 Ammonia Fiber Expansion 162
        8.4.2.5 Steam Explosion 163
        8.4.2.6 Hot-Water Extraction 166
    8.4.3 Biological Pre-treatment of Lignocellulose Biomass 167

DOI: 10.1201/9781003265597-8

| 124 | Biowaste and Biomass in Biofuel Applications |

8.5 Catalytic Pyrolysis of Pre-treated Biomass 168
8.6 Current Status, Challenges, and Future Recommendations........................177
8.7 Conclusions...182
8.8 Acknowledgments...183
References 183

Highlights

- Biomass pre-treatment methods for bio-oil upgrading are thoroughly discussed.
- Basic principles and key advantages of all the methods are highlighted.
- Thermal methods improve the biomass structure and energy content.
- Chemical treatments remove undesirable inorganic species from the biomass.
- Catalytic pyrolysis with pre-treated biomass increases aromatics in the bio-oil.

Abbreviations: AFE, Ammonia Fiber Expansion; Btu, British Thermal Unit; C, Carbon; Ca, Calcium; Ca $(OH)_2$, Calcium Hydroxide; CH_4, Methane; CO, Carbon Monoxide; CO_2, Carbon Dioxide; cP, Centipoise; cSt, Centistokes; Cu, Copper; DT, Dry Torrefaction; FTIR, Fourier-Transform Infrared Spectroscopy; g, Gram; GC-MS, Gas Chromatography-Mass Spectroscopy; H, Hydrogen; h, Hour; HCl, Hydrochloric Acid; HH, Higher Heating Value; HNO_3, Nitric Acid; H_3PO_4, Phosphoric Acid; H_2SO_4, Sulfuric Acid; HWE, Hot Water Extraction; K, Potassium; kg, Kilogram; kJ, Kilo Joule; kW, Kilo Watt; kWth, Kilo Watt Thermal; L, Liter; m, Meter; M, Molar; MJ, Mega Joule; mg, Milligram; Mg, Magnesium; MPa, Mega Pascal; min, Minute; mm, Millimeter; mL, Milliliter; mPa.s, Milli Pascal Second; MW, Mega Watt; N, Nitrogen; Na, Sodium; NaOH, Sodium Hydroxide; NH_4OH, Ammonium Hydroxide; nm, Nanometer; NO_x, Nitrogen Oxides; O, Oxygen; OECD, Organisation for Economic Co-operation and Development; P, Phosphorous; ppm, Parts Per Million; s, Second; S, Sulfur; SO_x, Sulfur Oxides; SE, Steam Explosion; WT, Wet Torrefaction; μm, Micrometer; °C, Degree Celsius

8.1 INTRODUCTION

The total world energy demand is rising each year and is expected to increase by nearly 28% by 2040, estimated to be approximately 739 quadrillion Btus [1]. Figure 8.1 shows historical and predicted energy consumption by non-OECD (Organisation for Economic Co-operation and Development) countries and the estimation of world energy consumption by energy source. Most of the energy demand is expected to originate from countries with strong economic growth. It has been predicted that by 2040, non-OECD countries would account for 64% of the total increase in energy consumption, which has been predicted to amount to approximately 473 quadrillion

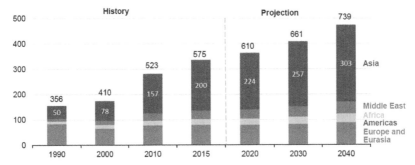
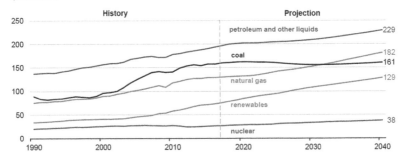

FIGURE 8.1 (a) History and predicted energy consumption by non-OECD (Organisation for Economic Co-operation and Development) countries. (b) Estimation of world energy consumption by energy source [1].

Btus, while the OPEC countries are assumed to consume about 266 quadrillion Btus of energy by 2040 [1]. Currently, most of the energy is produced by fossil fuels which release greenhouse gases, air toxics, and criteria pollutants, consequently leading to environmental pollution and adverse climate change impacts. Therefore, to mitigate environmental concerns and meet the increasing energy demand, it is highly indispensable to find alternative renewable and low-emission fuels. In this regard, developing and developed countries are striving to engineer novel and innovative ways to generate clean and environmentally friendly energy and fuels [2,3]. From this perspective, lignocellulose biomass is considered among the most valuable and sustainable energy resources. Recently, it has been estimated that approximately 550 gigatonnes of biomass carbon are present on the planet, where plants contribute to approximately 450 gigatonnes of carbon [4]. Figure 8.2 shows the graphical representation of the global biomass distribution by taxa.

Many technologies can utilize lignocellulose biomass or biomass waste as feedstock to produce a variety of energy fuels or energy resources that can be utilized to generate energy, as shown in Figure 8.3. Alternatively, biomass can also be used

126   Biowaste and Biomass in Biofuel Applications

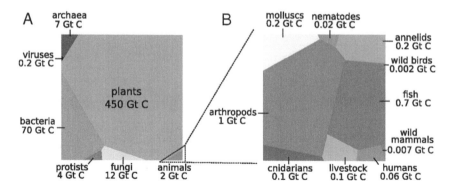

FIGURE 8.2 Graphical representation of the global biomass distribution by taxa. (A) Absolute biomasses of different taxa are represented using a Voronoi diagram, with the area of each cell being proportional to that taxa global biomass. (B) Absolute biomass of different animal taxa. Reproduced from reference [4].

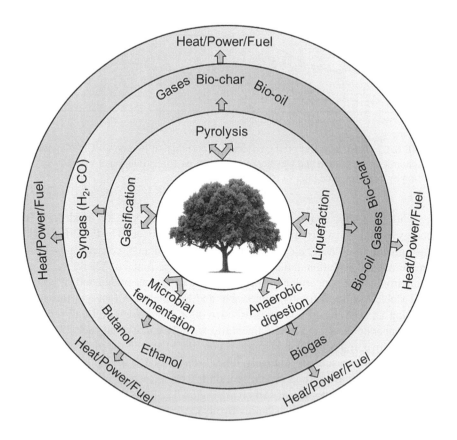

FIGURE 8.3 Technologies that can convert biomass into different fuels.

to produce various high-value-added chemicals of great agricultural and industrial importance. In this regard, pyrolysis has been considered an efficient, cost-effective, and significant process to convert organics into energy-rich products [5–7]. Pyrolysis can use various types of lignocellulosic biomass or contaminated biomass to produce bio-oil, bio-char, and pyrolytic gases [5,8]. Alternatively, it can also be applied to produce valuable chemicals, such as levoglucosenone, which is generally produced during the thermal degradation of cellulose [9]. The yield of the resultant pyrolytic products mainly depends on the type of biomass used, and the variables applied during the pyrolysis process. Generally, the pyrolysis of wood biomass at 500–550 °C results in a bio-oil yield in the range of 60–80 wt%, bio-char-20–30 wt%, and pyrolytic gases in a range of 20–25 wt% [5,10]. Among all the pyrolytic products, bio-oil is considered of great importance and foreseen as the future drop-in fuel, while the mixture of pyrolytic gases (CO_2, CO, CH_4, H_2, etc.) can be directly used for energy applications and the produced bio-char can be used as a soil amendment in the agriculture or as a solid fuel [8,11]. Bio-oil can be considered a clean and renewable fuel compared to conventional fossil fuels since its combustion releases a very low amount of acidic SO_x and NO_x emissions. Bio-oil can be potentially used in turbines and boilers for power and heat generation, and the upgraded bio-oil with enhanced higher heating values (HHV) can also be utilized as a transportation fuel. Besides, the pyrolysis bio-oils can be used as a promising resource to produce various chemicals with high-added values. However, bio-oil is currently considered an unsuitable drop-in fuel because of its poor properties, such as high oxygen content, low carbon and hydrogen content, acidic pH, high instability, and low HHVs. Various physical, thermal, chemical, and catalytic strategies can substantially improve the bio-oil properties. The strategies can be applied at different stages of the pyrolysis, such as pre-pyrolysis, during pyrolysis, and post-pyrolysis. For example, different physical methods such as grinding, thermal treatment at mild temperatures (torrefaction), and chemical treatment with an acidic solution or alkali metals can be utilized for pre-treatment of biomass to remove moisture and impurities in the biomass, increasing H/C ratios and energy content, and can also be ameliorated, thereby improving the overall fuel property of biomass for pyrolysis application. The bio-oil can be upgraded during pyrolysis using advanced and highly active catalysts. The catalysts can be mixed with the biomass and heated together, known as *in-situ* pyrolysis, or the catalyst bed can be placed downstream of the biomass, and the pyrolytic vapors are passed through a catalytic bed, termed *ex-situ* pyrolysis [10]. The catalytic pyrolysis in both modes has shown significant improvement in the bio-oil properties and, currently, is the most widely accepted and demonstrated approach for bio-oil upgrading.

Several methods have been developed to improve the bio-oil properties applicable to different types of biomass. While a considerable amount of literature has been devoted to review of the catalytic upgrading of bio-oils [12–17], there is a limitation of the reviews of physicochemical methods for biomass upgrading, which have been overviewed only in certain sections of review articles [8,16,18]. Some published review articles are focused on a particular upgrading method, such as dry torrefaction and wet torrefaction [19–22]. Hence, a critical review article focused on physicochemical methods of biomass upgrading is still lacking in the literature. Therefore, this article comprehensively reviews the various physicochemical

128   Biowaste and Biomass in Biofuel Applications

methods applicable for biomass pre-treatment and, consequently, for bio-oil upgrading, providing comprehensive information on the basic principles of the methods and important parameters that affect biomass properties. This article also highlights the key challenges involved in each treatment method and suggests possible future recommendations of the work that can be carried out to further understand the influence of pre-treatment methods on bio-oil upgrading. The last section provides the effect of integrated catalytic pyrolysis and pre-treatment methods on bio-oil upgrading.

8.2 BIOMASS PYROLYSIS

Biomass is a renewable energy source, generally referred to as biological organic materials derived from living organisms, which can originate from various sources, such as terrestrial forests, agricultural crops, aquatic plants, manures, and different wastes [6,23]. Photosynthesis is the primary process that makes biomass energy-rich. In this process, plants convert the radiant energy from the sun into chemical energy in the form of glucose or any other sugar. This chemical energy stored in the biomass is released as heat or can be converted using various technologies to produce liquid and gaseous fuels. Figure 8.3 presents the technologies that can be employed to generate various fuels from different types of biomass. The solid biomass can be utilized as a potential feedstock to generate various fuels (bio-oil, gases, char) using thermochemical technologies, such as pyrolysis, liquefaction, and gasification, while wet biomass (organic waste, manure, etc.) can be converted to renewable fuels, through biochemical processes like fermentation and anaerobic digestion [24,25]. Pyrolysis is the most studied thermochemical technology because of its ability to produce gas, liquid, and solid biofuels in a process that involves the degradation of biomass components in an oxygen-less atmosphere at specific heating conditions [6]. The yields of generated pyrolytic products primarily depend on the structure and complexity of biomass composition (fraction of cellulose, hemicellulose, and lignin) and secondly on the pyrolysis variables [6,8]. The complete thermal decomposition of biomass involves a complex array of multiple reactions, such as dehydration, decarboxylation, decarbonylation, hydrogenation, isomerization, aromatization, depolymerization, and charring, resulting in liquid, solid, and gaseous pyrolytic products [5,23]. Mechanism of biomass pyrolysis can be described based on the decomposition of its main three components, that is, cellulose, hemicellulose, and lignin, into subsequent organic compounds, which have been reviewed in the previously published review articles [26,27], hence is not discussed in this article. Figure 8.4 shows main pyrolytic pathways during the fast pyrolysis of cellulose, hemicellulose, and lignin.

The distribution of pyrolysis products depends on the interaction between these components during the pyrolysis process of lignocellulose biomass and other factors. Figure 8.5 shows the pyrolytic behavior of biomass with mixed components. Generally, in the biomass structure, lignin is present in the outer cell wall of the biomass, while cellulose is present within a lignin shell, and hemicellulose is either located within the cellulose or present between the cellulose and lignin.

Lignocellulose Biomass Pyrolysis for Bio-Oil Production

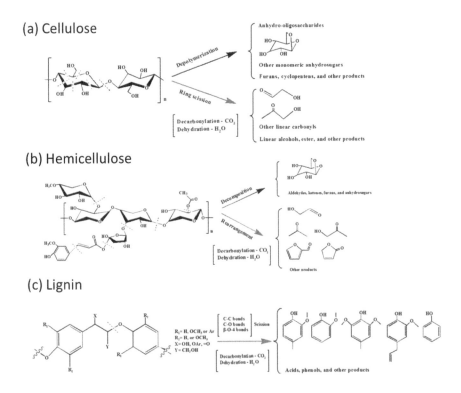

FIGURE 8.4 Pyrolytic pathways during the fast pyrolysis of cellulose, hemicellulose, and lignin.

Source: Reproduced with permission from reference [28]. Copyright © 2018, American Chemical Society.

All these components, for example, cellulose and lignin, cellulose, and hemicellulose, are mainly linked via hydrogen bonds, whereas covalent bonds are also present between cellulose and lignin [29]. Thus, these linkages affect the pyrolytic behavior of biomass and, consequently, the production and distribution of pyrolytic products. A number of studies have demonstrated the influence of the interaction of three components of biomass on the pyrolytic behavior of the biomass and pyrolytic products [30–33]. For example, a study demonstrated the effect of cellulose-xylan-lignin interactions on the distribution of pyrolytic products during fast pyrolysis at 525 °C, a heating rate of 1000 °C/s, and a holding time of 15s [34]. The experimental and predicted results of thermogravimetric analysis and pyrolysis product yields were compared to estimate the possible interactions between the components. The important results of the study are shown in Table 8.1. Figure 8.6 shows the pyrolysis mechanism of cellulose linked with lignin. The study showed that at 325 °C, no interactions between the components were observed, which could be ascribed to the insignificant degradation of cellulose that occurs at this temperature. Above 375 °C, mild interactions were estimated between levoglucosan and

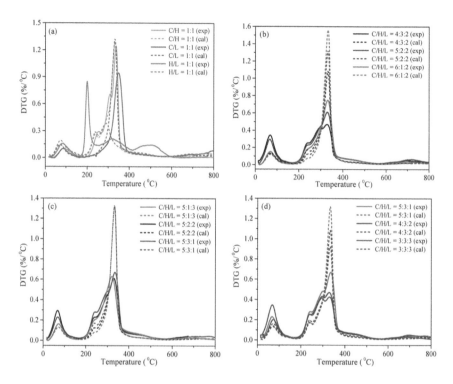

FIGURE 8.5 Pyrolytic behavior of biomass with mixed components, showing the expected and calculated DTG curves.

Source: Reproduced with permission from reference [28]. Copyright © 2018, American Chemical Society.

the pyrolysis products of xylan and lignin, leading to significant changes in product yields. However, at 525 °C, significant interactions were present between cellulose and xylan, cellulose, and lignin, but no obvious interactions between xylan and lignin were observed [34]. Volpe et al. [33] recently demonstrated the synergetic effect between lignin and cellulose during slow pyrolysis at varying temperatures (400–600 °C) with a heating rate of 150 °C/min. The pyrolytic results of the model synthetic mixtures (cellulose/lignin) were compared with real feedstocks, which revealed that the presence of lignin in the synthetic mixture behaved differently than the real feedstocks during the pyrolysis process. The results showed that the addition of lignin increased the char yield and decreased the tar yield from the pyrolysis of the synthetic mixture, while it was also responsible for the increased concentration of CO_2 in both synthetic and real biomass samples, attributing to the involvement of water molecules released from the pyrolysis of cellulose and lignin to facilitate water gas shift reaction. However, the presence of lignin in the synthetic mixtures inhibited the production of H_2 in the gas, whereas the pyrolysis of real biomass samples showed a higher concentration of H_2, ascribed to the presence of higher moisture content in the biomass samples that enhanced the breakdown

TABLE 8.1

Solid, Liquid, and Gas Yields from Pyrolysis of Individual Cellulose, Xylan, Lignin, and Mixture of These Three Components and Real Biomass Samples at 525 °C, Heating Rate of 1000 °C/S, and Holding Time of 15 s.

Sample	Pyrolysis products (wt%)		
	Solid	Liquid	Gas
Cellulose	2	82.3	15.7
Xylan	20.5	24.2	55.3
Lignin	34.8	46.3	18.9
Cellulose/xylan (1:1)	16.2	39.7	44.1
Cellulose/lignin (1:1)	17.5	54.1	28.4
Xylan/lignin (1:1)	27.9	35.4	36.7
Cellulose/xylan/lignin (1:1:1)	21.6	43.6	34.8
Oak[a]	9.6	65.6	24.8
Spruce[b]	7.8	62.5	29.7
Pine[c]	7.7	67.5	28.4

[a] Oak (Cellulose: 43 wt%, Hemicellulose: 22 wt%, Lignin: 35 wt%)
[b] Pine (Cellulose: 46wt%, Hemicellulose: 24 wt%, Lignin: 27 wt%)
[c] Spruce (Cellulose: 47wt%, Hemicellulose: 22 wt%, Lignin: 29 wt%)
Source: Data taken from Reference [36].

and degradation of the intermediate pyrolysis molecules and also water gas shift reaction to promote the formation of H_2 [33]. It was also noticed that significant interactions were found between cellulose and lignin during the pyrolysis of herbaceous biomass, estimated by the decreased yield of levoglucosan and increased yield of furans and light weight molecular compounds, while these interactions were not observed for woody biomass [31]. More recently, Zhao et al. [30] studied the interactions of three biomass components during their co-pyrolysis process. The results suggested that considerable interactions existed between the components that influenced the production of pyrolytic products. The study found that increasing the cellulose content in the biomass enhanced the production of levoglucosan, while increasing the hemicellulose content slightly increased the yield of furfural and acetic acid, and the presence of higher lignin content promoted the formation of phenolic compounds and inhibited the production of furan substances in the pyrolysis of cellulose and hemicellulose. The presence of cellulose and hemicellulose may promote the pyrolysis of lignin to produce phenolic compounds by favoring the deoxidation of polymer in the lignin structure or by cracking the polymer to produce C_2-C_6 olefins, which may undergo aromatization reactions to produce phenolic compounds [35]. Moreover, it has been noticed that hemicellulose has an inhibitory effect on the formation of carbohydrates, such as levoglucosan from cellulose pyrolysis [30].

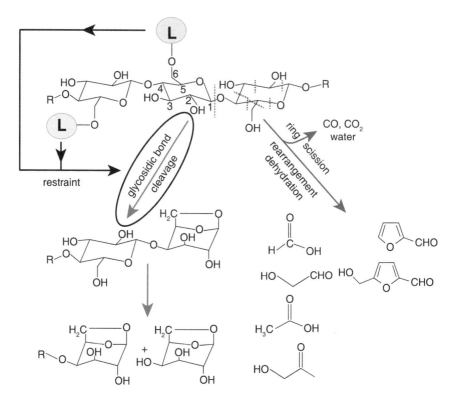

FIGURE 8.6 Postulated pyrolysis mechanisms of cellulose covalently linked with lignin. L in picture represents lignin.

Source: Reproduced with permission from reference [28]. Copyright © 2015, American Chemical Society.

Overall, it could be suggested that the presence and the content of each major component in the biomass plays a significant role in the production of pyrolytic products. Firstly, the higher content of cellulose is responsible to obtain higher liquid products, while high hemicellulose favors the production of higher gas products, and higher lignin content results in more solid residues. Previous studies have shown that cellulose-hemicellulose interactions are less prevalent as compared to cellulose-lignin and hemicellulose-lignin linkages. Moreover, it has been found that the interactions between the biomass components may vary the distribution of pyrolytic products, where the presence of lignin may promote the production of phenolic compounds, and cellulose and hemicellulose may favor the production of levoglucosan and furfural substances, respectively.

8.3 BIO-OIL PROPERTIES

Table 8.2 compares the properties of bio-oil and conventional petroleum fuel (heavy fuel oil) and Table 8.3 presents the physiochemical properties of bio-oil produced

TABLE 8.2
Comparative Properties of Bio-Oil and Heavy Fuel Oil.

Physical properties	Value	
	Bio-oil	Heavy fuel oil
pH	2.5	
Specific gravity	1.2	0.94
Moisture content (wt%)	15–30	0.1
Carbon (wt%)	54–58	85
Hydrogen (wt%)	5.5–7.0	11
Oxygen (wt%)	35–55	1.0
Nitrogen (wt%)	0–0.2	0.3
Ash (wt%)	0–0.2	0.1
HHV (MJ/kg)	16–19	40
Viscosity, at 500 °C (cP*)	40–100	180
Solids (wt%)	0.2–1.0	1
Distillation residue (wt%)	Up to 50	1

Source: Data taken from Reference [37] with permission. Copyright © 2004, American Chemical Society

* cP: centipoise

from different biomass materials without using any upgrading technique. It can be observed from both tables that the bio-oil needs significant upgrading to compete with petroleum fuels. As shown in Table 8.2, the water content in bio-oil is generally between 15% and 30%, which affects its heating and ignition properties. The high-water content decreases adiabatic flame temperature (the temperature in the combustion process if no heat is lost) and combustion temperature and reduces combustion reaction rates. Besides, it delays the bio-oil's ignition by reducing the droplet's vaporization rate, which may pose serious concerns if used in compression ignition engines. The presence of water decreases the heating value but could also help increase the bio-oil's pH. Higher oxygen content in the bio-oil also has a detrimental effect on its applications. The presence of highly reactive oxygen species, such as carboxylic acids and aldehydes, responsible for their acidic pH, and their reaction with other reactive organic compounds affect the stability of the bio-oil, consequently resulting in more concerns for storage. The acidic pH of bio-oil is responsible for its corrosive nature, making it unsuitable for use in turbines or combustion engines. The ash content in bio-oil is also slightly higher than the desired value. The ash contains some alkali metals, such as sodium and potassium, which are also responsible for their corrosive nature. The metals and other inorganic particles may agglomerate, subsequently leading to the formation of a sludge layer on the base of the container.

Another major concern is the chemical and thermal stability of bio-oils. Usually, the bio-oil exhibits lower chemical or thermal stability when compared to heavy fuel

TABLE 8.3
Physiochemical Properties of Bio-Oil Produced from Different Biomasses without Using Any Upgrading Technique.

Biomass	Reactor type	T (°C)	Bio-oil elemental analysis (wt%)				Bio-oil fuel properties						References
			C	H	N	O	Viscosity	Water content (wt%)	HHV (MJ/kg)	pH	Density (g/mL)	Acid value (mg of KOH/g)	
Softwood	-	600	39.96	7.74	0.11	52.19	67.39[a]	28.05	15.27	-	1.20	79.23	[38]
Oak wood	-	600	59.99	7.18	0.92	31.91	173.35[a]	15.15	24.87	-	-	-	[39]
Pine wood	-	500	42.60	8.47	0.08	48.85	175[a]	-	19.5	-	-	-	[40]
Hardwood	Fluidized bed	500	61.35	6.34	0.24	32.07	715[b]	8.93	23.5	-	-	-	[36]
Saccharina japonica	Fluidized bed	300	60.15	7.74	5.77	16.48	-	1.76	28.63	5.9	-	-	[41]
Pine wood	Auger reactor	450	-	-	-	-	55.2[c]	16.9	22.49	3.08	1.18	69.5	[42]
Pine wood	Auger reactor	450	-	-	-	-	6.49[c]	20.83	16.1	2.65	1.17	90.06	[43]
Sweetgum	Auger reactor	450	-	-	-	-	8.26[c]	38.3	2.65	2.65	1.16	119.2	[44]
Switchgrass	Auger reactor	450	-	-	-	-	1.51[c]	61.7	2.98	2.98	1.08	88.4	
Corn stover	Auger reactor	450	-	-	-	-	1.60[c]	54.7	2.66	2.66	1.08	85.8	
Saccharina japonica	Fixed bed batch	470	69.2	8.3	3.7	15.4	-	34.7	35.0	-	1.13	43	[45]
Pine nuts	Continuous fixed bed	550	58	8.2	0.3	33.5	1244[d]	9.36	19.31	4.84	1.09	-	[46]
Eucalyptus bark	Free-fall pyrolysis unit	550	-	-	-	-	-	26.07	12.45	2.78	1.13	-	[47]
Rice husk	Fluidized bed	600	-	-	-	-	58.16[d]	15.82	22.99	3.59	1.15	-	[48]
Pine wood	Pilot-scale reactor	500	42.64	7.55	0.22	49.59	178.2[c]	23.5	18.9	-	1.21	-	[49]
Walnut shell	-	550	-	-	-	-	7.98[d]	18.87	-	4.38	0.94	-	[50]

Lignocellulose Biomass Pyrolysis for Bio-Oil Production

Biomass	Reactor	Temp											Ref
Loblolly pine chips	Fluidized bed	500	50.1	6.65	0.53	42.7	16.4[b]	19.8	-	-	-	-	[51]
Rice straw	Fluidized bed	-	34.53	6.17	1.01	57.63	-	27.20	15.62	-	-	-	[52]
Walnut shell	Spouted bed	550	37.91	8.78	1.19	25.02	3.29[d]	23.29	-	4.28	0.95	-	[53]
Pine sawdust	Fluidized bed	500	57.82	7.13	0.04	32.33	-	-	23.83	3.57	1.23	-	[54]
Oak	Fluidized bed	500	54.9	6.28	0.07	38.7	57[d]	20.3	-	-	1.24	110	[55]
Switchgrass	Fluidized bed	500	60.9	5.73	1.07	32.3	9[d]	37.6	-	-	1.15	98	
Corn stover	Fixed bed	400	-	-	-	-	2.6[b]	-	15.3	2.67	1.25	-	[56]
Prairie cord grass	Fixed bed	400	-	-	-	-	2.5[b]	-	15.2	2.59	1.25	-	
Switchgrass	Fixed bed	400	-	-	-	-	2.1[b]	-	14.9	2.77	1.25	-	
Napier grass	Fixed bed	600	45.32	7.17	0.81	46.60	2.71[b]	26.01	20.97	2.95	1.05	-	[57]

Units of viscosity: [a] mPa.s; [b] cP; [c] cSt; [d] mm^2/s.

oil due to the abundance of highly active oxygenated compounds, such as carboxylic acids, aldehydes, and phenols, and low boiling point volatiles [58]. Therefore, due to low stability, some chemical reactions continue to occur between the highly active organic compounds with a change in temperature, which fluctuates the physical and chemical properties of the bio-oil. A higher amount of solid residues leads to changes in the viscosity and molecular weight of bio-oil, which further increases the problems with its storage and transportation. The HHV of the bio-oil produced from the pyrolysis process is very low as compared to crude oil or heavy fuel oil. This is mainly because the bio-oil contains a lower proportion of carbon and hydrogen that possess higher HHVs. The magnitude of HHV of fuel indicates its heat generation potential after combustion. Therefore, in the current scenario, it could be suggested that bio-oil would produce less heat in the combustion engine compared to heavy fuel oil. Overall, it can be concluded that bio-oil is a highly unsuitable fuel and require significant upgrading to make it a drop-in fuel, which can be either obtained by biomass pre-treatment methods or downstream bio-oil upgrading. In further sections, this article thoroughly discusses the various physicochemical methods to improve the bio-oil properties, mainly based on biomass pre-treatment. Physical and thermal methods, including grinding, densification, and dry torrefaction (DT), and chemical methods, such as acid and alkali pre-treatment, wet torrefaction (WT), ammonia fiber expansion (AFE), steam explosion (SE), hot water extraction (HWE), and biological pre-treatment of lignocellulose biomass have been comprehensively reviewed.

8.4 PRE-TREATMENT OF BIOMASS

8.4.1 PHYSICAL AND THERMAL METHODS

8.4.1.1 Grinding

Grinding biomass feedstock is an important process to achieve a high yield of quality pyrolysis products, but size reduction is an energy-intensive process and non-trivial operation which requires a considerable amount of cost and resources. The purpose of reducing feedstock size is to improve the heat flow between the substrates and decrease the degree of polymerization and crystallinity of the biomass components during the pyrolysis process, which, in turn, affects the yield and composition of the bio-oil compounds [59]. The effect of biomass particle size on the quality and yield of the bio-oil compounds is more significant for larger particle sizes [60]. For example, the bio-oil yield was observed to decrease as the particle size increased from 0.3 to 1.5 mm in the pyrolysis of mallee wood, which could be attributed to the particle size impact on the heating process and depolymerization of lignin-derived oligomers to bio-oil compounds. However, no change was observed in the yields of bio-oil, biochar, and pyrolytic gases when the particle size was increased from 1.5 to 5.2 mm. The change in bio-oil yields with increasing particle size (0.3–1.5 mm) could be attributed to the intra-particle reactions or the pyrolysis factors that influence the intra-particle reactions. In addition, the heating rate remains uniform in the smaller particles compared to

Lignocellulose Biomass Pyrolysis for Bio-Oil Production   137

the larger particles, which ultimately affects the thermal degradation of biomass constituents and, subsequently, the yields of pyrolytic products and bio-oil composition. In the case of small particles, high heating rates may also favor bond scission reactions that could lead to the formation of volatiles and, consequently, the higher bio-oil yield. In the case of larger particles, comparatively slower heating rates could favor recombination reactions that could lead to charring instead of volatile formation, thereby decreasing the bio-oil yield. Another reason for lower bio-oil yield with larger particle size could be the enhanced mass resistance of bio-oil precursors to diffuse out of the larger particles, which is greatly affected by the cellular structure of the biomass [61].

Particle size of the feedstock plays a pivotal role in the pyrolysis behavior of the biomass and, consequently, affects the energy content, physical properties, and organic composition of the bio-oil. It has been observed that the bio-oil composition is significantly changed with smaller biomass particles. Shen et al. [61] demonstrated decreasing yields of heavy bio-oil compounds with increasing particle sizes from 0.3 to 1.5 mm. In the same study, the yield of lightweight bio-oil compounds was observed to increase with increasing biomass particle size. This could be attributed to the high heating rates in the smaller particles that promoted the bond-breaking reactions at the higher temperatures and favored the diffusion of organic compounds due to the increased mass transport, while in the case of larger particles, bond-breaking reactions occur at a slower rate and the simultaneous bond formation reactions could take place, leading to the decrease in the mass transport. Figure 8.7 shows the composition of mallee oil expressed as a percentage of the initial weight of biomass (on a dry basis) as a function of average particle size and pyrolysis temperature of 500 °C. The impact of particle size on the yield and composition of bio-oil compounds was further demonstrated in a separate study during fast pyrolysis of different types of biomass materials consisting of herbaceous, waste, residue, and different blends of feedstocks, with a particle size range of 2–6 mm, treated at 600 °C and 14.2 °C/s. The study showed slight increments in the yield of the bio-oil compounds, indicating that pyrolysis reactions are slightly affected by sample size in these ranges of particle sizes [62]. Similar bio-oil yields were obtained from the pyrolysis of different sizes of corn stoves ranging from 1 to 4 mm. On the other hand, Abnisa et al. [62] observed a decrease in the liquid yield as the particle size increased from 0.5 to 2 mm during the pyrolysis of the palm shell, which was attributed to the improved heating and mass transfers in the smaller particles while the heat and mass transfer restrictions greatly affect the bio-oil yield for larger particles. Kang et al. [63] also observed increasing yield of bio-oil yields with decreasing particle sizes in the pyrolysis of pine wood and babool seeds at 500 °C, respectively. The highest bio-oil yield was 24.2% but significantly increased to 54% as the particle size decreased from 2 to 1 mm. Similarly, the bio-oil yield was observed to increase to 32%, decreasing the babool seed diameter from 1 to 0.4 mm. The bio-oils produced from the pyrolysis of babool seed at 500 °C and particle sizes >0.4 mm had a heating value of 36.45 MJ/kg, which is close to the transportation grade diesel or kerosene fuels [63]. The decrease in bio-oil yield with increasing particle size is mostly associated with the non-uniform heating of particles during the heating process. It has

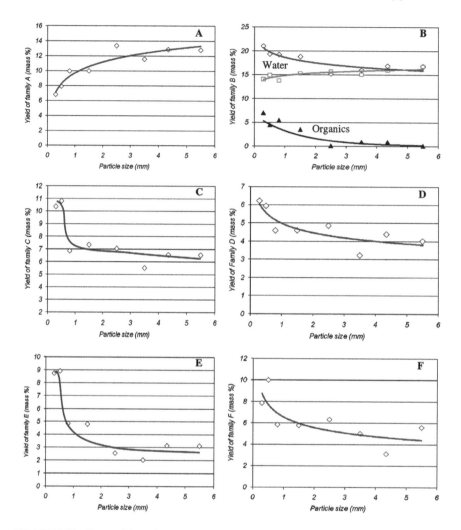

FIGURE 8.7 Composition of mallee oil (A, B, C, D, E, F) expressed as a percentage of the initial biomass mass (on a dry basis) as a function of average particle size at pyrolysis temperature of 500 °C. A–F show six families/groups of chemical compounds in the bio-oil. Peak A represents highly volatile organic compounds, mainly hydroxyacetaldehyde, formic acid, and methanol. Peak B represents water but also contains other organic compounds with boiling points close to water, such as acetic acid, acetol, and propionic acid. Peak C shows phenols and furans. Peak D is mainly due to sugars with a thermal behavior similar to levoglucosan and some polyaromatics. Peak E represents the oligomeric compounds insoluble in water but soluble in CH_2Cl_2. Peak F represents oligomeric compounds (for example, oligosugars) soluble in water.

Source: Reproduced from reference [61] with permission from Elsevier.

been demonstrated that smaller particles allow an efficient heat flow between the particles and have shown positive results in increasing the bio-oil yield, while the larger particles may result in non-uniform heating of the particles and could result

Lignocellulose Biomass Pyrolysis for Bio-Oil Production 139

in decreased bio-oil yield and low-quality bio-oil. Moreover, the interactions between the produced volatiles and other particles during the pyrolysis process could enhance the secondary pyrolytic reactions, resulting in enhanced gas yield and decreased bio-oil yield [64]. However, one should be careful to compare the effect of particle size of different biomass samples reported by different researchers in their studies because the particle sizes of varying biomass samples could possess dissimilar fibrous natures and elongated shapes. In addition to this, the studies might have used different milling and sieving methods that could result in particle sizes of different diameter and length ratios. Therefore, a fair comparison of the effects of particle size on biomass pyrolysis could only be made when the biomass particles are prepared using the same milling and sieving methods for the same type of biomass sample.

The effect of particle size on the yield and quality of the pyrolysis oil may vary depending on the type of biomass, heating rate, temperature, and other conditions. Thus, all parameters should be evaluated to identify the optimum particle size at each operating condition for higher pyrolysis oil yield and quality. In addition, the biomass particle size requirement could vary depending on the type of reactor used in the pyrolysis process. For instance, the particle size of <200 µm, <2 mm, and <6 mm is suitable to achieve higher heating rates in rotating cone reactor, fluidized bed reactor, and circulating fluidized bed reactor, respectively [65]. Although grinding could be a useful technique to prepare favorable particle sizes for biomass pyrolysis, the process requires energy input adds to the cost of processing. It has been estimated that grinding biomass could cost around $11/t, and requires approximately 50kWh of energy to grind 1 tonne of biomass [66]. However, the energy requirement and, subsequently, the total cost for the process may vary depending on the feedstock type and the equipment used (refer to Figure 8.8).

8.4.1.2 Densification

One of the major limitations of using biomass as feedstock for biofuel production is its low density, which is typically around 40–200 kg/m^3 for agricultural straws and 150–250 kg/m^3 for woody biomass [22,68]. The low density could make the biomass slightly difficult to store and transport and could lead to slow heat transfer through the particles during pyrolysis. The low density of biomass could be improved through the densification technique to increase the density up to 10 times and make the biomass more suitable for pyrolysis. Biomass densification is generally referred to as the compaction process of biomass by applying mechanical force to produce uniformly sized solid pellets (or briquettes). The compaction mechanism could vary depending on the type of feedstock and machine used for densification. Compaction using a screw extruder generally contains the following three steps: 1) Removal of air from void spaces increases the contacts between the particles, which results in heat generation. 2) As a result of heat generation, the compact biomass becomes soft, and further application of high-pressure results in the formation of local bridges and interlocking of particles. 3) Compression in tapered die forms the briquettes with uniform density. Densification changes the bulk density (generally increases), moisture content, durability index, and energy contents of the

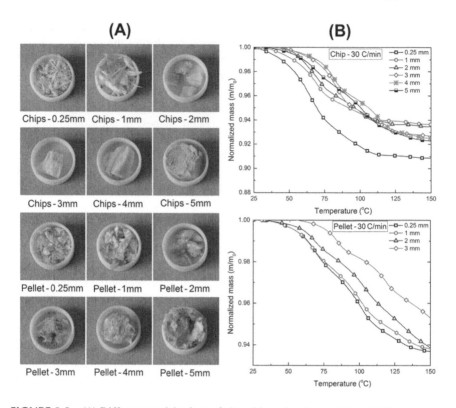

FIGURE 8.8 (A) Different particle sizes of pine chip and pellet particles. (B) Drying mass loss curve for chip and pellet particles; heating rate of 30 °C/min and temperature of up to 150 °C.

Source: Reproduced from reference [67] with permission from Wiley.

biomass, which can also affect the pyrolysis product distribution, heating, and mass transfer efficiencies of the pyrolysis process [69]. However, the quality of the densified biomass greatly depends on various process parameters, such as pre-heating of the biomass, the diameter of the die used to make pellets, pressure, and binders. In addition, the energy required for the densification process also depends on the biomass properties, such as the moisture content, particle size and distribution, biomass composition (levels of cellulose, hemicellulose, lignin, protein, and fat), and the process parameters [22]. All these factors play an important role in the quality of densified biomass.

The effect of biomass density on the yields of pyrolysis products and bio-oil composition has been studied by several researchers. A study on the pyrolysis of beech wood of different sizes of pellets and particles with varying densities (290–640kg/m^3) performed in external heat flux of 36.5 and 26.5 kW/m^2 showed subtle changes in the yields of pyrolytic products and bio-oil composition [70]. However, the results showed that heat flux had a significant effect on pyrolytic product yields and bio-oil composition. Noticeably, the bio-oil yields using external heat flux of 26.5 and

Lignocellulose Biomass Pyrolysis for Bio-Oil Production 141

36.5kW/m² of nearly 56 and 60 wt% were obtained using biomass pellets or particles with a bulk density of 290–640kg/m³. However, small changes were observed in the yields of individual organic compounds in bio-oil composition when the bulk density of the biomass was varied from 290 to 640kg/m³. For example, hydroxyacetaldehyde, acetic acid, and hydroxypropane were the most abundant bio-oil compounds with yields of 6.6, 18.5, and 4.3 wt%, respectively. As the packing density decreased to 290kg/m³, the yields slightly decreased to 5.3, 17.1, and 4.2 wt%, respectively [70]. In a separate study, Rezaei et al. [67] investigated the pyrolysis of a pine chip and a pine pellet three to four times denser than the pine chip and found that the rate of heat transfer in the pellets was low compared to the pine chip. The results are shown in Figure 8.8. It has been suggested that heat transfer in the central parts of larger particles is slow compared to the peripheral part of the particles and, subsequently, shows larger conductive heat resistance [71]. Besides, the larger particles show longer diffusion paths and lower specific surface areas. In another study, a solar-assisted pyrolysis experiment on beech wood demonstrated that pelletizing the feedstock can increase tar residence time, enhancing the formation of gaseous products at the expense of the tar secondary reactions [72].

In summary, densification could be highly advantageous to decrease the biomass's moisture content and increase the biomass's durability index and energy content, which could affect the pyrolysis kinetics but does not show any significant change in bio-oil composition. However, the densification technique uses expensive instruments for the compaction process, and their further maintenance may increase the overall cost of bio-oil upgrading.

8.4.1.3 Dry Torrefaction

Dry torrefaction (DT) is a thermal pre-treatment process of biomass performed at 200–300 °C and low heating rates under inert atmospheric conditions, which advances the biomass structure to produce better quality biofuels and improves the economic feasibility of the pyrolysis process. During the torrefaction process, the fibrous structure and tenacity of the biomass are changed, which could help in decreasing the activation energy for the pyrolysis process [73]. DT can be further classified into three categories based on the temperature selection for this biomass pre-treatment process: light, mild, and severe torrefaction performed at 200–235 °C, 235–275 °C, and 275–300 °C, respectively [74,75]. The light torrefaction (200–235 °C) mainly affects the degradation of the hemicellulose component in the biomass, which might constitute an array of reactions. For example, it may result in the breakdown of methenyl groups from the side chains and aldose groups from the main chain of the hemicellulose structure, breaking the glycosidic bonds and causing the dehydration of hydroxyl groups of the monosaccharides [76,77]. The mild torrefaction (235–275 °C) depolymerizes the hemicellulose to a large extent, while several bonds of the cellulose structure are also degraded. Torrefaction of cellulose mainly breaks the glycosidic bonds and hydrogen bonds and depolymerizes free hydroxyl groups on the glucose ring of the cellulose structure [76,78]. On the other hand, the severe torrefaction (275–300 °C) degrades hemicellulose almost completely and cellulose to a large extent, while the lignin part starts degrading at this temperature.

Torrefaction of lignin generally results in the breakdown of ether bonds (β-O-4 type) and promotes demethoxylation reaction in a benzene ring structure [76,79].

Oxygen migration and carbon migration are two important pathways that affect the oxygen removal and carbon content of the biomass during the DT process. Both pathways could significantly affect the energy content of the biomass, where the removal of oxygen could improve the energy content, while the carbon migration could result in energy loss [101]. Torrefaction temperature and content of biomass constituents play a pivotal role in oxygen removal and carbon migration. It has been suggested that the increase in torrefaction temperature (200–300 °C) showed higher oxygen removal during the torrefaction of hemicellulose compared to cellulose and lignin, while more carbon was retained in cellulose and lignin compared to hemicellulose [76]. The dominant deoxygenation pathway during DT is dehydration, while the generation of gaseous products, such as CO_2 and CO, contributes to oxygen removal. On the other hand, torrefaction temperature also influences the structural properties of biomass constituents, which could further affect their pyrolysis behavior. It has been observed that the temperature of 200–250 °C increases the crystallinity of cellulose, while further increase in torrefaction temperature has been shown to decrease the crystallinity of cellulose [78], which could be attributed to recrystallization of amorphous cellulose or conversion of crystalline cellulose to amorphous cellulose at a higher temperature. During torrefaction of hemicellulose at lower temperatures, dehydration and degradation of the branches are dominant reactions, while the higher temperatures promote depolymerization of hemicellulose and fragmentation of the monosaccharide units [77]. In addition, torrefaction of lignin has been shown to favor demethoxylation and polycondensation reactions [101]. The biomass torrefied at different temperatures with improved characteristics has been applied in pyrolysis to obtain the bio-oil with upgraded physiochemical properties. However, it has been noticed that the selection of temperature is a very important parameter that decides the fate of oxygen and carbon content in the biomass and could vary depending on the composition of the biomass constituents. Overall, torrefaction has been shown to decrease the oxygen and increase the carbon content in the biomass, consequently increasing its HHV.

DT could be an advantageous approach to improve biomass properties. It can alter its structural properties and enhance the carbon content. The utilization of torrefied biomass in the pyrolysis process could help obtain bio-oil with enhanced aromatics and calorific value. DT has been shown to improve the bio-oil quality, reduce the oxygen content, increase the heating value and enhance the content of hydrocarbons in the bio-oil. Table 8.4 summarizes the effects of DT on the yield and composition of the pyrolytic oils. However, it has also been observed that DT decreases the bio-oil yield, which can be compensated with the increased quality of the bio-oil. The decrease in the bio-oil yield can be attributed to the torrefaction-induced crosslinking reactions, charring of the biomass, and increase in gaseous products during pyrolysis [102]. More importantly, DT increases the amount of atomic carbon and decreases the biomass's oxygen content, which improves the biomass's energy conversion capacity during pyrolysis [81]. For example, Gogoi et al. [82,85,86] compared the oxygen content of bio-oils obtained from the pyrolysis of torrefied and raw arecanut husk (*Areca catechu*), and found lower oxygen content from the pyrolysis of

TABLE 8.4

Summary of Effect of Torrefaction on the Composition of Pyrolytic Oils.

Feedstock	Torrefaction temperature	Time	Pyrolysis temperature	Reactor type	Key results	References
Fruit bunches	493–573 K; 10 K/min	30 min		Electric furnace	Bio-oil yield decreased from 92% to 81%; calorific value increased by 18%	[81]
Loblolly pine	273–330 °C	2.5 min	500 °C; feeding rate 150 g/h	Fluidized-bed reactor	Oxygen-to-carbon ratio of bio-oil decreased from 0.63 to 0.31; heating value increased from 20 to 26.3 MJ/kg	[74]
Arecanut husk	200–300 °C; 10 °C/min	30 min	300 to 600 °C; 40 °C/min	Fixed bed reactor	Bio-oil yield decreased from 21 to 32 wt%; reduced O/C ratio of bio-oil from 0.36 to 0.28	[82]
Douglas Fir Sawdust Pellets	250–300 °C	20 min		Microwave	Bio-oil with increased yield of hydrocarbon (3.21–7.5 area%) and phenols; reduced concentration of acids, guaiacols, furans	[83,84]
Cotton stalk	220–280 °C	30	500 °C	Fixed-bed	Phenol-derived (0.53–8.25 peak area%)- and ketone-derived (0.59–6.41 peak area%) bio-oils increased. Acids and furnace decreased.	[73]
Yunnan pine	210–300 °C	30 min	500 °C	Fixed bed reactor	Bio-oil yield decreased from 37 to 20 wt%. Phenols and hydrocarbons in bio-oil increased. Aldehydes, acids, and ketones decreased	[85]
Rice straw	225–275 °C	30 min	450 to 500 °C and 1000 °C/s	Micro pyrolysis reactor	Water, acid, and oxygenated species of the bio-oil decreased. Acids, aldehydes, ketones, furans and sugar contents also decreased	[86]
Corncobs feedstock	210–300 °C	20 to 60 min	600 °C; 20000K/s	Semi-batch pyroprobe reactor	Bio-oil yield increased from 51% to 82%. Aromatic yield decreased from 29% to 16% with torrefaction temperature	[87]

(Continued)

TABLE 8.4 (Continued)

Feedstock	Torrefaction temperature	Time	Pyrolysis temperature	Reactor type	Key results	References
Rice straw	240 °C	1 h	550 °C	Vertical drop fixed-be	Phenols increased from 28 to 42 area%. Acids, aldehydes, ketones and furans decreased	[88]
Animal waste; Sewage sludge	220–300 °C	100 to 160 min	300 °C, 10 °C/min	/	Torrefaction improved hygroscopicity and heating value of the products. Bio-oil yield increased with temperature from 2.2 to 20.4 wt% for the animal waste and 12.6 to 23.3 wt% for the sludge.	[89]
Oak and scrublands	200–300 °C; at 3 °C/min		300 °C for 30 min	/	Acids, furans, alcohols, aldehydes, and phenols were the main bio-oil compounds that were observed to increase with torrefaction temperature	[90]
Empty fruit bunch and mesocarp fibers	220–270 °C	60 min	300 °C	Standard retort	Liquid fraction, composed of alcohols, acids, and phenols, were in the range of 6 to 26 wt% and contained 26 to 42 wt% of water and LHV up to 11 MJ/kg	[91]
Pigeon peak stalk	225–275 °C at 15 °C/min	15 to 45 min	Upto 275 °C	Split tube furnace with quartz tube reactor	Liquid yield increased from 8.84 to 35.44 wt% with torrefaction temperature and residence time	[92]
Douglas fir sawdust	250 °C	10 min	300 °C for 20 min	Microwave	Bio-oil yields increased with torrefaction temperature from 21.73 to 37.77 wt%. Produced bio-oils were phenols, cyclooctene, furan, furfural, levoglucosan, and others	[93]
Agricultural residues (rice straw, cotton stalk)	200–300 °C at 10 °C/min	60 min	300 °C	Fixed-bed reactor	The highest bio-oil yields were 19.4% for the rice straw and 15% for the cotton stalk, obtained for the biomasses torrefied at 250 °C and 275 °C, respectively	[94]

Corn stalk (wet torrefaction)	160–220 °C	30 min	550 °C	Fixed-bed reactor	Bio-oil yield from the torrefied sample increased by 3 to 5 wt% from the un-torrefied (raw) sample. Main bio-oil components were acids (up to 40 area%), phenols (up to 20 area%), sugars (up to 75 area%), cyclopentanes (5 area%), furans (up to 8 area%), and ketones (16 area%).	[95]
Corn stalk (dry torrefaction)	200–290 °C	30 min	550 °C	Fixed-bed reactor	Bio-oil yield obtained from the torrefied sample decreased from the un-torrefied biomass. Compositional distribution of the dry torrefied bio-oil compounds were similar to the wet torrefied bio-oils except the sugars component that substantially reduced to ~1 area%	[95]
Cotton stalk with Mg-based additives	200–350 °C at 50 °C/min	50 min	550 for 10 min	Fixed-bed reactor	The bio-oil compounds from pyrolysis decreased with rising torrefaction temperature from ~6 to 10 wt%. The highest yields of aromatic hydrocarbon (~59 area%), phenols (~51 area%), and ketones (~29 area%) were obtained for 350 °C, 260 °C, and 230 °C torrefied samples, respectively	[96]
Prosopis Julifloar	250 °C	30 min	300 to 600 watts	Microwave	Guaiacols, syringols, and other phenols were the major components of the bio-oil, making >50%	[97]
Food waste	225–300 °C at 15 °C/min	1 to 3 h	Up to 300 °C for 3 h	/	Torrefaction at 275 °C was optimal while severe torrefaction at 300 °C was efficient in terms of producing bio-products with high energy contents	[98]
Herbaceous residues	210–280 °C	60 min	600 °C at 50 °C/min	/	Phenols, acids, ketones, esters, and furans were the main bio-oil compounds, which account for approximately 72.1% of the total detected compounds	[99]
Rubber wood	200–300 °C at 6 °C/min		500 °C for 10 min	/	Aldehydes (coniferyl aldehyde; 3,5-dimethoxy-4-hydroxycinnamaldehyde), phenols (2,6-dimethyxy-4-allylphenol; isoeugenol), and esters (diethyl phthalate) were the most prominent products	[100]

the torrefied arecanut husk. Two studies by Ren et al. [83,84] reported that yields of aromatic hydrocarbons were greatly improved from the pyrolysis of torrefied woody biomass. Compared to the pyrolytic oils from the raw biomass, the bio-oils obtained from pyrolysis of the torrefied feedstock contained 3.21–7.5% more hydrocarbons and reduced concentration of organic acids, guaiacols, and furans. The increased production of aromatics could be attributed to enhanced deoxygenation reactions, such as dehydration, decarboxylation, decarbonylation, aromatization, and rearrangement reactions. The increase of hydrocarbons in the bio-oil also improves other physiochemical properties of the bio-oil, and the HHV is significantly increased. In addition, the bio-oil properties and organic composition obtained from the pyrolysis of biomass are greatly affected by the temperature used to pre-treat the biomass during torrefaction. For instance, a study showed that the bio-oil obtained using biomass torrefied at 240 °C had a pH of 2.49 and HHV of 15.61 MJ/kg, which increased to pH 2.69 and HHV of 18.58 MJ/kg with the biomass torrefied at 320°C. The effect of torrefied biomass on bio-oil composition has also been investigated in several other studies. For example, DT pre-treatment was conducted on Yunnan pine biomass at different temperatures (210–300 °C) [85]. The torrefied biomass was then pyrolyzed at 450 °C and analyzed the bio-oil for its yield, energy, and production composition. Results showed that with increasing the torrefaction temperature, phenol and hydrocarbon contents in the bio-oil markedly increased while aldehydes, acids, and ketones were generally observed to decrease. During torrefaction, the cellulose and hemicellulose components of the feedstock are cracked, increasing the lignin concentration for pyrolysis, which results in an increase in the hydrocarbon and phenolic contents of the bio-oil [103]. In a separate study, Zheng et al. [104] performed two-stage pine chips pyrolysis consisting of torrefaction at 240–320 °C and subsequent fast pyrolysis in a fluidized bed reactor at 520 °C. The results showed that the total bio-oil yield, water, and acetic acid contents in the bio-oil decreased with elevated torrefaction temperature, whereas the total aromaticity, higher heating value and density of the bio-oil increased. The highest bio-oil yield (55 wt%) was obtained at 240 °C and decreased to its lowest yield (23 wt%) at 320 °C (as shown in Figure 8.9), whereas the highest aromatic yield and heating value, which occurred at the highest temperature, were 30 wt% and 19 MJ/kg, respectively.

Besides bio-oil upgrading, DT effectively enhances the contents of high-value chemicals in the bio-oils. For example, all the phenolic and ketone-derived bio-oil compounds obtained from the pyrolysis of a torrefied cotton stalk at 500 °C were substantially increased from 0.53% to 8.25% peak area; and from 0.59% to 6.41% peak area, respectively; while acetic acid and furans were observed to decrease from 37% to 1.8% peak area; and from 5% to 1% peak area, respectively [73]. A recent study by Dong et al. [88] compared the bio-oil chemical composition from the pyrolysis of raw and torrefied rice straw samples. The sample was torrefied at 240 °C for 1 h in a tubular furnace reactor and pyrolyzed at 550 °C in a vertical drop fixed bead reactor. Relative contents of oxygenated compounds, such as acids, aldehydes, and ketones, decreased while the relative contents of phenols increased from 28 to 42 area% in the bio-oils from the pyrolysis of the torrefied sample, which could be associated with the enriched concentration of lignin after torrefaction which favors the production of phenols and low weight hydrocarbon compounds [102].

Lignocellulose Biomass Pyrolysis for Bio-Oil Production   147

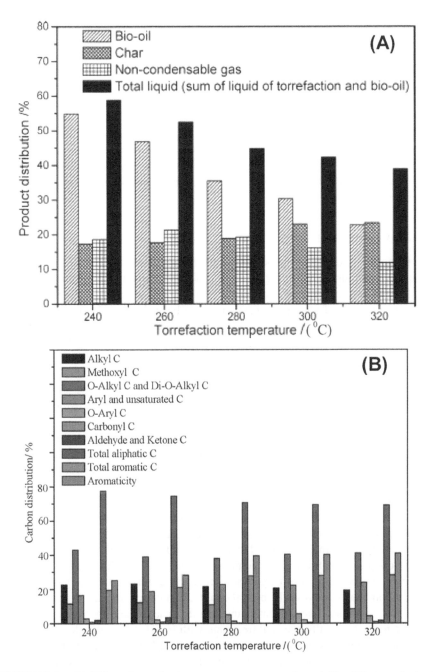

FIGURE 8.9 (A) Effect of torrefaction temperatures on product yields of fast pyrolysis of torrefied pine. (B) Percentage of carbon distribution from ^{13}C NMR spectra of the bio-oil influenced by torrefaction temperature.

Source: Reprinted with permission from reference [80]. Copyright © 2012, American Chemical Society.

The above discussion suggests that DT is a useful technique to improve the quality of biomass as well as bio-oil composition. On the one hand, it can increase the amount of atomic carbon in the biomass and decrease the activation energy for pyrolysis. On the other hand, it can increase the number of aromatic hydrocarbons in the bio-oil and its heating value. However, it has also been noticed that the pyrolysis of torrefied biomass may result in a decreased bio-oil yield and increased content of ash in the bio-oil, while the biomass with poor pelletability could be obtained after the DT process. Therefore, applying suitable temperature and residence time conditions is important to obtain torrefied biomass with desirable properties for the pyrolysis process. Moreover, the pyrolysis parameters and reactor configurations also play an important role in the pyrolysis behavior of torrefied biomass and subsequent bio-oil upgrading.

8.4.2 CHEMICAL METHODS

Due to the recalcitrance of lignocellulose, chemical pre-treatment is one of the most important methods for achieving desirable pyrolytic products. To destruct the lignocellulosic structure, decrease the thermal stability and alter the components in the biomass, a variety of chemical treatments have been developed prior to pyrolysis, including acid and alkali pre-treatments, hydrothermal pre-treatment, ammonia fiber expansion, and steam explosion, which are discussed in the following sections.

8.4.2.1 Acid Treatment of Biomass

Lignocellulose biomass used as the feedstock in the pyrolysis process generally contains inorganic minerals, which may be in the form of phosphates, carbonates, sulfates, or chlorides. These minerals exhibit some catalytic activity and hence may influence the biomass's pyrolysis behavior; consequently, a certain change in the pyrolytic products could be observed. In addition, some soluble inorganic species may be retained in the produced bio-oil, which would negatively affect the bio-oil's physical properties. For example, if present in the bio-oil, the inorganics can initiate polymerization or condensation reactions that are highly unfavorable for bio-oil stability, aging, and viscosity, and they can also increase the corrosion activity, which may limit its application as a transportation fuel. Therefore, it is important to eliminate the inorganic minerals to avoid their further influence on the pyrolysis behavior and bio-oil quality. In this regard, biomass pre-treatment with dilute acidic chemicals has been considered an advantageous approach to eliminate the inorganic species and simultaneously improve the bio-oil quality. In addition, the acidic pre-treatment of biomass also causes significant changes in its structure and increases its average pore diameter. Generally, the acid treatment with H_2SO_4 favors the cleavage of C-O bonds in the biomass structure, which are present in all the connections between cellulose, hemicellulose, and lignin and the breaking of alkyl-aryl ether bonds in lignin [80]. Consequently, the removal of extractives and some portions of all three biomass constituents leads to a decrease in the mass yield after the acid treatment. On the other hand, the energy density of the treated biomass increases due to the increase in the heating value, which is mainly attributed to the removal of ash content. It has been indicated that the ash content of even0.1% in the biomass has a significant

Lignocellulose Biomass Pyrolysis for Bio-Oil Production

catalytic effect during pyrolysis, which could lead to a decrease in the bio-oil yield [105]. However, the results of acid pre-treatment of biomass have been shown to lower the ash content considerably, which could help obtain higher yield and better quality of the bio-oil [57,106]. Certain minerals in the ash, such as silicon, do not affect the pyrolysis process, but alkali metals, including sodium and potassium, and alkali earth metals, such as calcium and magnesium, are well known to catalyze the thermal decomposition of biomass [107–108]. The ash content in the biomass could vary depending on the uptake of minerals during plant growth. The acid treatment of biomass generally removes the soluble metals or insoluble minerals that are physiologically not attached to the plant tissue. The leaching of the minerals and metals has been observed to be improved with an increase in the concentration of the acidic solvent [57,105].

Table 8.5 summarizes various studies that investigated the effect of acid and alkali pre-treatments on the physiochemical properties of pyrolytic bio-oil. Among the acids, H_2SO_4 is the most widely used acid for biomass pre-treatment [57,109–111]. For instance, Mohammed et al. [57] investigated the application of different proportions of H_2SO_4 on the removal of alkali metals and bio-oil properties. They treated Napier grass feedstock with 0.5–2.5 wt% of H_2SO_4 at 70 °C for 1 h, and the pyrolysis of the pre-treated biomass samples was carried out in a fixed bed reactor at 600 °C at a heating rate of 30 °C/min. The acid pre-treatment results revealed that H_2SO_4 decreased the concentration of all inorganic species in the biomass, and this decrease was found to be proportional to the increase in the concentration of H_2SO_4. For example, treatment with 0.5 wt% of H_2SO_4 resulted in 4.10 mg/kg of Na (12.85 mg/kg in raw biomass) and 988.2 mg/kg of K (3079.5 mg/kg in raw biomass) in the biomass, which further decreased to 0.47 and 142.88 mg/kg for Na and K, respectively. Consequently, the pyrolysis results showed that the acid-treated biomass produced bio-oil with enhanced quality as compared to the untreated biomass, producing bio-oil with a higher HHV of 27.96 MJ/kg and increased carbon content of 48.95 wt%, while the bio-oil produced from untreated biomass had an HHV of 20.97 MJ/kg and C content of 45.32 wt% [57]. Similarly, other acids have also been explored for biomass pre-treatment that have shown promising results for bio-oil upgrading. For example, recently, Cao et al. [111] treated *Enteromorpha clathrate* (microalga biomass) with different acids, such as 7% H_2SO_4, 7% HCl, and 7% H_3PO_4, for 12 h, and these treated biomass samples were pyrolyzed in a fixed bed reactor at 550 °C. Acid-washing resulted in a significant increase in bio-oil yield. Reportedly, pyrolysis of H_2SO_4-, H_3PO_4-, and HCl-treated biomass increased the bio-oil yield by 11.5%, 9.7%, and 9.6%, respectively, when compared with the untreated biomass. On the other hand, the char yield was significantly reduced, which is attributed to the removal of inorganic minerals that otherwise could have promoted char formation. Further, the gas chromatography-mass spectroscopy (GC-MS) results suggested that the acid-washing resulted in a reduction in acids and other oxygenated species, while a substantial increase in aliphatic hydrocarbons was observed in the bio-oil samples. For instance, HCl pre-treatment decreased approximately 37% acids and 52.6% other oxygenated compounds in the bio-oil, attributing to the disruption of hydroxyl bonds as indicated by Fourier Transform Infrared (FT-IR) spectroscopic results that showed a significant reduction in O-H stretching vibration, while the content of aromatic

TABLE 8.5
Effect of Acid and Alkali Pre-treatment on Physiochemical Properties of Bio-Oil.

Feedstock	Pre-treatment (concentration in wt% to dry biomass)	Reactor configuration	T (°C)	Biomass composition (%)			Yield (%)	Properties of pyrolytic bio-oil			References
				lignin	cellulose	hemi-cellulose		HHV (MJ/kg)	Water content (%)	pH	
Loblolly Pine	untreated	Auger	450	39.9	33.55	27.34	54	16.10	20.83	2.65	[119]
	0.5% H_2SO_4			45.23	34.6	24.25	63	15.00	29.51	2.52	
	1% H_2SO_4			44.26	32.1	24.58	63	16.53	27.45	2.77	
	0.5% NaOH			38.26	31.62	24.80	49	/	55.57	3.15	
Loblolly Pine	untreated	Auger	450	/	/	/	/	22.49	16.9	3.08	[120]
	14% H_3PO_4			/	/	/	/	22.70	17.8	2.92	
	10.4% H_2SO_4			/	/	/	/	23.83	18.9	2.81	
	10.6% NaOH			/	/	/	/	24.4	17.6	3.76	
	10.0% $Ca(OH)_2$			/	/	/	/	21.9	17.9	3.55	
	34.4% NH_4OH			/	/	/	/	19.66	19.4	3.49	
	14.3% H_2O_2			/	/	/	/	7.28	24.0	3.62	
Sweetgum	untreated	Auger	450	37.8	/	/	51	/	38.3	2.65	[121]
	1% H_2SO_4			40.6	/	/	56	/	52.2	1.99	
Switchgrass	untreated			20.4	/	/	31	/	61.7	2.98	
	1% H_2SO_4			25.1	/	/	46	/	46.2	2.38	
corn stover	untreated			22.6	/	/	35	/	54.7	2.66	
	1% H_2SO_4			28.4	/	/	51	/	41.6	1.87	
Coir pith	untreated	Packed bed	500	31.2	28.6	15.3	29.4	18.66	/	/	[122]
	10% HCl + 5% NaOH			/	/	/	36.2	22.33	/	/	
Corn cob	untreated			16.6	40.3	28.7	37.4	23.81	/	/	

Biomass	Treatment	Reactor	Temp.									Ref.
	10% HCl + 5% NaOH			/	/	/	43.4	24.19		/	/	
Ground nut shell	untreated			30.2	35.7	18.7	40.5	23.62		/	/	
	10% HCl + 5% NaOH			/	/	/	45.9	26.15		/	/	
Rice husk	untreated			14.3	31.3	24.3	41.2	22.45		/	/	
	10% HCl + 5% NaOH			/	/	/	57.4	23.72		/	/	
Subabul wood	untreated			24.7	39.8	24.0	22.6	24.94		/	/	
	10% HCl + 5% NaOH			/	/	/	40.1	28.54		/	/	
mallee wood	untreated	Fluidized bed	500	24.7	42.4	23.8	~61	/	~22	/	/	[108]
	water wash for 1h			/	/	/	~61	/	~21	/	/	
	water wash for 24h			/	/	/	~61	/	~20	/	/	
	water wash for 48h			/	/	/	~61	/	~20	/	/	
	0.1% HNO_3 wash			/	/	/	~61	/	~16	/	/	
red maple wood	untreated	Pyro-probe	600	24.9	/	/	66.7	/		/	/	[123]
	hot water wash			/	/	/	45.9	/		/	/	
	hot water wash + enzymatic hydrolysis			/	/	/	10.2	/		/	/	
Empty palm fruit bunches	untreated	Semi-batch	300	18.1	59.7	22.1	30	/		/	/	[124]
	80% $Ca(OH)_2$			~16.5	/	/	/			/	/	
	80% NaOH			~6.5	/	/	/			/	/	
	80% $Ca(OH)_2$ + H_2O_2 simultaneously			~12.5	/	/	/			/	/	
	80% NaOH + H_2O_2 simultaneously			~5	/	/	/			/	/	
	80% $Ca(OH)_2$, H_2O_2 consecutively			~10	/	/	/			/	/	
	80% NaOH, H_2O_2 consecutively			~1	/	/	/			/	/	

(Continued)

TABLE 8.5 (Continued)

Feedstock	Pre-treatment (concentration in wt% to dry biomass)	Reactor configuration	T (°C)	Biomass composition (%)			Properties of pyrolytic bio-oil				References
				lignin	cellulose	hemi-cellulose	Yield (%)	HHV (MJ/kg)	Water content (%)	pH	
Corn stalks	untreated (water added)	Auger	450	/	/	/	35	/	27.3	3.29	[125]
	2% H_2SO_4 (water added)			/	/	/	46	/	21	3.09	
	untreated (fed dry)	Auger	400	18.1	/	/	35	/	54.7	2.66	
	2% H_2SO_4 (fed dry)						51	/	41.6	2.87	
Switchgrass	untreated	Fluidized bed	500	8.6	/	/	63.8	16.4	24.7	0.69	[126]
	water wash			8.6	/	/	67.1	16	17.2	2.8	
Festuca arundinacea	untreated			3.6	/	/	47.2	16.7	34.1	0.18	
	water wash			3.6	/	/	50.4	21.7	29.2	3	
Sugarcane bagasse	untreated	Packed bed	500	21.8	31	23.3	19.5	23.3	12	2.6	[127]
	water wash			21.2	43.4	22.2	25.6	22.2	11.2	2.5	
	50% HCl			19.9	61.8	4.4	21	21.6	8.3	2.3	
	3% HF			23.3	40.4	16.2	33.0	23.2	2.4	2.4	
Pinus radiate wood	untreated	Fluidized bed	500	28	43	26	~47	/	24	/	[128]
	1% acetic acid			28	43	26	54.6	/	17.4	/	
	torrefaction at 270 °C			44	44	10	~38	/	6.1	/	
	1% acetic acid + torrefaction at 270 °C			40	46	12	58.7	/	7.1	/	

Cotton stalk	untreated	Downdraft fixed bed	500	/	/	/	41.53	11.34	58.19	2.95 [129]
	washing with torrefaction liquid			/	/	/	41.97	12.57	55.22	3.04
	torrefaction at 150 ℃			/	/	/	27.09	14.83	41.39	3.23
	washing + torrefaction			/	/	/	24.40	15.56	37.08	3.34
rick husk	untreated	Vertical drop fixed-bed	550	/	/	/	~40	~12.3	~44	~2.4 [130]
	torrefaction at 210 ℃			/	/	/	~36	~13	~42	~2.5
	torrefaction at 240 ℃			/	/	/	~31	~13.5	~39	~2.8
	torrefaction at 270 ℃			/	/	/	~15	~15.2	~35	~3.1
	raw biomass + organic acid leaching			/	/	/	~45	~14	~37	~3
	torrefaction at 210 ℃ + organic acid leaching			/	/	/	~41	~14.5	~36	~3.1
	torrefaction at 240 ℃ + organic acid leaching			/	/	/	~33	~15.3	~33	~3.3
	torrefaction at 270 ℃ + organic acid leaching			/	/	/	~17	~16.2	~32	~3.5
Napier grass	untreated	Fixed bed	600	/	/	/	~32	20.97	26.01	2.95 [57]
	water wash			/	/	/	~33	22.22	20.52	2.92
	5% H_2SO_4			/	/	/	~38	27.96	17.36	2.68
	5% NaOH			/	/	/	~29	21.94	27.47	3.26

hydrocarbons was increased by 1.5 times, mainly producing toluene (15.5%), styrene (2.5%), and ethylbenzene (1.4%) [111]. In a separate study, Hassan et al. [42] treated pine wood biomass with dilute H_2SO_4 and H_3PO_4 at 100°C for 1 h and investigated its influence on the physiochemical properties of the bio-oil produced at 450°C in a stainless steel auger reactor. The results showed a positive effect of the acid pre-treatment on HHV of the bio-oil, which increased to 23.83 MJ/kg with H_2SO_4 and 22.70 MJ/kg with H_3PO_4 compared to untreated pine wood of 22.49 MJ/kg. However, a slight decrease in the pH values and an increase in the acidic values of the bio-oils were observed, attributing to the removal of inorganic minerals and alkali metals from the biomass post-acid pre-treatments [42]. Furthermore, Tan and Wang [112] demonstrated the effect of acid pre-treatments of pine wood and rice husk biomass on the removal of inorganic species and, subsequently, on the bio-oil properties. The results revealed that the acid pre-treatments significantly decreased the concentration of metal ions in the biomass and increased the bio-oil yield during the pyrolysis process. For example, HCl pre-treatment of pine wood decreased the K content to ~116 ppm and increased the bio-oil yield to 52.8 wt% in comparison to the untreated biomass that showed a K content of ~984 ppm and bio-oil yield of 41.74 wt%, respectively [112]. In addition to bio-oil upgrading, acid pre-treatments can also be used to enhance the production of certain chemicals and anhydrosugars (for example, levoglucosan) by suppressing or eliminating the effect of alkali and alkaline earth metals from biomass pyrolysis. Evidently, David et al. [113] showed a significant increase of about seven times in the formation of anhydrosugars from the pyrolysis of combined acid treatment (0.1 wt% of HNO_3 and 0.2 wt% of H_2SO_4) of sugarcane bagasse biomass pyrolyzed at 350 °C. This increase in the concentration of sugars was attributed to the alkali and alkaline earth metal passivation after acid pre-treatment [113]. Acid treatment of lignocellulose biomass has also been shown to promote the formation of certain organic compounds, such as 4-vinyl guaiacol and 2,3-dihydrobenzofuran, which are mainly derived from thermal degradation of lignin component, indicating the breaking of $\alpha C - \beta C$ bonds and $\beta - 5$ bonds in the lignin structure post acidic treatment [114]. It should be noted that the yield of organic compounds in the pyrolytic bio-oil is greatly influenced by the concentration of acidic solvent and its ratio with biomass used in the pre-treatment process.

Overall, it can be suggested that the treatment of biomass with dilute acid solutions could be highly beneficial to improve the biomass structure and, consequently, physiochemical properties of the bio-oil. It can effectively remove the inorganic species from the biomass, solubilize hemicellulose, improve cellulose digestibility, and increase the amount of atomic carbon and energy conversion capacity of the biomass. The acid treatment of biomass could also prove useful to achieve a higher bio-oil yield in the pyrolysis process. The main challenge of this process could be the disposal of the highly acidic leachate that may contain hazardous heavy metals. However, the acidic leachate might contain a higher proportion of sugars which can be subjected to a biochemical conversion processes to produce some value-added products or bioethanol that can be used as a liquid fuel [57]. Alternatively, the ethanol produced from the biochemical process could also be used for bio-oil stabilization during its storage as ethanol addition to the bio-oil has been shown to increase bio-oil stability [115]. Another challenge of acid pre-treatment is it causes corrosion to the reactor

Lignocellulose Biomass Pyrolysis for Bio-Oil Production   155

used for the pre-treatment process, which necessitates the use of non-corrosive construction materials that are usually expensive, thus increasing the overall operational and maintenance cost of the process. Less information is available about the possible reactions between the acid chemicals and biomass constituents (cellulose, hemicellulose, lignin) and inorganic species (Na, K, Ca, etc.) present in the biomass. Therefore, more studies should be conducted to examine the chemical reactions and kinetics during the process, which could help to understand the removal mechanism of inorganic species and the effect of chemicals on biomass structure.

8.4.2.2 Alkali Treatment of Biomass

Similar to acid pre-treatments, alkaline pre-treatments (such as NaOH, Ca (OH)$_2$, NH$_4$OH) of biomass have also been carried out to improve the biomass structure, especially to remove the lignin component and improve cellulose digestibility. The alkali treatment of lignocellulose biomass has been found to disrupt the ester and glycosidic bonds between lignin and hemicellulose, which consequently leads to the solubilization of lignin and hemicellulose, keeping most part of the cellulose intact [57]. The alkali treatment of lignocellulose biomass could also result in cellulose swelling, leading to its partial decrystallization and decrease in the degree of polymerization, which helps improve the treated biomass's internal surface area [116].

Several alkali reagents, such as NaOH, KOH, Ca(OH)$_2$, and NH$_4$OH, have been extensively used for biomass pre-treatment and, subsequently, the treated biomass was pyrolyzed to investigate the effect on different pyrolytic products, bio-oil composition, and its physiochemical properties. Generally, during the alkali pre-treatment, the hydroxide ion and metal ion (for example, Na$^+$) dissociate, and the increase in hydroxide ion concentration is directly proportional to the hydrolysis reaction rate [117]. It has been observed that, unlike acid pre-treatments, during the alkaline pre-treatment, some of the alkali may convert into salts or may incorporate into the biomass as salts which in turn can inhibit the bio-oil production and increase the char formation. In addition, the alkaline treatments have also been shown to reduce the mass yield as well as the energy density of the treated biomass, attributing to the removal of a higher amount of lignin, while the increase in ash content could lower the heating value of the biomass [57,105]. As a result, the alkaline pre-treatment decreases the bio-oil yield as well as the concentration of anhydrosugars in the bio-oil, where the acid pre-treatment usually increases the bio-oil yield and promotes the formation of anhydrosugars. Noticeably, a study by Wang et al. [43] demonstrated the pre-treatment of pinewood biomass with 0.5% NaOH and its pyrolysis in an auger reactor at 450 °C. The authors reported approximately a 5% decrease in the bio-oil with treated biomass compared to the untreated biomass, while some other physical properties were also observed to be altered after NaOH treatment. For example, the higher ash and moisture contents in the bio-oil of 2.49% and 55.57%, respectively, were obtained, while a lower viscosity of 1.49 cSt was observed compared to the untreated biomass (6.49 cSt). It was also noticed that the bio-oil produced from the alkaline pre-treatment had a lower concentration of levoglucosan and other anhydrosugars. This could be because the pre-treatment resulted in the attachment of the alkali metals in pinewood biomass and their catalytic effect changed the bio-oil composition, leading to a lower concentration of levoglucosan [106]. The results also revealed that NaOH treatment decreased the amount of hemicellulose and lignin pyrolyzed compounds in the bio-oil, indicating the removal of hemicellulose and lignin in the biomass following the pre-treatment [43]. This study concluded that NaOH was not advantageous for the treatment of pine wood biomass as it could not show noticeable improvement in the bio-oil yield and removal of ash content. However, other studies suggested that NaOH could be useful for pine wood treatment. The difference in the results could be due to the different pre-treatment methods and dissimilar pyrolysis operating conditions. For example, Hassan et al. [42] demonstrated alkaline pre-treatment of pine wood with NaOH, $Ca(OH)_2$, and NH_4OH and its pyrolysis at 450°C in a stainless steel auger reactor. The bio-oil produced from all the pre-treatments showed improved physical properties, such as the pH and HHV was increased with NaOH, while $Ca(OH)_2$ and NH_4OH exhibited lower viscosities in the produced bio-oils. The higher pH of the bio-oil could be attributed to the removal of acidic groups from the hemicellulose structure. In addition, GC-MS results revealed that NaOH and NH_4OH pre-treated biomass produced a lower content of levoglucosan in the bio-oil, while it increased with $Ca(OH)_2$ and the concentration of hydrocarbons improved with all the alkaline treatments, also confirmed by more pronounced C-H stretching vibrations in FTIR results [42]. The treatment with $Ca(OH)_2$ was found to depolymerize the lignin into phenolic monomers and dimers and prevents its agglomeration during the pyrolysis process, hence improving the pyrolytic behavior of lignin and the biomass containing a large proportion of lignin component [118]. Usually, the presence of phenolic hydroxyl, aldehyde, and carboxylic acid groups in lignin results in the agglomeration behavior of lignin, while the pre-treatment with $Ca(OH)_2$ reduces phenol-, hydroxyl-, and carbonyl-containing groups by forming phenolic alcohols, hydroxylcalcium phenoxides, and phenolic carboxylate salts [118]. A possible reaction mechanism of $Ca(OH)_2$ with lignin during pre-treatment and pyrolysis has been depicted in Figure 8.10.

The alkali pre-treatment has shown positive results for certain lignocellulose biomass, while few studies suggested that the alkali pre-treated biomass could not prove a suitable feedstock for pyrolysis as the resultant treated biomass is obtained with lower mass yield and higher ash content. Consequently, a lower bio-oil yield is obtained from the pyrolysis process with the treated biomass. However, alkali pre-treatment improves the biomass structure by promoting the breaking of ester and glycosidic linkages in the lignin structure. In addition, the pre-treatment method could be highly advantageous to produce specific high-value-added products through pyrolysis. Noticeably, NaOH has been shown to increase the yield of methanol and benzene using corncob as the biomass 114]. On the other hand, post-treatment requires washing and drying of the biomass, which requires energy input, making the process more uneconomical. Like acidic leachate, alkaline leachate also contains a small amount of sugars, probably resulting from the solubilization of the biomass's hemicellulose part. Subsequently, the downstream biochemical processing of the alkaline leachate could be used to produce valuable fuels like bioethanol. Less attention has been paid to understanding the possible reactions between the alkali solvents, such as NaOH and biomass constituents and reactions involved in removing minerals, alkali, and alkali earth metals. Therefore, more studies should

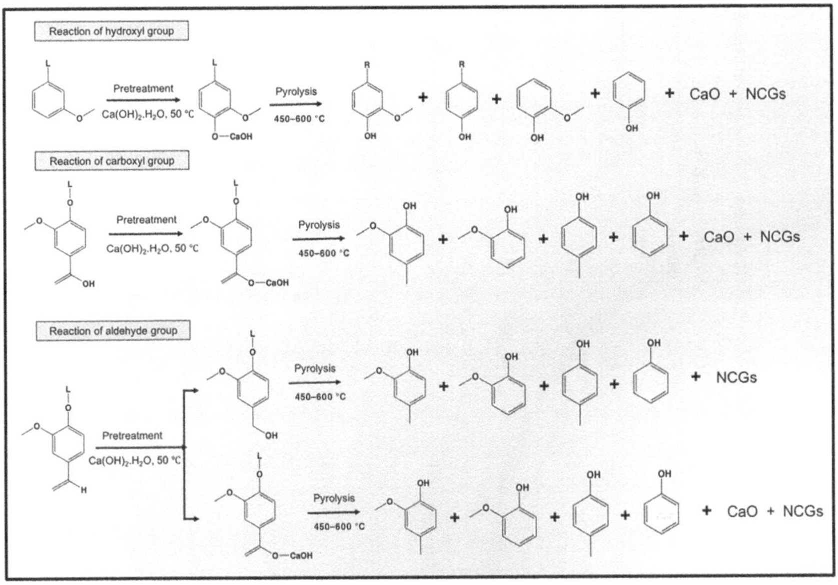

Lignocellulose Biomass Pyrolysis for Bio-Oil Production

FIGURE 8.10 Proposed reaction mechanism of lignin and calcium hydroxide during pretreatment and pyrolysis.

Source: Adapted from reference [118] with permission from The Royal Society of Chemistry.

be conducted to examine the chemical reactions and mechanisms involved in the removal of inorganic species.

8.4.2.3 Wet Torrefaction

Wet torrefaction (WT) (sometimes also termed hydrothermal carbonization or hot compressed water pre-treatment) is usually defined as the biomass treatment in hydrothermal media/hot-compressed water or subcritical water at a mild temperature range of 180–260 °C [95,131–133]. A pressure higher than the saturated vapor pressure of water is applied to keep the water in the liquid phase, and the heat of vaporization could increase the required energy for the process [134]. Very high pressures are usually not preferred for the WT process as they do not improve the reaction rate. The WT process results in three main products: hydrochar (the solid product), a mixture of gases, and a liquid product [134,135]. In WT, hydrochar is considered the primary product, which contains approximately 89.1% of the energy and 88.3% of the mass of the raw biomass, while in the gas mixture, CO_2 is the main gas, constituting nearly 95% of the total volume. The liquid product is usually rich in phenolic compounds, organic acids, furans, furfurals, and sugars [134,135]. The hydrochar, which is considered as the treated biomass, could be further subjected to the pyrolysis process to produce quality bio-oil. Table 8.6 shows some of the studies that examined the effect of WT on the physiochemical properties of pyrolytic bio-oil.

TABLE 8.6

Effect of Wet Torrefaction and Steam Explosion on Physiochemical Properties of Bio-Oil.

Feedstock	Pre-treatment	Reactor configuration	T (°C)	Biomass composition (%)			Properties of pyrolytic bio-oil				References
				Lignin	Cellulose	Hemi-cellulose	Bio-oil yield (%)	HHV (MJ/kg)	Water content (%)	pH	
Eucalyptus wood	untreated	Fluidized bed	500	28.25	44.08	24.02	~59	16.62	26	3.13	[136]
	wet torrefaction 160 °C			27.74	45.28	21.85	~62	17.68	21	3.15	
	wet torrefaction 170 °C			28.07	47.90	18.02	~64	17.91	19	3.14	
	wet torrefaction 180 °C			30.60	50.39	8.82	~67	18.35	18	3.17	
	wet torrefaction 190 °C			31.86	52.59	3.47	~68	18.42	18	3.15	
Sweetgum	untreated	Auger	450	37.8	/	/	51	/	38.3	2.65	[121]
	steam explosion			39.0	/	/	33	/	55.4	2.65	
Switchgrass	untreated			20.4	/	/	31	/	61.7	2.98	
	steam explosion			27.8	/	/	28	/	64.8	3.07	
Corn stover	untreated			22.6	/	/	35	/	54.7	2.66	
	steam explosion			41.0	/	/	34	/	58.7	2.47	
Loblolly Pine	untreated	Auger	450	39.9	33.55	27.34	54	16.10	20.83	2.65	[43]
	steam explosion			45.16	46.21	0	44	/	29.32	2.78	
Rice husk	untreated	Vertical drop fixed-bed	550	/	/	/	38.2	~12.2	~41	2.3	[137]
	wet torrefaction 150 °C			/	/	/	45.4	~12.9	~35	~2.4	
	wet torrefaction 180 °C			/	/	/	~44	~13.2	~33	~2.5	
	wet torrefaction 210 °C			/	/	/	42.7	~13.6	~31	~2.5	
	wet torrefaction 240 °C			/	/	/	30.2	~14	~27	2.7	

Cultivar willow	untreated	Microwave	460	~25	~41.6	~19.3	40.1	29.5	47.4	/	[138]
	wet torrefaction 160 °C		580	/	/	/	22.1	31.1	46.6	/	
Beech wood	untreated	Fixed bed	500	/	/	/	60.23	/	21.40	/	[139]
	wet torrefaction 190 °C			/	/	/	68.28	/	16.51	/	
Trembling aspen	untreated	Auger	450	24.4	52.2	23.4	56.1	13.10	41.0	2.3	[140]
	wet torrefaction 195°C			20.0	72.0	8.0	56.2	15.33	32.0	2.2	
Corncob	untreated	Pyro-probe	500	14.34	38.49	35.36	/	/	/	/	[141]
	wet torrefaction 175°C			18.09	47.51	26.71	/	/	/	/	
	wet torrefaction 185°C			20.92	54.11	20.05	/	/	/	/	
	wet torrefaction 195°C			24.39	64.72	4.52	/	/	/	/	
Corn stalk	untreated	Fixed bed	550	/	/	/	41.45	/	/	/	[142]
	wet torrefaction 230°C			/	/	/	~38	/	/	/	
	wet torrefaction 260°C			/	/	/	~33	/	/	/	
	wet torrefaction 290°C			/	/	/	18.7	/	/	/	
Rice husk	untreated	Vertical drop fixed bed	500	/	/	/	40.78	/	/	/	[143]
	wet torrefaction 170°C			/	/	/	47.70	/	/	/	

A number of studies reported the biomass pre-treatment in WT using varying operating conditions (temperature, pressure, and residence time) and their effect on the fuel properties and, consequently, on the bio-oil production in the pyrolysis process [142–145]. WT of lignocellulose biomass generally solubilizes the hemicellulose part almost completely, breaks the lignin linking interactions, and leaves the cellulose part nearly retained in the solid product. Therefore, it could be predicted that WT decreases the formation of water and light compounds in the bio-oil mainly produced from the pyrolysis of hemicellulose, while increasing the concentration of compounds derived from cellulose and lignin. Zheng et al. [141] demonstrated the application of WT of corncobs in a high-pressure reactor at three different temperatures of 175, 185, and 195 °C. The results showed that the concentration of hemicellulose significantly decreased from 26.71% at 175 °C to 4.52% at 195 °C, while the content of cellulose increased with rising temperature from 47.51% to 64.72% at 175 and 195 °C, respectively. Subsequently, the pyrolysis results were consistent with the composition of biomass, which revealed that the bio-oil had a higher proportion of compounds derived from the pyrolysis of cellulose. For instance, the yields of hydroxyacetaldehyde and levoglucosan were found to be maximum with the biomass torrefied at 195 °C, producing 1.89% and 12.13%, respectively. The enhanced production of levoglucosan was also attributed to the removal of undesirable inorganic species, which were significantly reduced after the WT process [141]. Similarly, Bach et al. [146] investigated the effect of temperature (175, 200, and 225 °C) and residence time (10, 30, and 60 min) on Norway spruce and birch woods during the WT and subsequently their effect on the pyrolysis kinetics. The results showed that WT for all the biomass samples decreased the pyrolysis temperature. However, the kinetic analysis further revealed that activation energy decreased for hemicellulose for both types of biomass. For spruce biomass, it reduced from 95.67 to 26.63 kJ/mol, and for birch wood, it decreased from 106.80 to 34.18 kJ/mol. It is known that WT promotes the degradation and cracking of hemicellulose into simpler or smaller molecules, which exhibit a lower degree of polymerization, and thus, lower activation energy is observed for hemicellulose [147]. However, WT increased the activation energy of cellulose and lignin. Actually, cellulose is a semi-crystal polymer, and WT increases its crystallinity [148]. During WT treatment, the number of intermolecular crosslinks increases, and the crystalline region is widened [148]. The resultant higher crystallinity shows more thermal resistance, and hence higher activation energy is obtained for cellulose after WT. Similarly, lignin is an amorphous and highly complex polymer, and its hydrothermal treatment promotes condensation and re-polymerization reactions between the decomposed products of hemicellulose and lignin [147], resulting in higher activation energy after WT. The temperature of 200 °C and residence time of 30 min (70 bar) was found optimal for WT to achieve the maximum pyrolysis rate. Further increase in the temperature and residence time decreased the pyrolysis rate [146]. A recent study by Zhang et al. [132] also suggested that temperatures higher than 200 °C are not suitable for WT, as higher ash contents were observed in the solid char at the higher temperatures of WT.

Apart from water, some other media, such as HCl [149], acetic acid [150], and aqueous ammonia [151], have also been utilized for WT of biomass, which showed significant enhancement in the fuel properties of the produced solid char. For example, Lynam et al. [150] studied the effect of acetic acid of various concentrations (0.25–0.75g/g of biomass) on WT of loblolly pine biomass in a Parr Series 4560 bench-top reactor using varying temperatures. The results revealed that the increasing concentration of acetic acid decreased the mass yield of the resultant char, while 200 °C was the optimum temperature to obtain the maximum mass yield which was 88.7%. During WT, acetic acid acts as a catalyst for the decomposition of the biomass components, resulting in lower activation energy. However, the addition of acetic acid increased the biomass calorific value. 0.4 g of acetic acid with 1 g of biomass was found to be the suitable ratio for achieving the maximum HHV of 22.09 MJ/kg, nearly 30% higher than the raw biomass. The increase in HHV with the addition of acetic acid was correlated with the removal of cellulose and the presence of higher lignin content in the solid char [150]. In a separate study, Li et al. [149] carried out microwave-assisted WT of bamboo biomass with varying concentrations of HCl at 180 °C at different residence times of 5–30 min. The results revealed that WT with 0.4 M HCl and a residence time of 30 min produced solid char with the highest carbon content of 67.03%, while 0.2 M HCl resulted in the highest HHV of 24.86 MJ/kg [149]. It was further reported that the addition of HCl with a higher concentration removed almost completely the hemicellulose part, and the content of cellulose was also decreased, while the lignin was increased with the residence time. The solid residue was found rich in complex condensed aromatic substances, including aromatic, carbonyl, and methoxy groups, as FTIR confirmed the signals for C–H, C=, C=O, and C–O–C stretching vibrations [149]. More recently, Hu et al. [144] examined microwave-assisted WT of corn stalks in aqueous ammonia (15 wt%) at 180 °C for 30 min and a pressure of up to 2 MPa, which substantially improved the fuel properties of the biomass. Noticeably, the addition of ammonia reduced the ash content from 9.87 wt% (of untreated corn stalk) to 2.19 wt%, while the carbon content and HHV values increased from 41.93 to 48.15 wt% and 14.85 to 17.05 MJ/kg, respectively. The surface area and porosity of the biomass were also increased after pre-treatment with ammonia. The pyrolysis of the pre-treated biomass was carried out at 800 °C, and the results showed that the concentration of acids and phenols was reduced in the liquid product, while the proportion of furans, esters, and ketones increased after the treatment [144]. WT of biomass with ammonia is believed to disrupt the O-acetyl groups and uronic acid on hemicellulose, consequently producing acetic acids which further promotes the cracking of the ester bonds in oligosaccharides and other molecules of hemicellulose and lignin [110].

WT can be considered an effective approach to improve the fuel properties of the biomass, especially to remove the inorganic species present in the biomass and increase the calorific value of the biomass. WT can be applied to diverse types of lignocellulosic biomass, including wet or dry biomass. However, WT could be a complex process compared to DT, which needs specific reactor materials to maintain the required temperature and pressure. DT has been commercialized, while WT has been used only at the laboratory scale because of the unsuitable reactor design that requires fast heating and rapid cooling. Therefore, an advanced WT reactor is required to improve the reaction efficiency and address the challenges related to reactor fouling. Moreover, compared to DT, WT of biomass results in wastewater that might contain toxic metals removed from the biomass during the treatment.

Therefore, proper solubilization of the toxic metals using specific solvents is pivotal before the final disposal of the wastewater. In addition, the downstream recovery of biomass further requires a drying process prior to pyrolysis, which is an energy-intensive step and would increase the overall cost of the WT process.

8.4.2.4 Ammonia Fiber Expansion

Ammonia fiber expansion (AFE) is another effective pre-treatment technique to improve the biomass structure and its fuel properties. This approach has been widely used for biomass pre-treatment and its conversion for biofuel production using various techniques [152–154]. AFE process is usually carried out in a special reactor equipped with a temperature and pressure controller and an inflow for liquid ammonia. Figure 8.11 shows the AFE setup. The process can be applied to a variety of biomass. Generally, the biomass is mixed with liquid ammonia in a 1:1 or 1:2 at a temperature of 60–120 °C and a pressure of ~2 MPa for 10–60 min in a closed vessel. The mixture of biomass and ammonia is heated to the required temperature with a holding time of approximately 5 min, and then the

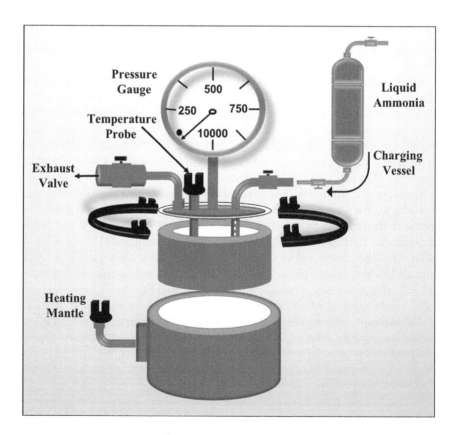

FIGURE 8.11 Picture showing AFEX reactor setup and heating system.

Source: Adapted from reference [153].

Lignocellulose Biomass Pyrolysis for Bio-Oil Production

pressure is rapidly released by opening the vent valve. This rapid release of pressure results in the evaporation of ammonia, and the temperature of the system starts decreasing. AFE pre-treatment promotes the removal of acetyl groups on hemicellulose, cleavage of C−O−C bonds, and lignin-carbohydrate complex linkages in lignin, and decrystallization of cellulose molecules in the lignocellulose biomass. Consequently, it affects the biomass structure considerably, which may result in enhanced thermal stability, pellet durability, and bulk and particle density [56]. It has also been suggested that AFE is not very effective for pre-treatment biomass with higher lignin content. Several studies have been conducted to determine the optimum operating conditions, such as temperature or pressure, for the pre-treatment of biomass in the AFE process, but the resultant pre-treated biomass has been utilized for other biofuel production, such as ethanol instead of pyrolysis, for bio-oil production. Since AFE pre-treated biomass has shown positive results for other biofuel production, it could also be used for pyrolysis. However, scarce information is available in the literature about the effect of AFE pre-treatment on the pyrolysis process or bio-oil composition. Sundaram et al. [56] demonstrated the effect of AFE pre-treatment on different biomass (corn stover, prairie cord grass, and switchgrass) and their effect on the composition of bio-oil during pyrolysis. The pre-treatment was carried out at 100 °C at varying loadings of ammonia and residence time, while the pyrolysis of the pre-treated biomass was carried out in a cylindrical stainless-steel reactor (batch mode) at 400 °C with a heating rate of 30 °C/min. The results revealed that AFE pre-treatment has a significant effect on the physical properties of all biomass samples used in the study, but it did not affect the properties of bio-oil produced after their pyrolysis. Noticeably, the pre-treated biomass showed enhanced pellet durability, thermal stability, and bulk and particle density. On the other hand, the yields of pyrolytic products, such as bio-oil, bio-char, and pyrolytic gases, were almost similar to the untreated biomass, as well as the bio-oil properties, such as pH, viscosity, and heating value, which did not show any noticeable changes after the AFE treatment [56]. Therefore, it can be indicated that AFE pre-treatment has less effect on biomass pyrolysis mechanism or kinetics; however, more studies should be conducted to understand its effect on the pyrolysis process and bio-oil upgrading.

8.4.2.5 Steam Explosion

Steam explosion (SE) is a commonly used biomass pre-treatment technique to improve the biomass structure for its further applications in various processes to generate biofuels. SE could be preferred over AFE due to its low energy consumption and could prove more cost-effective or economical as it does not require any chemical addition. In the first step of the SE process, the biomass is loaded in a steam explosion vessel and water is added at different water-to-biomass ratios [121,155]. The vessel is then heated to obtain a temperature nearly in the range of 160–260 °C and a pressure in the range of 0.69–4.83 MPa. The mixture of biomass and steam is held for a certain period of time to stimulate the hydrolysis of the hemicellulose component of the biomass, followed by a reduction in the pressure that allows the mixture to undergo explosive decompression. The resultant biomass or SE-treated biomass is then collected through the discharge valve

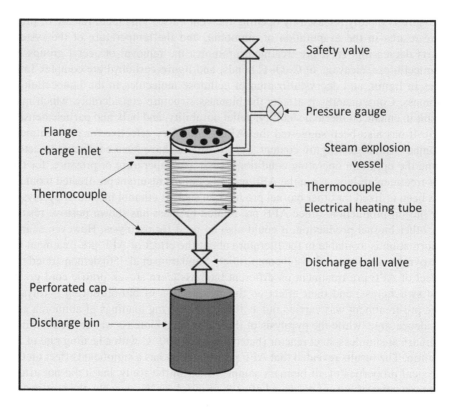

FIGURE 8.12 Schematic of steam explosion equipment.

Source: Adapted with permission from reference [43]. Copyright © 2011, American Chemical Society.

and dried in the oven at nearly 105–110 °C for 10–12 h, which can be further used in the pyrolysis process for bio-oil production [152]. Figure 8.12 shows the schematic diagram of an explosive steam vessel. This technique also works in the similar way as WT and AFE, resulting in the degradation of the hemicellulose and lignin components of the biomass by promoting the removal of the acetyl group on hemicellulose, which produces acetic acids that further promote cracking of the ester bonds in oligosaccharides and other molecules of hemicellulose and lignin. The reduction of the hemicellulose part results in the creation of large pores in the biomass structure, which enhances the accessibility of the cellulose part [132,148]. Evidently, a study showed that after SE treatment of banana fibers, the cellulose content significantly increased from 64% to 95%, and the content of hemicellulose and lignin considerably decreased to 0.4% and 1.9%, respectively [156]. SE can also lead to higher crystallinity of the cellulose and higher thermal stability due to the removal of hemicellulose and lignin [155,156]. In addition, SE pre-treatment has shown a significant decrease in the concentration of alkali and alkaline earth metals [152].

The pyrolysis of SE pre-treated biomass could show noticeable changes in the pyrolysis kinetics and also in the bio-oil composition and bio-oil physical properties. Biswas et al. [147] demonstrated the SE pre-treatment of Salix wood chips at different temperatures (approximately 205, 220, and 228 °C) and residence time of 6–12 min. Further, they examined their pyrolysis behavior in a thermogravimetric analyzer, heating the biomass sample from 100 to 750 °C at a heating rate of 10 °C/min. The results reported that SE had a significant effect on the biomass structure. They decreased the content of hemicellulose in the biomass. At the same time, the crystallinity of cellulose was increased as X-ray diffraction analysis revealed the narrowing of peaks at 2θ of 15° and 22° that represent the crystalline cellulose in the biomass. It was further noticed that the pyrolysis of the pre-treated biomass initiated at a lower temperature compared to the untreated biomass, attributing to the removal of hemicellulose and lignin content after the SE treatment. In a separate study, Wang et al. [43] investigated the influence of SE pre-treated pine wood biomass on the composition and physical properties of the bio-oil. SE process of the biomass was carried out in a vertical stainless-steel reactor at a temperature of 173–193 °C, a pressure of 1.3 MPa, and a residence time of 10 min, while the pyrolysis of the pre-treated biomass was conducted in an auger reactor at a temperature of 450 °C. The results indicated considerable changes in the bio-oil properties after SE pre-treatment. For example, the viscosity and acid value of the bio-oil decreased from 6.49 to 3.93 cSt and 90.06 to 64.16, respectively; however, the water content increased from 20.83% to 29.32%. GC-MS analysis further revealed that the pre-treated biomass produced the bio-oil with an enhanced concentration of phenols that were mainly produced from the pyrolysis of lignin and cellulose and reduced concentration of hemicellulose-derived compounds, suggesting the removal of hemicellulose component during the SE process. Wang et al. [44] conducted another study demonstrating the SE pre-treatment of three biomass samples (sweetgum, switchgrass, and corn stover) using almost similar operating conditions for SE and pyrolysis and the trend of the results was also similar to the previous study. The authors reported that some of the bio-oil properties, such as viscosity and acid value, decreased, and the bio-oil was enriched with phenols after the SE pre-treatment. Although SE pre-treated biomass could not produce high-quality oil during pyrolysis, certain undesirable oxygenated compounds can be removed, and more valuable compounds can be produced.

Overall, it can be suggested that SE is an efficient technique for improving biomass structure. It can result in the formation of large pores in the biomass and increase the accessibility of the cellulose component. SE has shown a remarkable decrease in the concentration of alkali and alkaline earth metals in the biomass and a decrease in viscosity and acid value of the resultant bio-oil. Besides, the technique requires low energy input. However, the process requires expensive reactor materials and higher temperatures to generate the steam, which can make the process slightly expensive compared to the other techniques. Another disadvantage of SE could be the incomplete dissociation of lignin-cellulose or lignin-hemicellulose matrix, which may result in the precipitation of soluble lignin constituents.

8.4.2.6 Hot-Water Extraction

Hot-water extraction (HWE) is one of the simplest and most cost-effective routes for biomass pre-treatment. It does not require any special reactor and severe temperature and pressure conditions like WT. HWE could be carried out at a temperature range of 160–230 °C. In the pre-treatment process, the biomass and water are kept in contact for nearly 15 min around 200 °C, which usually results in the breaking of hemiacetal linkages, further promoting the cleavage of ether linkages in the biomass. Consequently, HWE is useful for removing a large extent of the hemicellulose part and a small part of lignin, leaving a water-resistant solid residue with higher content of lignin and cellulose. HWE is considered highly useful in improving the biomass structure to obtain a better-quality bio-oil [157]. HWE has shown substantial removal of inorganic metal species from the biomass that could negatively affect the pyrolysis chemistry. Their catalytic reactions may enhance the formation of char and gas and result in low bio-oil yield [42,158]. HWE technique has been shown to promote the production of high-value-added chemicals, such as levoglucosan [158,159].

Several studies have reported the application of hot water pre-treatment of different biomass types to improve the biomass composition and its subsequent use in the pyrolysis process to ameliorate the quality of bio-oil or produce some high-value-added chemicals [57,159,160]. For instance, a study demonstrated the significant reduction in the concentration of alkali and alkaline earth metals in the biomass after treating with water at different retention times from 30 min to 6 h and pyrolysis at 600 °C, producing bio-oils with varying composition and physical properties [57]. Noticeably, the concentrations of Na, K, and Ca significantly reduced, while an increase in HHV of the bio-oil was noticed with the treated biomass. In a separate study, Le Roux et al. [159] carried out fast pyrolysis of hot water pre-treated (at 175–215 °C) trembling aspen (*Populus tremuloides*) and white spruce (*Picea glauca*), and the results revealed that the pre-treated biomass produced higher bio-oil yield, while the concentration of anhydrosugars was also higher compared to the untreated biomass. Furthermore, Tarves et al. [138] demonstrated the HWE of shrub willow and examined its effect on the pyrolysis product distribution. HWE was carried out using 0.5 kg oven-dried biomass with a water-to-biomass ratio of 4:1 at 160 °C for 2 h, and the pyrolysis process was performed at 500 °C. The results showed that the pre-treatment affected the physical properties of the biomass and altered its elemental composition. There was a significant reduction in the concentration of inorganic minerals, such as Ca, K, Mg, P, and S, while the mass fraction of hemicellulose remarkably decreased from 20.1% to 8.4% for Owasco shrub willow and the mass fraction of cellulose increased significantly from 40.2% to 54.7%. The pre-treatment also improved the surface area of the biomass by approximately twice compared to the untreated biomass. The pyrolysis results suggested some variations in the product yields, where the bio-oil yield was slightly affected, and the gas yield decreased from 7.8 to 5.6wt%, mainly attributing to the decrease in CO_2 yield that suggests the removal of carbonyl functional groups in the biomass following the hot water pre-treatment. The authors further reported that the concentration of acetic acid and phenols significantly decreased in the bio-oil, while the content of levoglucosan increased approximately four times with the pre-treated biomass [158].

Lignocellulose Biomass Pyrolysis for Bio-Oil Production

HWE technique could be more effective for biomass pre-treatment in combination with other techniques, such as ultrasonication. A combined process could be highly advantageous to increase the bio-oil yield and can reduce the residence time for HWE. Evidently, Shi et al. [157] demonstrated the application of HWE with ultrasonic pre-treatment of cellulose (at a temperature range of 240–340 °C and pressure of 12–20 MPa), and the results showed an increase of nearly 22% in the bio-oil yield, while the residence time of the process was also reduced.

Overall, it can be suggested that HWE is an efficient and cost-effective technique for biomass pre-treatment and can be applied to improve the biomass structure and remove the inorganic minerals or alkali metals in the biomass. Consequently, a higher bio-oil yield and better bio-oil quality could be obtained. However, the downstream processing of the treated biomass and its subsequent drying process requires high energy input to convert into a suitable feedstock for pyrolysis, which ultimately could increase the overall cost of bio-oil upgrading.

8.4.3 BIOLOGICAL PRE-TREATMENT OF LIGNOCELLULOSE BIOMASS

Biological pre-treatment of lignocellulose biomass is considered one of the most economical and eco-friendly treatment methods since it is carried out under ambient temperature and pressure and requires no energy or chemical inputs. It makes the process more cost-effective as compared to the physical or chemical methods and improves the biomass composition for the production of high-value-added chemicals and energy-rich pyrolytic products [161,162]. The ultimate goal of biological treatment of lignocellulose biomass is to degrade or depolymerize complex compounds, such as lignin, into their monomer units. Biological treatment of biomass can also decompose the main linkages between lignin and hemicellulose or lignin and cellulose, consequently decreasing the activation energy and increasing the rate of reaction during the thermochemical conversion of biomass at lower temperatures [162]. The microorganisms are used for the biomass pre-treatments that exhibit the ligninolytic enzyme system, mainly comprising laccases and peroxidases with a high reduction potential that oxidize the lignin polymer structure [163]. Some low molecular weight organic compounds act as mediators (2,4,6-tri-tert -butylphenol, 4-tert -butyl-2,6-dimethylphenol, and 3-hydroxyanthranilic acid) can be used to enhance the oxidation of lignin [164]. These small-sized mediators can diffuse through the cell wall pores and help the enzymes, such as laccases, to oxidize the bonds in the lignin structure, which otherwise could not be accessed by the enzymes due to their large size and selectivity. There are several microorganisms, including bacteria and fungi, that have shown the remarkable ability to degrade the lignocellulose biomass, but only fungi, mainly white rot fungi [163,165] and brown rot fungi [166], have been utilized for biomass pre-treatment, which has been further applied for the pyrolysis process.

White rot fungi are considered the most effective microorganisms for lignin degradation due to their ability to produce an adequate amount of laccases and peroxidases that effectively help in lignin oxidation, thereby, have been widely used for biomass pre-treatment [163,165]. For example, Yang et al. [165] demonstrated the application of white rot fungus *Echinodontium taxodii* for the pre-treatment of corn stover biomass and analyzed its effect on the distribution of pyrolytic products. Approximately 10 g of dry biomass was pre-treated with 10 mL of the fungus seed culture at 28 °C and cultivated for 30 days. Subsequently, the biomass was pyrolyzed at 340 °C for 1 min. The results revealed that the fungal treatment of biomass improved the pyrolysis of cellulose, hemicellulose, and lignin, demonstrating its degrading effect on all the components. Noticeably, the production of pyrolytic products from cellulose and hemicellulose was greatly enhanced. The treated biomass produced an enhanced number of polycyclic aromatic hydrocarbons and long-chain hydrocarbons as compared to untreated biomass, indicating the effect of white rot fungus on lignin degradation. In addition, the kinetic analysis in the study showed that the biological treatment decreased the activation energy and increased the reaction rate during low-temperature pyrolysis [165]. More recently, a combination of white rot fungus (*Trametesorientalis*) and brown rot fungus (*Fomitopsispinicola*) was applied for corncob lignin treatment at 28 °C for 25 days, and the pyrolysis was carried out at 600 °C for 1 min [166]. The study showed that the white rot fungus performed efficient degradation of lignin into its constituent compounds, while the brown rot fungus further promoted the breakdown of guaiacyl units. It was also noticed that the proportions of phenols and alkyl phenols were significantly increased in the case of treated biomass. These compounds are mainly produced from the pyrolysis of lignin, indicating a synergetic effect of the fungi in lignin degradation [166]. In a separate study, lignin pre-treated with *E. taxodii* (at 28 °C for 30 days) was investigated for the generation of pyrolytic products at 600 °C [167]. FTIR results confirmed that the fungus had a significant effect on lignin degradation, especially the aromatic skeletal carbon, and side chain of lignin was distorted after the treatment. The pyrolysis results showed that the formation of lignin-derived pyrolytic compounds increased using the treated biomass as compared to the untreated biomass [167]. The above discussion specifies that the biological treatment of biomass improves the pyrolysis process and kinetics of all biomass components. The enhanced production of pyrolytic products derived from cellulose, hemicellulose, and lignin indicates the degrading effect of biological treatment on all these constituents. Therefore, it could be suggested that an increased number of organic compounds and a higher liquid yield can be obtained with the treated biomass under favorable pyrolysis variables. However, the process could be time-consuming as microorganisms take longer to decompose the biomass. Another challenge of this approach is the requirement of a large amount of space to carry out the microbial pre-treatment at the pilot scale application. Microorganisms could also consume some part of the carbohydrate for their growth, which could decrease the mass yield of the treated biomass [168]. Since limited microorganisms have been used for biomass pre-treatment and its subsequent thermal degradation process, there is a need to further explore the application of microorganisms for biomass pre-treatment and its effect on pyrolytic behavior as well as bio-oil upgrading.

8.5 CATALYTIC PYROLYSIS OF PRE-TREATED BIOMASS

The different biomass pre-treatment methods discussed in the previous sections suggest that certain pre-treatment methods improve the biomass properties, which

Lignocellulose Biomass Pyrolysis for Bio-Oil Production

consequently significantly impact the distribution of pyrolysis products and bio-oil properties. However, it has also been noticed that biomass pre-treatment methods, except DT, have very less or negligible effect on improving the selectivity of hydrocarbons in the bio-oil, making the bio-oil highly rich with oxygenated compounds and hence resulting in the bio-oil with low energy density. For instance, torrefaction of biomass could increase the content of phenols in the bio-oil composition [169], while the acid treatment of biomass could increase the amount of anhydrosugars, such as levoglucosan, in the bio-oil [170]. Therefore, the conversion of different low-energy-density oxygenated compounds into high-energy-density hydrocarbons is very important to transform the bio-oil into a gasoline-like liquid fuel. This can be achieved by coupling the biomass-treatment methods and the catalytic pyrolysis approach. The application of different catalysts, such as zeolites, metal-zeolite-based catalysts, and metal oxides, can successfully convert the oxygenated compounds (phenols, alcohols, acids, ketones, furans) into various desirable hydrocarbons (olefins, paraffin, monocyclic aromatic hydrocarbons, and polycyclic aromatic hydrocarbons) [171–175]. The catalytic pyrolysis of pre-treated biomass samples could be carried out mainly *via* two pyrolysis modes, *in-situ* (a catalyst is mixed with biomass) and *ex-situ* catalytic pyrolysis (catalyst is placed separately downstream of the biomass and the produced pyrolytic vapors are passed through the catalyst bed) [176,177]. However, more pyrolysis configurations, like two-stage or three-stage *ex-situ* pyrolysis and combined *in-situ* and *ex-situ* pyrolysis, could also be applied for bio-oil upgrading [176,178,179]. The catalytic pyrolysis in all modes could significantly improve bio-oil quality by converting the oxygenated compounds into hydrocarbons. Still, it also decreases the bio-oil yield and increases the gaseous products. Generally, the application of catalysts promotes the various deoxygenation reactions, such as dehydration, decarboxylation, decarbonylation, hydrogen transfer, aldol condensation, Diels-Alder reaction, aromatization, and rearrangement reactions to convert the oxygen containing compounds into different hydrocarbons [180–183]. These deoxygenation reactions are believed to be catalyzed primarily by the Brønsted (proton donating species) and Lewis acid (electron accepting species) sites present inside the pores as well as on the surface of the catalysts [184–186]. More critical information about the role of catalysts and pathways involved in the conversion of oxygenated compounds to hydrocarbons could be found elsewhere [182,187,188].

A number of studies have demonstrated the application of coupled biomass pre-treatment and catalytic pyrolysis, which have shown considerably enhanced bio-oil upgrading. Table 8.7 summarizes a few studies that utilized catalytic pyrolysis of pre-treated biomass for bio-oil upgrading. Generally, the acidic catalysts that show a high number of strong Brønsted acid sites, shape selectivity, and micro and mesoporous properties are highly desirable for bio-oil upgrading. It has been found that the catalysts with a greater number of Brønsted acid sites have achieved a higher proportion of aromatic hydrocarbons in the bio-oil and, subsequently, higher carbon yield [189,190]. Although various thermal and chemical methods can be used to pre-treat the biomass, only a few methods, such as dry torrefaction, wet torrefaction, and acid treatment, have been coupled with catalytic pyrolysis to investigate their effect on bio-oil upgrading. For example, torrefied biomass catalytic pyrolysis has been extensively demonstrated

TABLE 8.7

Effect of Catalytic Pyrolysis of Pre-treated Biomass on Selectivity of Aromatic Hydrocarbons in Bio-Oil Samples.

| No. | Biomass | Pre-treatment | | Non-catalytic pyrolysis | | | | Catalyst | Catalytic pyrolysis | | | References |
		Technique	Conditions	Reactor	T (°C)	HR (°C/s)	Bio-oil composition		Mode	C/B or FR	Bio-oil composition	
1.	Loblolly pine	DT	225 °C, 15 min	Pyroprobe	550	2000	AR-0.13%, PH-1.44%	ZSM-5	In-situ	9	AR-27.05%, PH-0.17%, BTX-14.44%	[190]
2.	Loblolly pine	DT	225 °C, 30 min	Pyroprobe	550	2000	AR-0.15%, PH-2.64	ZSM-5	In-situ	9	AR-38.25%, PH-0.26%, BTX-17.82%	[190]
3.	Loblolly pine	DT	225 °C, 45 min	Pyroprobe	550	2000	AR-0.18%, PH-2.57	ZSM-5	In-situ	9	AR-26.68%, PH-0.28%, BTX-13.13%	[190]
4.	Loblolly pine	DT	250 °C, 15 min	Pyroprobe	550	2000	AR-0.18%, PH-2.67	ZSM-5	In-situ	9	AR-37.34%, PH-0.43%, BTX-16.97%	[190]
5.	Loblolly pine	DT	250 °C, 30 min	Pyroprobe	550	2000	AR-0.20%, PH-3.26	ZSM-5	In-situ	9	AR-35.51%, PH-0.61%, BTX-16.33%	[190]
6.	Loblolly pine	DT	250 °C, 45 min	Pyroprobe	550	2000	AR-0.20%, PH-3.16	ZSM-5	In-situ	9	AR-22.05%, PH-0.14%, BTX-11.65%	[190]
7.	Loblolly pine	DT	275 °C, 15 min	Pyroprobe	550	2000	AR-0.19%, PH-3.22	ZSM-5	In-situ	9	AR-29.81%, PH-0.3%, BTX-15.72%	[190]

8.	Loblolly pine	DT	275 °C, 30 min	Pyroprobe	550	2000	AR-0.32%, PH-3.45	ZSM-5	In-situ	9	AR-19.30%, PH-0.21%, BTX-9.61%	[190]
9.	Loblolly pine	DT	275 °C, 45 min	Pyroprobe	550	2000	AR-0.32%, PH-2.94	ZSM-5	In-situ	9	AR-8.57%, PH-0.04%, BTX-4.30%	[190]
10	Corncobs	DT	210°C, 40 min	Pyroprobe	600	20000	AR-27.14%	HZSM-5	In-situ	9	PAH-32.7%, BTX-40.0%	[87]
11.	Corncobs	DT	240°C, 40 min	Pyroprobe	600	20000	AR-25.35%	HZSM-5	In-situ	9	PAH-30.1%, BTX-43.9%	[87]
12.	Corncobs	DT	270°C, 40 min	Pyroprobe	600	20000	AR-20.0%	HZSM-5	In-situ	9	PAH-31.4%, BTX-45.7%	[87]
13.	Corncobs	DT	300°C, 40 min	Pyroprobe	600	20000	AR-12.67%	HZSM-5	In-situ	9	PAH-26.0%, BTX-51.1%	[87]
14.	Corncobs	DT	270°C, 20 min	Pyroprobe	600	20000	AR-22.18%	HZSM-5	In-situ	9	PAH-28.2%, BTX-47.8%	[87]
15.	Corncobs	DT	270°C, 40 min	Pyroprobe	600	20000	AR-20.18%	HZSM-5	In-situ	9	PAH-31.4%, BTX-45.7%	[87]
16.	Corncobs	DT	270°C, 60 min	Pyroprobe	600	20000	AR-16.72%	HZSM-5	In-situ	9	PAH-25.5%, BTX-49.0%	[87]
17.	Pine wood	DT	225 °C, 30 min	Pyroprobe	650	2000	AR-8.64%, TCY-18.15%	ZSM-5	In-situ	9	[a]AR-9.57%, PH-1.18%	[189]
18.	Pine wood	DT	225 °C, 30 min	Pyroprobe	650	2000	AR-8.64%, TCY-18.15%	ZSM-5	In-situ	9	[b]AR-15.27%, PH-2.45%	[189]

(Continued)

TABLE 8.7 (Continued)

No.	Biomass	Pre-treatment		Non-catalytic pyrolysis				Catalyst	Catalytic pyrolysis			References
		Technique	Conditions	Reactor	T (°C)	HR (°C/s)	Bio-oil composition		Mode	C/B or FR	Bio-oil composition	
19.	Pine wood	DT	225 °C, 30 min	Pyroprobe	650	2000	AR-8.64%, TCY-18.15%	ZSM-5	In-situ	9	cAR-18.68%, PH-6.17%	[189]
20.	Pine wood	DT	225 °C, 30 min	Pyroprobe	650	2000	AR-8.64%, TCY-18.15%	ZSM-5	In-situ	9	dAR-24.22%, 7.67%	[189]
21.	E. globulus	DT	304 °C, 15 min	Micropyrolysis unit	500	2000	AR-9.21%, PH-22.48%	HZSM-5	In-situ	5	BTX-26%, PAH-29%, PH-8%	[198]
22.	E. globulus	DT	304 °C, 15 min	Micropyrolysis unit	500	2000	AR-9.21%, PH-22.48%	Ni/CAG	In-situ	5	BTX-6.7%, PAH-0%, PH-10%	[198]
23.	E. globulus	DT	304 °C, 15 min	Micropyrolysis unit	500	2000	AR-9.21%, PH-22.48%	Fe/CAG	In-situ	5	BTX-5.6%, PAH-0%, PH-8%	[198]
24.	Rice husk	Acid + DT	Acetic acid-30 °C, 4 h DT-210 °C, 1 h	Fixed bed	550	/	PH-23.9%, AC-4.24%	ZSM-5	Ex-situ	5	BTX-45.79%, PAH-3.01%	[192]
25.	Rice husk	Acid + DT	Acetic acid-30 °C, 4 h DT-240 °C, 1 h	Fixed bed	550	/	PH-24.51%, AC-3.15%	ZSM-5	Ex-situ	5	BTX-48.88%, PAH-2.59%	[192]

Lignocellulose Biomass Pyrolysis for Bio-Oil Production

No.	Feedstock	Pretreatment	Conditions	Reactor	Temp.		Products	Catalyst	Mode		Products	Ref.
26.	Rice husk	Acid + DT	Acetic acid-30 °C, 4 h DT-270 °C, 1 h	Fixed bed	550	/	PH-29.00%, AC-1.94%	ZSM-5	Ex-situ	5	BTX-53.99%, PAH-1.75%	[192]
27.	Rice husk	Acid	Acetic acid-30 °C, 4 h	Fixed bed	550	/	PH-23.17%, AC-5.33%	ZSM-5	Ex-situ	5	BTX-43.86%, PAH-3.34%	[192]
28.	Lignin pine	DT	150 °C, 15 min	Tandem microreactor	500	/	PH-11.2%, TCY-82.2%	HZSM-5	In-situ	4	BTX-51.4%, TCY-91.8%	[199]
29.	Lignin pine	DT	175 °C, 15 min	Tandem microreactor	500	/	PH-13.1%, TCY-77.2%	HZSM-5	In-situ	4	BTX-56.3%, TCY-91.7%	[199]
30.	Lignin pine	DT	200 °C, 15 min	Tandem microreactor	500	/	PH-15.7%, TCY-77.91%	HZSM-5	In-situ	4	BTX-58.9%, TCY-92.2%	[199]
31.	Lignin pine	DT	225 °C, 15 min	Tandem microreactor	500	/	PH-18.1%, TCY-76.9%	HZSM-5	In-situ	4	BTX-61.4%, TCY-93.4%	[199]
32.	Lignin switchgrass	DT	150 °C, 15 min	Tandem microreactor	500	/	PH-13.5%, TCY-78.3%	HZSM-5	In-situ	4	BTX-50.2%, TCY-89.5%	[199]
33.	Lignin switchgrass	DT	175 °C, 15 min	Tandem microreactor	500	/	PH-15.1%, TCY-78.2%	HZSM-5	In-situ	4	BTX-52.9%, TCY-91.5%	[199]
34.	Lignin switchgrass	DT	200 °C, 15 min	Tandem microreactor	500	/	PH-16.2%, TCY-76.7%	HZSM-5	In-situ	4	BTX-56.8%, TCY-92.2%	[199]
35.	Lignin switchgrass	DT	225 °C, 15 min	Tandem microreactor	500	/	PH-16.8%, TCY-76.0%	HZSM-5	In-situ	4	BTX-59.4%, TCY-91.9%	[199]
36.	Pine wood	DR	220 °C, 30 min	Fixed bed	550	/	AR-24.38%, PH-40.17%	HZSM-5	Ex-situ	0.5	AR-21.29%, PH-32.51%	[200]
37.	Pine wood	DR	250 °C, 30 min	Fixed bed	550	/	AR-29.33%, PH-42.29%	HZSM-5	Ex-situ	0.5	AR-23.06%, PH-35.84%	[200]
38.	Pine wood	DR	280 °C, 30 min	Fixed bed	550	/	AR-30.15%, PH-44.76%	HZSM-5	Ex-situ	0.5	AR-26.18%, PH-37.71%	[200]

(Continued)

TABLE 8.7 *(Continued)*

| No. | Biomass | Pre-treatment | | Non-catalytic pyrolysis | | | | Catalytic pyrolysis | | | | References |
		Technique	Conditions	Reactor	T (°C)	HR (°C/s)	Bio-oil composition	Catalyst	Mode	C/B or FR	Bio-oil composition	
39.	Lignocel HBS	WT	190 °C, 8 min, water	Fixed bed	500	/	PH-20.51%, AC-5.76%	HZSM-5	Ex-situ	0.46	AR-41.31%, PAH-22.56%, PH-17.93%	[197]
40.	Lignocel HBS	WT	190 °C, 8 min, water	Fixed bed	500	/	PH-20.51%, AC-5.76%	Al-MCM-41	Ex-situ	0.46	AR-7.77%, PAH-11.73%, PH-32.82%	[197]
41.	Lignocellulose biomass	Acid	Acetic acid-85 °C, 30 min	Fixed bed	600	/	High acids and sugars	HZSM-5	Ex-situ	1	High BTX yield	[201]

C/B, Catalyst to biomass; FR, Feed rate; DT, Dry torrefaction; WT, Wet torrefaction; AC, Acids; AR, Aromatics; PH, Phenols; BTX, Benzene, toluene, xylene; PAH, Polycyclic aromatic hydrocarbons; Oxy, Oxygenates; TCY, Total carbon yield; CAG, Cellulose-derived carbon aerogels
a: catalytic pyrolysis was carried out at 450 °C; b: catalytic pyrolysis was carried out at 500 °C; c: catalytic pyrolysis was carried out at 550 °C; d: catalytic pyrolysis was carried out at 600 °C

Lignocellulose Biomass Pyrolysis for Bio-Oil Production

using zeolite-based catalysts like ZSM-5 [189,191,192]. On the one hand, sole pyrolysis of torrefied biomass could generate a small amount of aromatics while considerably increasing the content of phenolics in the bio-oil. The increase in phenolic compounds could be attributed to the significant changes in the lignin structure post-torrefaction process [76,101], and the subsequent thermal degradation could result in the phenolic compounds *via* cleavage of ether linkages and demethoxylation reactions [193]. The incorporation of an acidic catalyst could convert the phenolic compounds into various aromatic hydrocarbons *via* dehydration, hydrogen transfer, and cracking reactions, thereby increasing the total carbon yield [169,194]. Neupane et al. [190] carried out *in-situ* catalytic pyrolysis of torrefied pine wood using HZSM-5 catalyst at 550 °C with a catalyst-to-biomass ratio of 9. The results showed that the noncatalytic pyrolysis of pine wood torrefied at 250 °C (for 15 min) resulted in the bio-oil with approximately 0.18% aromatics and 2.67% phenolics, while the catalytic pyrolysis of the torrefied biomass substantially increased the aromatic yield to 37.34% and reduced the phenolic yield to 0.43%. Besides selecting a particular catalyst, several other factors, such as pyrolysis reactors, pyrolysis temperature, heating rate, catalyst-to-biomass ratio, residence time, and biomass composition, affect the selectivity of hydrocarbons and other organic compounds in the bio-oil. It has been found that higher pyrolysis temperature of 600 °C compared to 450 °C produce a greater concentration of aromatic hydrocarbons; however, they also promote the formation of phenolic compounds, which could be attributed to the cleavage of ether bonds in lignin structure at higher temperatures [189]. Similarly, the higher catalyst-to-biomass ratios favor monocyclic and polycyclic aromatic hydrocarbons but decrease the bio-oil yield and increase the gas yield [195]. A higher amount of the catalyst could provide an increased number of active sites to carry out the different deoxygenation reactions, thereby increasing the kinetics of the pyrolysis process and conversion of oxygenated compounds into hydrocarbons at the expense of the bio-oil yield. It has been observed that *in-situ* catalytic pyrolysis mode requires higher catalyst-to-biomass ratios compared to the *ex-situ* mode as the biomass and catalyst are heated together during the *in-situ* mode and the produced pyrolytic vapors could not access the required amount of active sites of the catalyst due to less interaction time between the pyrolytic vapors and the catalyst [176]. Although the higher catalyst-to-biomass ratios could increase the overall yield of aromatic hydrocarbons, this could result in the selectivity of different hydrocarbons. For example, Srinivasan et al. [189] carried out the catalytic pyrolysis of torrefied biomass using ZSM-5 at different catalyst-to-biomass ratios (4, 9, 14) and suggested that the overall yield of aromatic hydrocarbons increased with increase in catalyst to biomass ratio. However, it was noticed that the increase in catalyst-to-biomass ratios lightly increased the selectivity of toluene and xylenes while the selectivity of benzene and naphthalene decreased [189]. Collectively, it could be inferred that the integration of catalytic pyrolysis with torrefaction has proved to improve the quality of bio-oil, particularly by increasing the content of monocyclic hydrocarbons, like benzene, toluene, and xylenes, and improving the overall carbon yield in the bio-oil.

Catalytic pyrolysis of torrefied biomass has been widely explored; however, limited studies have been conducted on catalytic pyrolysis of biomass pre-treated with other thermal, chemical, and biological methods. The pre-treatment of biomass with WT mainly causes the hydrolysis of the hemicellulose component of the biomass and breaks the lignin-linking interactions, and leaves the cellulose part nearly retained in the solid product. Subsequently, pyrolysis increases the formation of organic compounds (mainly oxygenated compounds like phenols, sugars, and furans) that are primarily derived from the thermal degradation of lignin and cellulose [133,196]. These oxygen-containing compounds can be successfully converted to energy-rich hydrocarbons using acidic catalysts. For example, a study demonstrated the catalytic pyrolysis of biomass pre-treated with the WT approach using HZSM-5 and Al-MCM-41 catalysts [197]. The results showed that the catalytic pyrolysis of the pre-treated biomass using both catalysts produced a better quality of bio-oil compared to the non-catalytic pyrolysis, with bio-oil rich in monocyclic and polycyclic hydrocarbons, while the bio-oil produced by the non-catalytic pyrolysis of the pre-treated biomass contained higher proportions of furans, sugars, and phenols [197]. Similarly, the integration of catalytic pyrolysis using acidic catalysts and acid or alkali biomass pre-treatment approaches can substantially improve the content of aromatic and aliphatic hydrocarbons and remove the oxygenated compounds, owing to the improved pyrolysis kinetics and deoxygenation reactions (like dehydration, decarboxylation, decarbonylation, aromatization, oligomerization, and cracking reactions) carried out by the Brønsted acid sites on the catalysts.

Biological pre-treatment of biomass could be highly useful to decompose the main linkages between lignin and hemicellulose, or lignin and cellulose, decreasing the activation energy while increasing the rate of reaction during the pyrolysis process. It has shown that biological pre-treatment increases the bio-oil yield and enhances the content of hydrocarbons in the bio-oil. The application of fast catalytic pyrolysis of biologically treated biomass could help convert these compounds into valuable hydrocarbons with improved bio-oil quality. Yu et al. [163] investigated the effect of ZSM-5 catalyst on the conversion of pyrolytic vapors generated from corn stover pre-treated with *Irpex lacteus*. Firstly, it was observed that the fungal treatment increased the production of volatile products that mainly contained oxygenated compounds, compared to non-treated corn stover, and secondly, the use of ZSM-5 converted the oxygenated compounds into aromatic hydrocarbons, with a maximum percentage of 11.49 wt% obtained in the bio-oil. In addition, a decrease in the char yield was observed with the treated biomass, indicating degradation of the lignin component and its successful conversion to volatile products [163].

It can be suggested that coupling catalytic pyrolysis and other pre-treatment methods are highly advantageous approaches to enhance bio-oil quality. The application of catalysts improves the kinetics of pyrolysis by decreasing the activation energy. The active sites on the catalysts (mainly inside the pores) carry out various deoxygenation reactions to convert the low-energy-density oxygenated compounds into high-energy-density aromatic and aliphatic hydrocarbons, hence improving the calorific value of the bio-oil. However, the use of catalysts decreases the bio-oil yield considerably and enhances the gaseous products compared to the non-catalytic pyrolysis of pre-treated biomass feedstocks. Moreover, the catalysts are highly prone to deactivation due to the deposition of coke/carbonaceous species produced during catalytic pyrolysis. Therefore, the development of advanced catalysts that reduce coke deposition would be required to make catalytic pyrolysis more efficient and cost-effective. On the other hand, negligible research has been conducted using the catalytic pyrolysis of biomass pre-treated with SE, AFE, and HWE, and limited studies have demonstrated the application of catalytic pyrolysis of biologically pre-treated biomass.

8.6 CURRENT STATUS, CHALLENGES, AND FUTURE RECOMMENDATIONS

The physicochemical pre-treatment of lignocellulosic biomass has shown significant advantages to improve the biomass properties, which converts the biomass into a more suitable feedstock for pyrolysis, especially for improved pyrolysis kinetics, generation of a better-quality bio-oil, and production of desirable high value-added products. The pre-treatment methods, such as DT, acid, and alkali treatment, could help to disrupt the recalcitrant structure of lignocellulosic biomass, by breaking different chemical bonds or linkages present between three biomass components (cellulose, hemicellulose, and lignin) and also reducing the crystallinity of cellulose and degree of polymerization. As a result, the treated biomass shows lower activation energy for its thermal degradation compared to the untreated biomass. The other methods, SE, HWE, and WT, are highly effective in removing undesirable minerals, alkali metals, and alkali earth metals that, if present in the biomass, could significantly affect the pyrolysis process. Overall, all the pre-treatment methods have certain advantages to improve the biomass properties, which affect the pyrolysis process and, consequently, the bio-oil composition. However, among all the pre-treatment methods, only a few techniques, such as DT, have been used on a pilot scale so far, while most of them are still in the development stages. Estimating and comparing the efficacy of pre-treatment methods is difficult due to the noticeable differences in total capital investment and operating and maintenance costs. Therefore, the economic analysis of each pre-treatment process using a particular biomass feedstock could be carried out to better understand the efficacy of the pre-treatment methods. A number of studies have demonstrated techno-economic analysis of different biomass pre-treatment techniques for different fuel production and separate economic analyses of biomass pyrolysis for bio-oil production as well as catalytic biomass pyrolysis for bio-oil upgrading [66,202–205], but very limited studies have been conducted to determine the economic analysis of integrated biomass pre-treatment techniques and their effect on bio-oil upgrading. Recently, Chai et al. [206] estimated the cost of integrated torrefaction of spent coffee grounds and its catalytic pyrolysis for bio-oil upgrading, mainly focusing on BTEX (benzene, toluene, ethyl benzene, xylenes) yield. The study applied a range of torrefaction temperatures of 200–300 °C and residence time of 15–50 min, while the cost for BTEX production was predicted using a surface response model. The authors suggested that a temperature of 239 °C and a residence time of 34 min was economical, producing approximately 9.65 wt% BTEX per tonne of biomass, costing $1246 [206]. It was further indicated that increasing torrefaction temperature as well as residence time or decreasing both parameters increases the overall cost for BTEX production, which could be attributed to the severe mass loss at higher torrefaction temperatures with high residence time and lower BTEX yield at lower torrefaction temperatures with low residence time, thereby making the process expensive for BTEX production.

Although biomass pre-treatment techniques could be useful to improve the physiochemical properties of the bio-oil, there are several challenges related to each technique. Table 8.8 summarizes the advantages and challenges of each method used for biomass pre-treatment. The major challenge for the physical methods of biomass

TABLE 8.8

Advantages and Challenges of Methods Used for Bio-Oil Upgrading.

No.	Method	Advantages	Challenges
1	Grinding	• Improves heat flow between feedstock particles • Decreases the degree of polymerization and crystallinity of the biomass components during the pyrolysis process • A higher bio-oil yield and enhanced calorific value bio-oil could be achieved with smaller size particles	• It is an energy-intensive process • Increases cost
2	Densification	• Decreases moisture content of biomass • Increases durability index and energy content of biomass	• Requires energy input, for example, in screw extruder-60 kWh/ ton. • High maintenance cost for the instrument used in compaction.
3	Dry-torrefaction	• Lowers the activation energy for pyrolysis process • Increases the amount of atomic carbon in biomass and hence the energy conversion capacity • Improves the quality of bio-oil by decreasing the oxygenated compounds • Increases the content of hydrocarbons and heating value of bio-oil	• Decreases bio-oil yield • Higher ash content • Results in the biomass with poor pelletability • It is an energy-intensive process • Increases overall cost
4	Acid and alkali treatment	• Removes undesirable inorganic species from the biomass • Decreases viscosity of bio-oil • Enhances heating value of bio-oil • Improves carbon content in the biomass • Acid treatment can increase the bio-oil yield • Decreases the content of acids and increases the amount of hydrocarbons in the bio-oil • Improves cellulose digestibility • Acid treatment can enhance the production of certain chemicals and anhydrosugars, such as levoglucosan	• Alkali treatment can decrease the bio-oil yield • Alkali treatment can decrease the production of levoglucosan • Post-treatment requires washing and drying of the biomass, which requires energy input for the process • Use of expensive chemicals can make the process costly • Leachate contains toxic metals • Possible reaction of chemicals and inorganic species needs more investigation

5	Wet-torrefaction	• Can be applied to wet biomasses or biomass wastes • Removal of minerals and alkali metals • Increases calorific value, grindability, and pelletability of biomass • Requires less severe operating conditions, such as lower temperature and pressure • Decreases activation energy for hemicellulose, while increases for cellulose and lignin • Decreases the amount of light compounds in bio-oil • Increases the yield of levoglucosan	• Requires expensive reactor materials that can increase the overall cost for bio-oil upgrading • Inorganic precipitates produced during the process can cause clogging in the reactor • Requires a high-pressure slurry pump for feeding the biomass feedstock • Requires post-treatment of wastewater for resource recovery • After the downstream recovery of biomass, it further requires drying process prior to use in pyrolysis process
6	Ammonia fiber expansion	• Requires less severe temperature and pressure operating conditions (temperature of 60–120 °C and pressure of ~2 MPa) • Improves biomass thermal stability • Improves pellet durability, and bulk and particle density of biomass	• Not very effective for pre-treatment of biomass with higher content of lignin • Requires expensive reactor materials that can increase the overall cost for bio-oil upgrading • Has less effect on bio-oil properties • Requires more investigations to understand its effect on the pyrolysis process and bio-oil upgrading
7	Steam explosion	• Improves the biomass structure by creating large pores and increasing the accessibility of the cellulose part • Leads to higher crystallinity of the cellulose and higher thermal stability • Decreases the concentration of alkali and alkaline earth metals • Decreases viscosity and acid value of the bio-oil • Can increase the formation of high value-added chemicals	• Can increase the moisture content • Requires higher temperature • Requires expensive reactor materials • After the downstream recovery of biomass, it further requires drying of the biomass prior to use in pyrolysis process

(Continued)

TABLE 8.8 (*Continued*)

No.	Method	Advantages	Challenges
8	Hot-water extraction	• Very simple and cost-effective method • Improves surface area of biomass • Improves the bio-oil quality • Removes minerals and inorganic species • Enhances the production of high value-added chemicals • Increases bio-oil yield	• Drying process can make the process energy intensive
9	Biological pre-treatment	• Economic and eco-friendly treatment method • No energy or chemical inputs • Decomposes the main linkages between lignin and hemicellulose or lignin and cellulose • Decreases activation energy and increases the rate of reaction during pyrolysis process • Enhances the content of hydrocarbons in the bio-oil • Increases bio-oil yield and decreases char yield	• The process could be time consuming as microorganisms take longer time to decompose biomass • Selection of a certain microorganism could be a challenge for specific biomass due to difference in the biomass composition • Very less microorganisms have been explored so far, hence, more studies need to carry out to explore the application of microorganism for biomass treatment

pre-treatment is that they are energy-intensive, which makes the pre-treatment methods expensive. This can be alleviated by supplying the heat from a renewable energy source, which could make the overall process less expensive and self-sustainable. DT could lead to decreased bio-oil yield and increased ash content in the bio-oil, while biomass with poor pelletability could be obtained after the DT process. Optimization of different operating parameters during torrefaction, such as temperature, residence time, and heating rate is highly important to obtain biomass with improved properties. DT of biomass has been used on a pilot scale, but more studies are required to transform the technology into a commercial scale, especially, to obtain the torrefied biomass suitable for pyrolysis to achieve better-quality bio-oil. Commercialization of DT could also require the development of new reactors. On the other hand, WT is still in the developmental stage, and several challenges have been associated with this technology. The first challenge is the requirement of a high-pressure slurry pump for feeding the biomass feedstock. During WT process, inorganic precipitates could be formed that can cause clogging in the reactor, which ultimately could increase the maintenance cost. Furthermore, the development of reactors requires non-corrosive materials, which are usually expensive and makes the process highly uneconomical. Similarly, SE and AFE also need expensive reactor materials that can increase the overall cost of bio-oil upgrading. The treated biomass further requires drying of the biomass prior to pyrolysis, which is an energy-intensive step and increases the overall operating costs.

For chemical treatments, including acid and alkali treatments, the disposal of the leachate is a great challenge since it contains toxic metals. Therefore, further treatment of the leachate to remove toxic metals would increase the cost of the process. Alternatively, the leachate also contains a small amount of sugars, which could be converted into value-added chemicals or bioethanol using biochemical processes. In this regard, various microorganisms could be potentially applied for the conversion of sugars into bioethanol or other value-added chemicals. The acid and alkali treatment of biomass have shown significant changes in the biomass structure and removal of inorganic minerals, alkali, and alkali earth metals, but no studies have provided sufficient evidence to understand the reaction mechanisms between the acidic or alkaline chemical and different linkages present between the biomass constituents. Therefore, more studies should be conducted to examine the chemical reactions and kinetics during the process, which could help understand the removal mechanism of inorganic species and the effect of chemicals on the biomass structure. On the other hand, the biological pre-treatment of biomass could be time-consuming as microorganisms take a longer time to decompose the biomass. In addition, very few microorganisms have been known for pre-treatment of biomass. Hence, more studies are required to explore the application of microorganisms for biomass treatment and its effect on bio-oil upgrading.

To obtain the bio-oil with higher carbon and hydrogen content and higher calorific value, biomass pre-treatment methods have been combined with catalytic pyrolysis producing a substantial increase in the amount of aliphatic and aromatic hydrocarbons in the bio-oil and consequently in the total carbon yield. However, catalytic pyrolysis has been coupled with mainly DT and WT, while limited studies have been carried out using catalytic pyrolysis combined with SE and AFE, HWE, and biologically pre-treated biomass [207,208]. Thus, more studies should be carried out using an integrated process to optimize the process parameters of bio-oil upgrading.

As discussed in this article, a number of approaches and some other downstream upgrading methods, like emulsification and solvent addition, have been used for bio-oil upgrading [20,40,43]. Subsequently, the upgraded bio-oil has been tested for different applications, and the demonstrations suggest that the bio-oil has a great potential to serve as a fuel in turbines, boilers, and diesel engines for heat and power generation [37,209,210]. However, some modifications are still required in the combustion units or mixing the bio-oil with solvents, like ethanol, methanol, or diesel fuel, to avoid the ignition time delay. On the other hand, bio-oil application as a transport fuel needs further investigation. The lower heating values, chemical instability and other poor physical properties currently restrict its use in internal combustion engines. The bio-oil upgrading to a suitable transport fuel needs the complete removal of oxygenated compounds and the presence of naphthenes, paraffins, and aromatic hydrocarbons, and the other physical properties should also be improved to make it a realistic drop-in fuel. Besides, the production of bio-oil at a large scale, similar to the cost of conventional fuels, is one of the key challenges to overcome in order to make bio-oil economical and affordable to consumers.

8.7 CONCLUSIONS

This review article comprehensively discussed the various physicochemical methods to improve the bio-oil properties, mainly based on biomass pre-treatment. The physical and thermal methods are mainly employed to improve the biomass structure and increase the amount of atomic carbon, which plays a significant role in the pyrolysis kinetics, bio-oil yield, and bio-oil quality. For example, grinding is used to reduce the feedstock size to improve the heat flow between the substrates and decrease the degree of polymerization and crystallinity of the biomass components during the pyrolysis process, which, in turn, affects the yield and composition of the bio-oil compounds. Densification changes the density, moisture content, durability index, and energy contents of the biomass, which can also affect the pyrolysis product distribution, heating, and mass transfer efficiencies of the pyrolysis process. Torrefaction improves the biomass structure to produce better-quality biofuels and improves the economic feasibility of the pyrolysis process. During the torrefaction process, the fibrous structure and tenacity of the biomass are changed, which could help decrease the activation energy for the pyrolysis process and has shown positive results to improve the bio-oil quality, such as reduction in oxygen content, and increase in the heating value and amount of hydrocarbons in the bio-oil. Biomass pre-treatment with dilute acidic and alkaline chemicals and hot water extraction has shown advantageous results in eliminating the inorganic minerals and simultaneously improving the bio-oil quality. In addition, the acid pre-treatment of the biomass also causes significant changes in its structure and increases its average pore diameter and energy density. On the other hand, biological treatment with white rot fungi can improve the pyrolysis process's overall biomass conversion efficiency and has been shown to enhance the number of hydrocarbons in the bio-oil compared to the untreated biomass.

The integration of catalytic pyrolysis with pre-treatment techniques has proved to be a highly significant approach to converting the low-energy-density oxygenated compounds into high-energy-density aliphatic and aromatic hydrocarbons, thereby considerably increasing the bio-oil quality. Although biomass pre-treatment methods could prove advantageous for bio-oil upgrading, there are also certain challenges related to their applications. For example, the physical methods are energy-intensive, and chemical methods, such as SE and AFE, require expensive reactor materials, making the bio-oil upgrading an uneconomical approach. The chemical methods of acid and alkali biomass treatment result in toxic leachate and require another step in the process, while the biological methods are time-consuming. Therefore, more research should be carried out to overcome the key challenges related to the pre-treatment methods and make the bio-oil upgrading technique more efficient and cost-effective. Particularly, novel designs of reactors with less expensive materials should be invented for WT, SE and AFE, and different approaches should be adopted to convert the low-energy density oxygenated compounds into high-energy density hydrocarbons and make the bio-oil a realistic drop-in fuel.

8.8 ACKNOWLEDGMENTS

This article is reproduced from R. Kumar, V. Strezov, H. Weldekidan, J. He, S. Singh, T. Kan, B. Dastjerdi, Lignocellulose biomass pyrolysis for bio-oil production: A review of biomass pre-treatment methods for production of drop-in fuels, Renewable and Sustainable Energy Reviews, 123, 109763, 2020, with copyright license permission from Elsevier, license number 5334000377742.

REFERENCES

[1] Capuano DL. International Energy Outlook 2018 (IEO2018) 2000:21.
[2] Kumar R, Kumar P. Future microbial applications for bioenergy production: a perspective. *Frontiers in Microbiology* 2017;8. https://doi.org/10.3389/fmicb.2017.00450.
[3] Kumar R, Singh L, Zularisam AW, Hai FI. Microbial fuel cell is emerging as a versatile technology: a review on its possible applications, challenges and strategies to improve the performances: microbial fuel cell is emerging as a versatile technology. *International Journal of Energy Research* 2018;42:369–394. https://doi.org/10.1002/er.3780.
[4] Bar-On YM, Phillips R, Milo R. The biomass distribution on earth. *Proceedings of the National Academy of Sciences* 2018;115:6506–6511. https://doi.org/10.1073/pnas.1711842115.
[5] Kumar R, Strezov V, Lovell E, Kan T, Weldekidan H, He J, et al. Bio-oil upgrading with catalytic pyrolysis of biomass using Copper/zeolite-Nickel/zeolite and Copper-Nickel/zeolite catalysts. *Bioresource Technology* 2019. https://doi.org/10.1016/j.biortech.2019.01.067.
[6] Mohan D, Pittman, CU, Steele PH. Pyrolysis of wood/biomass for bio-oil: a critical review. *Energy & Fuels* 2006;20:848–889. https://doi.org/10.1021/ef0502397.
[7] Yang H, Yan R, Chen H, Lee DH, Zheng C. Characteristics of hemicellulose, cellulose and lignin pyrolysis. *Fuel* 2007;86:1781–1788. https://doi.org/10.1016/j.fuel.2006.12.013.

[8] Kan T, Strezov V, Evans TJ. Lignocellulosic biomass pyrolysis: a review of product properties and effects of pyrolysis parameters. *Renewable and Sustainable Energy Reviews* 2016;57:1126–1140. https://doi.org/10.1016/j.rser.2015.12.185.

[9] Wang L, Liao C. Mechanism study of cellulose rapid pyrolysis. *Industrial & Engineering Chemistry Research* 2004;43:5605–5610. https://doi.org/10.1021/ie030774z.

[10] Kumar R, Strezov V, Kan T, Weldekidan H, He J. Investigating the effect of Cu/zeolite on deoxygenation of bio-oil from pyrolysis of pine wood. *Energy Procedia* 2019;160:186–193. https://doi.org/10.1016/j.egypro.2019.02.135.

[11] Weldekidan H, Strezov V, Town G. Review of solar energy for biofuel extraction. *Renewable and Sustainable Energy Reviews* 2018;88:184–192. https://doi.org/10.1016/j.rser.2018.02.027.

[12] Alonso DM, Wettstein SG, Dumesic JA. Bimetallic catalysts for upgrading of biomass to fuels and chemicals. *Chemical Society Reviews* 2012;41:8075. https://doi.org/10.1039/c2cs35188a.

[13] Ennaert T, Van Aelst J, Dijkmans J, De Clercq R, Schutyser W, Dusselier M, et al. Potential and challenges of zeolite chemistry in the catalytic conversion of biomass. *Chemical Society Reviews* 2016;45:584–611. https://doi.org/10.1039/C5CS00859J.

[14] Kabir G, Hameed BH. Recent progress on catalytic pyrolysis of lignocellulosic biomass to high-grade bio-oil and bio-chemicals. *Renewable and Sustainable Energy Reviews* 2017;70:945–967. https://doi.org/10.1016/j.rser.2016.12.001.

[15] Rahman MdM, Liu R, Cai J. Catalytic fast pyrolysis of biomass over zeolites for high quality bio-oil – a review. *Fuel Processing Technology* 2018;180:32–46. https://doi.org/10.1016/j.fuproc.2018.08.002.

[16] Zacher AH, Olarte MV, Santosa DM, Elliott DC, Jones SB. A review and perspective of recent bio-oil hydrotreating research. *Green Chemistry* 2014;16:491–515. https://doi.org/10.1039/C3GC41382A.

[17] Wang S, Dai G, Yang H, Luo Z. Lignocellulosic biomass pyrolysis mechanism: a state-of-the-art review. *Progress in Energy and Combustion Science* 2017;62:33–86. https://doi.org/10.1016/j.pecs.2017.05.004.

[18] Iliopoulou EF, Triantafyllidis KS, Lappas AA. Overview of catalytic upgrading of biomass pyrolysis vapors toward the production of fuels and high-value chemicals. *Wiley Interdisciplinary Reviews: Energy and Environment* 2018;e322. https://doi.org/10.1002/wene.322.

[19] Chen D, Zhou J, Zhang Q, Zhu X. Evaluation methods and research progresses in bio-oil storage stability. *Renewable and Sustainable Energy Reviews* 2014;40:69–79. https://doi.org/10.1016/j.rser.2014.07.159.

[20] Leng L, Li H, Yuan X, Zhou W, Huang H. Bio-oil upgrading by emulsification/microemulsification: a review. *Energy* 2018;161:214–232. https://doi.org/10.1016/j.energy.2018.07.117.

[21] Dai L, Wang Y, Liu Y, Ruan R, He C, Yu Z, et al. Integrated process of lignocellulosic biomass torrefaction and pyrolysis for upgrading bio-oil production: a state-of-the-art review. *Renewable and Sustainable Energy Reviews* 2019;107:20–36. https://doi.org/10.1016/j.rser.2019.02.015.

[22] Tumuluru JS, Wright CT, Hess JR, Kenney KL. A review of biomass densification systems to develop uniform feedstock commodities for bioenergy application. *Biofuels, Bioproducts and Biorefining* 2011;5:683–707. https://doi.org/10.1002/bbb.324.

[23] Yao X, Zhang L, Li L, Liu L, Cao Y, Dong X, et al. Investigation of the structure, acidity, and catalytic performance of CuO/Ti0.95Ce0.05O2 catalyst for the selective catalytic reduction of NO by NH_3 at low temperature. *Applied Catalysis B: Environmental* 2014;150–151:315–329. https://doi.org/10.1016/j.apcatb.2013.12.007.

[24] Ennaert T, Schutyser W, Dijkmans J, Dusselier M, Sels BF. Conversion of biomass to chemicals. In: *Zeolites and Zeolite-Like Materials*, Elsevier, 2016; pp. 371–431. https://doi.org/10.1016/B978-0-444-63506-8.00010-0.

Lignocellulose Biomass Pyrolysis for Bio-Oil Production 185

[25] Neumann J, Meyer J, Ouadi M, Apfelbacher A, Binder S, Hornung A. The conversion of anaerobic digestion waste into biofuels via a novel thermo-catalytic reforming process. *Waste Management* 2016;47:141–148. https://doi.org/10.1016/j.wasman.2015.07.001.

[26] Liu W-J, Li W-W, Jiang H, Yu H-Q. Fates of chemical elements in biomass during its pyrolysis. *Chemical Reviews* 2017;117:6367–6398. https://doi.org/10.1021/acs.chemrev.6b00647.

[27] Dhyani V, Bhaskar T. A comprehensive review on the pyrolysis of lignocellulosic biomass. *Renewable Energy* 2018;129:695–716. https://doi.org/10.1016/j.renene.2017.04.035.

[28] Zhang J, Choi YS, Yoo CG, Kim TH, Brown RC, Shanks BH. Cellulose–hemicellulose and cellulose–lignin interactions during fast pyrolysis. *ACS Sustainable Chemistry & Engineering* 2015;3:293–301. https://doi.org/10.1021/sc500664h.

[29] Jin Z, Katsumata KS, Lam TBT, Iiyama K. Covalent linkages between cellulose and lignin in cell walls of coniferous and nonconiferous woods. *Biopolymers* 2006;83:103–110. https://doi.org/10.1002/bip.20533.

[30] Zhao S, Liu M, Zhao L, Zhu L. Influence of interactions among three biomass components on the pyrolysis behavior. *Industrial & Engineering Chemistry Research* 2018;57:5241–5249. https://doi.org/10.1021/acs.iecr.8b00593.

[31] Zhang J, Choi YS, Yoo CG, Kim TH, Brown RC, Shanks BH. Cellulose–hemicellulose and cellulose–lignin interactions during fast pyrolysis. *ACS Sustainable Chemistry & Engineering* 2015;3:293–301. https://doi.org/10.1021/sc500664h.

[32] Wu S, Shen D, Hu J, Zhang H, Xiao R. Cellulose-lignin interactions during fast pyrolysis with different temperatures and mixing methods. *Biomass and Bioenergy* 2016;90:209–217. https://doi.org/10.1016/j.biombioe.2016.04.012.

[33] Volpe R, Zabaniotou AA, Skoulou V. Synergistic effects between lignin and cellulose during pyrolysis of agricultural waste. *Energy & Fuels* 2018;32:8420–8430. https://doi.org/10.1021/acs.energyfuels.8b00767.

[34] Yu J, Paterson N, Blamey J, Millan M. Cellulose, xylan and lignin interactions during pyrolysis of lignocellulosic biomass. *Fuel* 2017;191:140–149. https://doi.org/10.1016/j.fuel.2016.11.057.

[35] Hosoya T, Kawamoto H, Saka S. Pyrolysis behaviors of wood and its constituent polymers at gasification temperature. *Journal of Analytical and Applied Pyrolysis* 2007;78:328–336. https://doi.org/10.1016/j.jaap.2006.08.008.

[36] Martin JA, Mullen CA, Boateng AA. Maximizing the stability of pyrolysis oil/diesel fuel emulsions. *Energy & Fuels* 2014;28:5918–5929. https://doi.org/10.1021/ef5015583.

[37] Czernik S, Bridgwater AV. Overview of applications of biomass fast pyrolysis oil. *Energy & Fuels* 2004;18:590–598. https://doi.org/10.1021/ef034067u.

[38] Jiang X, Ellis N. Upgrading bio-oil through emulsification with biodiesel: mixture production. *Energy & Fuels* 2010;24:1358–1364. https://doi.org/10.1021/ef9010669.

[39] Farooq A, Shafaghat H, Jae J, Jung S-C, Park Y-K. Enhanced stability of bio-oil and diesel fuel emulsion using Span 80 and Tween 60 emulsifiers. *Journal of Environmental Management* 2019;231:694–700. https://doi.org/10.1016/j.jenvman.2018.10.098.

[40] Zhang M, Yewe-Siang Lee Shee We M, Wu H. Direct emulsification of crude glycerol and bio-oil without addition of surfactant via ultrasound and mechanical agitation. *Fuel* 2018;227:183–189. https://doi.org/10.1016/j.fuel.2018.04.099.

[41] Choi JH, Kim S-S, Ly HV, Kim J, Woo HC. Effects of water-washing Saccharina japonica on fast pyrolysis in a bubbling fluidized-bed reactor. *Biomass and Bioenergy* 2017;98:112–123. https://doi.org/10.1016/j.biombioe.2017.01.006.

[42] Hassan EM, Steele PH, Ingram L. Characterization of fast pyrolysis bio-oils produced from pretreated pine wood. *Applied Biochemistry and Biotechnology* 2009;154:3–13. https://doi.org/10.1007/s12010-008-8445-3.

[43] Wang H, Srinivasan R, Yu F, Steele P, Li Q, Mitchell B. Effect of acid, alkali, and steam explosion pretreatments on characteristics of bio-oil produced from pinewood. *Energy & Fuels* 2011;25:3758–3764. https://doi.org/10.1021/ef2004909.

[44] Wang H, Srinivasan R, Yu F, Steele P, Li Q, Mitchell B, et al. Effect of acid, steam explosion, and size reduction pretreatments on bio-oil production from sweetgum, switchgrass, and corn stover. *Applied Biochemistry and Biotechnology* 2012;167:285–297. https://doi.org/10.1007/s12010-012-9678-8.

[45] Choi J, Choi J-W, Suh DJ, Ha J-M, Hwang JW, Jung HW, et al. Production of brown algae pyrolysis oils for liquid biofuels depending on the chemical pretreatment methods. *Energy Conversion and Management* 2014;86:371–378. https://doi.org/10.1016/j.enconman.2014.04.094.

[46] Xu X, Li Z, Sun Y, Jiang E, Huang L. High-quality fuel from the upgrading of heavy bio-oil by the combination of ultrasonic treatment and mutual solvent. *Energy & Fuels* 2018;32:3477–3487. https://doi.org/10.1021/acs.energyfuels.7b03483.

[47] Pidtasang B, Udomsap P, Sukkasi S, Chollacoop N, Pattiya A. Influence of alcohol addition on properties of bio-oil produced from fast pyrolysis of eucalyptus bark in a free-fall reactor. *Journal of Industrial and Engineering Chemistry* 2013;19:1851–1857. https://doi.org/10.1016/j.jiec.2013.02.031.

[48] Zhang L, Liu R, Yin R, Mei Y, Cai J. Optimization of a mixed additive and its effect on physicochemical properties of bio-oil. *Chemical Engineering & Technology* 2014;37:1181–1190. https://doi.org/10.1002/ceat.201300786.

[49] Zhang M, Wu H. Phase behavior and fuel properties of bio-oil/glycerol/methanol blends. *Energy & Fuels* 2014;28:4650–4656. https://doi.org/10.1021/ef501176z.

[50] Zhu L, Li K, Ding H, Zhu X. Studying on properties of bio-oil by adding blended additive during aging. *Fuel* 2018;211:704–711. https://doi.org/10.1016/j.fuel.2017.09.106.

[51] Meng J, Moore A, Tilotta D, Kelley S, Park S. Toward understanding of bio-oil aging: accelerated aging of bio-oil fractions. *ACS Sustainable Chemistry & Engineering* 2014;2:2011–2018. https://doi.org/10.1021/sc500223e.

[52] Li H, Xia S, Ma P. Upgrading fast pyrolysis oil: solvent–anti-solvent extraction and blending with diesel. *Energy Conversion and Management* 2016;110:378–385. https://doi.org/10.1016/j.enconman.2015.11.043.

[53] Zhu L, Li K, Zhang Y, Zhu X. Upgrading the storage properties of bio-oil by adding a compound additive. *Energy & Fuels* 2017;31:6221–6227. https://doi.org/10.1021/acs.energyfuels.7b00864.

[54] Mei Y, Liu R, Wu W, Zhang L. Effect of hot vapor filter temperature on mass yield, energy balance, and properties of products of the fast pyrolysis of pine sawdust. *Energy & Fuels* 2016;30:10458–10469. https://doi.org/10.1021/acs.energyfuels.6b01877.

[55] Elliott DC, Wang H, French R, Deutch S, Iisa K. Hydrocarbon liquid production from biomass via hot-vapor-filtered fast pyrolysis and catalytic hydroprocessing of the bio-oil. *Energy & Fuels* 2014;28:5909–5917. https://doi.org/10.1021/ef501536j.

[56] Sundaram V, Muthukumarappan K, Gent S. Understanding the Impacts of AFEX™ pretreatment and densification on the fast pyrolysis of corn stover, prairie cord grass, and switchgrass. *Applied Biochemistry and Biotechnology* 2017;181:1060–1079. https://doi.org/10.1007/s12010-016-2269-3.

[57] Mohammed IY, Abakr YA, Kazi FK, Yusuf S. Effects of pretreatments of Napier grass with deionized water, sulfuric acid and sodium hydroxide on pyrolysis oil characteristics. *Waste and Biomass Valorization* 2017;8:755–773. https://doi.org/10.1007/s12649-016-9594-1.

[58] Yang Z, Kumar A, Huhnke RL. Review of recent developments to improve storage and transportation stability of bio-oil. *Renewable and Sustainable Energy Reviews* 2015;50:859–870. https://doi.org/10.1016/j.rser.2015.05.025.

[59] Alvira P, Tomás-Pejó E, Ballesteros M, Negro MJ. Pretreatment technologies for an efficient bioethanol production process based on enzymatic hydrolysis: a review. *Bioresource Technology* 2010;101:4851–4861. https://doi.org/10.1016/j.biortech.2009.11.093.

[60] Kersten SRA, Wang X, Prins W, van Swaaij WPM. Biomass pyrolysis in a fluidized bed reactor. Part 1: literature review and model simulations. *Industrial & Engineering Chemistry Research* 2005;44:8773–8785. https://doi.org/10.1021/ie0504856.

[61] Shen J, Wang X-S, Garcia-Perez M, Mourant D, Rhodes MJ, Li C-Z. Effects of particle size on the fast pyrolysis of oil mallee woody biomass. *Fuel* 2009;88:1810–1817. https://doi.org/10.1016/j.fuel.2009.05.001.

[62] Abnisa F, Daud WMAW, Husin WNW, Sahu JN. Utilization possibilities of palm shell as a source of biomass energy in Malaysia by producing bio-oil in pyrolysis process. *Biomass and Bioenergy* 2011;35:1863–1872. https://doi.org/10.1016/j.biombioe.2011.01.033.

[63] Garg R, Anand N, Kumar D. Pyrolysis of babool seeds (Acacia nilotica) in a fixed bed reactor and bio-oil characterization. *Renewable Energy* 2016;96:167–171. https://doi.org/10.1016/j.renene.2016.04.059.

[64] Raja SA, Kennedy ZR, Pillai BC, Lee CLR. Flash pyrolysis of Jatropha oil cake in electrically heated fluidized bed reactor. *Energy* 2010;35:2819–2823. https://doi.org/10.1016/j.energy.2010.03.011.

[65] Yin C. Microwave-assisted pyrolysis of biomass for liquid biofuels production. *Bioresource Technology* 2012;120:273–284. https://doi.org/10.1016/j.biortech.2012.06.016.

[66] Wright MM, Satrio JA, Brown RC, University IS. Techno-economic analysis of biomass fast pyrolysis to transportation fuels. *Renewable Energy* 2010:73.

[67] Rezaei H, Yazdanpanah F, Lim CJ, Lau A, Sokhansanj S. Pyrolysis of ground pine chip and ground pellet particles. *The Canadian Journal of Chemical Engineering* 2016;94:1863–1871. https://doi.org/10.1002/cjce.22574.

[68] Mani S, Tabil LG, Sokhansanj S. Effects of compressive force, particle size and moisture content on mechanical properties of biomass pellets from grasses. *Biomass and Bioenergy* 2006;30:648–654. https://doi.org/10.1016/j.biombioe.2005.01.004.

[69] Karkania V, Fanara E, Zabaniotou A. Review of sustainable biomass pellets production – a study for agricultural residues pellets' market in Greece. *Renewable and Sustainable Energy Reviews* 2012;16:1426–1436. https://doi.org/10.1016/j.rser.2011.11.028.

[70] Di Blasi C, Branca C, Lombardi V, Ciappa P, Di Giacomo C. Effects of particle size and density on the packed-bed pyrolysis of wood. *Energy & Fuels* 2013;27:6781–6791. https://doi.org/10.1021/ef401481j.

[71] Demirbas A. Effects of temperature and particle size on bio-char yield from pyrolysis of agricultural residues. *Journal of Analytical and Applied Pyrolysis* 2004;72:243–248. https://doi.org/10.1016/j.jaap.2004.07.003.

[72] Zeng K, Soria J, Gauthier D, Mazza G, Flamant G. Modeling of beech wood pellet pyrolysis under concentrated solar radiation. *Renewable Energy* 2016;99:721–729. https://doi.org/10.1016/j.renene.2016.07.051.

[73] Chen D, Zheng Z, Fu K, Zeng Z, Wang J, Lu M. Torrefaction of biomass stalk and its effect on the yield and quality of pyrolysis products. *Fuel* 2015;159:27–32. https://doi.org/10.1016/j.fuel.2015.06.078.

[74] Meng J, Park J, Tilotta D, Park S. The effect of torrefaction on the chemistry of fast-pyrolysis bio-oil. *Bioresource Technology* 2012;111:439–446. https://doi.org/10.1016/j.biortech.2012.01.159.

[75] Bert V, Allemon J, Sajet P, Dieu S, Papin A, Collet S, et al. Torrefaction and pyrolysis of metal-enriched poplars from phytotechnologies: effect of temperature and biomass chlorine content on metal distribution in end-products and valorization options. *Biomass and Bioenergy* 2017;96:1–11. https://doi.org/10.1016/j.biombioe.2016.11.003.

[76] Chen D, Gao A, Cen K, Zhang J, Cao X, Ma Z. Investigation of biomass torrefaction based on three major components: hemicellulose, cellulose, and lignin. *Energy Conversion and Management* 2018;169:228–237. https://doi.org/10.1016/j.enconman.2018.05.063.

[77] Wang S, Dai G, Ru B, Zhao Y, Wang X, Zhou J, et al. Effects of torrefaction on hemicellulose structural characteristics and pyrolysis behaviors. *Bioresource Technology* 2016;218:1106–1114. https://doi.org/10.1016/j.biortech.2016.07.075.

[78] Wang S, Dai G, Ru B, Zhao Y, Wang X, Xiao G, et al. Influence of torrefaction on the characteristics and pyrolysis behavior of cellulose. *Energy* 2017;120:864–871. https://doi.org/10.1016/j.energy.2016.11.135.

[79] Zheng A, Jiang L, Zhao Z, Huang Z, Zhao K, Wei G, et al. Impact of torrefaction on the chemical structure and catalytic fast pyrolysis behavior of hemicellulose, lignin, and cellulose. *Energy & Fuels* 2015;29:8027–8034. https://doi.org/10.1021/acs.energyfuels.5b01765.

[80] Kumagai S, Matsuno R, Grause G, Kameda T, Yoshioka T. Enhancement of bio-oil production via pyrolysis of wood biomass by pretreatment with H_2SO_4. *Bioresource Technology* 2015;178:76–82. https://doi.org/10.1016/j.biortech.2014.09.146.

[81] Uemura Y, Omar W, Othman NA, Yusup S, Tsutsui T. Torrefaction of oil palm EFB in the presence of oxygen. *Fuel* 2013;103:156–160. https://doi.org/10.1016/j.fuel.2011.11.018.

[82] Gogoi D, Bordoloi N, Goswami R, Narzari R, Saikia R, Sut D, et al. Effect of torrefaction on yield and quality of pyrolytic products of arecanut husk: an agroprocessing wastes. *Bioresource Technology* 2017;242:36–44. https://doi.org/10.1016/j.biortech.2017.03.169.

[83] Ren S, Lei H, Wang L, Bu Q, Wei Y, Liang J, et al. Microwave torrefaction of *Douglas fir* sawdust pellets. *Energy & Fuels* 2012;26:5936–5943. https://doi.org/10.1021/ef300633c.

[84] Ren S, Lei H, Wang L, Bu Q, Chen S, Wu J, et al. The effects of torrefaction on compositions of bio-oil and syngas from biomass pyrolysis by microwave heating. *Bioresource Technology* 2013;135:659–664. https://doi.org/10.1016/j.biortech.2012.06.091.

[85] Zheng Y, Tao L, Yang X, Huang Y, Liu C, Gu J, et al. Effect of the torrefaction temperature on the structural properties and pyrolysis behavior of biomass. *BioResources* 2017;12. https://doi.org/10.15376/biores.12.2.3425-3447.

[86] Ukaew S, Schoenborn J, Klemetsrud B, Shonnard DR. Effects of torrefaction temperature and acid pretreatment on the yield and quality of fast pyrolysis bio—oil from rice straw. *Journal of Analytical and Applied Pyrolysis* 2018;129:112–122. https://doi.org/10.1016/j.jaap.2017.11.021.

[87] Zheng A, Zhao Z, Huang Z, Zhao K, Wei G, Wang X, et al. Catalytic fast pyrolysis of biomass pretreated by torrefaction with varying severity. *Energy & Fuels* 2014;28:5804–5811. https://doi.org/10.1021/ef500892k.

[88] Dong Q, Zhang S, Ding K, Zhu S, Zhang H, Liu X. Pyrolysis behavior of raw/torrefied rice straw after different demineralization processes. *Biomass and Bioenergy* 2018;119:229–236. https://doi.org/10.1016/j.biombioe.2018.09.032.

[89] Isemin R, Klimov D, Larina O, Sytchev G, Zaichenko V, Milovanov O. Application of torrefaction for recycling bio-waste formed during anaerobic digestion. *Fuel* 2019;243:230–239. https://doi.org/10.1016/j.fuel.2019.01.119.

[90] González Martínez M, Dupont C, da Silva Perez D, Míguez-Rodríguez L, Grateau M, Thiéry S, et al. Assessing the suitability of recovering shrub biowaste involved in wildland fires in the South of Europe through torrefaction mobile units. *Journal of Environmental Management* 2019;236:551–560. https://doi.org/10.1016/j.jenvman.2019.02.019.

[91] Talero G, Rincón S, Gómez A. Biomass torrefaction in a standard retort: a study on oil palm solid residues. *Fuel* 2019;244:366–378. https://doi.org/10.1016/j.fuel.2019.02.008.

[92] Kumar SR, Sarkar A, Chakraborty JP. Effect of torrefaction on the physicochemical properties of pigeon pea stalk (Cajanus cajan) and estimation of kinetic parameters. *Renewable Energy* 2019;138:805–819. https://doi.org/10.1016/j.renene.2019.02.022.

Lignocellulose Biomass Pyrolysis for Bio-Oil Production

[93] Ren S, Lei H, Zhang Y, Wang L, Bu Q, Wei Y, et al. Furfural production from microwave catalytic torrefaction of Douglas fir sawdust. *Journal of Analytical and Applied Pyrolysis* 2019;138:188–195. https://doi.org/10.1016/j.jaap.2018.12.023.

[94] Budde PK, Megha R, Patel R, Pandey J. Investigating effects of temperature on fuel properties of torrefied biomass for bio-energy systems. *Energy Sources, Part A: Recovery, Utilization, and Environmental Effects* 2019;41:1140–1148. https://doi.org/10.1080/15567036.2018.1544992.

[95] Wang X, Wu J, Chen Y, Pattiya A, Yang H, Chen H. Comparative study of wet and dry torrefaction of corn stalk and the effect on biomass pyrolysis polygeneration. *Bioresource Technology* 2018;258:88–97. https://doi.org/10.1016/j.biortech.2018.02.114.

[96] Zeng K, Yang Q, Zhang Y, Mei Y, Wang X, Yang H, et al. Influence of torrefaction with Mg-based additives on the pyrolysis of cotton stalk. *Bioresource Technology* 2018;261:62–69. https://doi.org/10.1016/j.biortech.2018.03.094.

[97] Natarajan P, Suriapparao DV, Vinu R. Microwave torrefaction of Prosopis juliflora: experimental and modeling study. *Fuel Processing Technology* 2018;172:86–96. https://doi.org/10.1016/j.fuproc.2017.12.007.

[98] Rago YP, Surroop D, Mohee R. Assessing the potential of biofuel (biochar) production from food wastes through thermal treatment. *Bioresource Technology* 2018;248:258–264. https://doi.org/10.1016/j.biortech.2017.06.108.

[99] Xin S, Mi T, Liu X, Huang F. Effect of torrefaction on the pyrolysis characteristics of high moisture herbaceous residues. *Energy* 2018;152:586–593. https://doi.org/10.1016/j.energy.2018.03.104.

[100] Chen W-H, Wang C-W, Kumar G, Rousset P, Hsieh T-H. Effect of torrefaction pretreatment on the pyrolysis of rubber wood sawdust analyzed by Py-GC/MS. *Bioresource Technology* 2018;259:469–473. https://doi.org/10.1016/j.biortech.2018.03.033.

[101] Zheng A, Jiang L, Zhao Z, Huang Z, Zhao K, Wei G, et al. Impact of torrefaction on the chemical structure and catalytic fast pyrolysis behavior of hemicellulose, lignin, and cellulose. *Energy Fuels* 2015;29:8027–8034. https://doi.org/10.1021/acs.energyfuels.5b01765.

[102] Chen Y, Yang H, Yang Q, Hao H, Zhu B, Chen H. Torrefaction of agriculture straws and its application on biomass pyrolysis poly-generation. *Bioresource Technology* 2014;156:70–77. https://doi.org/10.1016/j.biortech.2013.12.088.

[103] Branca C, Di Blasi C, Galgano A, Broström M. Effects of the torrefaction conditions on the fixed-bed pyrolysis of Norway spruce. *Energy & Fuels* 2014;28:5882–5891. https://doi.org/10.1021/ef501395b.

[104] Zheng A, Zhao Z, Chang S, Huang Z, He F, Li H. Effect of torrefaction temperature on product distribution from two-staged pyrolysis of biomass. *Energy & Fuels* 2012;26:2968–2974. https://doi.org/10.1021/ef201872y.

[105] Carpenter D, Westover TL, Czernik S, Jablonski W. Biomass feedstocks for renewable fuel production: a review of the impacts of feedstock and pretreatment on the yield and product distribution of fast pyrolysis bio-oils and vapors. *Green Chemistry* 2014;16:384–406. https://doi.org/10.1039/C3GC41631C.

[106] Scott DS, Paterson L, Piskorz J, Radlein D. Pretreatment of poplar wood for fast pyrolysis: rate of cation removal. *Journal of Analytical and Applied Pyrolysis* 2001;57:169–176. https://doi.org/10.1016/S0165-2370(00)00108-X.

[107] Arora JS, Chew JW, Mushrif SH. Influence of alkali and alkaline-earth metals on the cleavage of glycosidic bond in biomass pyrolysis: a DFT study using cellobiose as a model compound. *The Journal of Physical Chemistry A* 2018;122:7646–7658. https://doi.org/10.1021/acs.jpca.8b06083.

[108] Mourant D, Wang Z, He M, Wang XS, Garcia-Perez M, Ling K, et al. Mallee wood fast pyrolysis: effects of alkali and alkaline earth metallic species on the yield and composition of bio-oil. *Fuel* 2011;90:2915–2922. https://doi.org/10.1016/j.fuel.2011.04.033.

[109] Garrido R, Reckamp J, Satrio J. Effects of pretreatments on yields, selectivity and properties of products from pyrolysis of Phragmites australis (common reeds). *Environments* 2017;4:96. https://doi.org/10.3390/environments4040096.

[110] Zhang S, Chen T, Xiong Y. Effect of washing pretreatment with aqueous fraction of bio-oil on pyrolysis characteristic of rice husk and preparation of Amorphous silica. *Waste and Biomass Valorization* 2018;9:861–869. https://doi.org/10.1007/s12649-017-9845-9.

[111] Cao B, Wang S, Hu Y, Abomohra AE-F, Qian L, He Z, et al. Effect of washing with diluted acids on Enteromorpha clathrata pyrolysis products: towards enhanced bio-oil from seaweeds. *Renewable Energy* 2019;138:29–38. https://doi.org/10.1016/j.renene.2019.01.084.

[112] Tan H, Wang S. Experimental study of the effect of acid-washing pretreatment on biomass pyrolysis. *Journal of Fuel Chemistry and Technology* 2009;37:668–672. https://doi.org/10.1016/S1872-5813(10)60014-X.

[113] David GF, Perez VH, Rodriguez Justo O, Garcia-Perez M. Effect of acid additives on sugarcane bagasse pyrolysis: production of high yields of sugars. *Bioresource Technology* 2017;223:74–83. https://doi.org/10.1016/j.biortech.2016.10.051.

[114] Wang X, Leng S, Bai J, Zhou H, Zhong X, Zhuang G, et al. Role of pretreatment with acid and base on the distribution of the products obtained via lignocellulosic biomass pyrolysis. *RSC Advances* 2015;5:24984–24989. https://doi.org/10.1039/C4RA15426F.

[115] Mei Y, Chai M, Shen C, Liu B, Liu R. Effect of methanol addition on properties and aging reaction mechanism of bio-oil during storage. *Fuel* 2019;244:499–507. https://doi.org/10.1016/j.fuel.2019.02.012.

[116] Baruah J, Nath BK, Sharma R, Kumar S, Deka RC, Baruah DC, et al. Recent trends in the pretreatment of lignocellulosic biomass for value-added products. *Frontiers in Energy Research* 2018;6:141. https://doi.org/10.3389/fenrg.2018.00141.

[117] Kim JS, Lee YY, Kim TH. A review on alkaline pretreatment technology for bioconversion of lignocellulosic biomass. *Bioresource Technology* 2016;199:42–48. https://doi.org/10.1016/j.biortech.2015.08.085.

[118] Zhou S, Brown RC, Bai X. The use of calcium hydroxide pretreatment to overcome agglomeration of technical lignin during fast pyrolysis. *Green Chemistry* 2015;17:4748–4759. https://doi.org/10.1039/C5GC01611H.

[119] Wang H, Srinivasan R, Yu F, Steele P, Li Q, Mitchell B. Effect of acid, alkali, and steam explosion pretreatments on characteristics of bio-oil produced from pinewood. *Energy & Fuels* 2011;25:3758–3764. https://doi.org/10.1021/ef2004909.

[120] Hassan EM, Steele PH, Ingram L. Characterization of fast pyrolysis bio-oils produced from pretreated pine wood. *Applied Biochemistry and Biotechnology* 2009;154:3–13. https://doi.org/10.1007/s12010-008-8445-3.

[121] Wang H, Srinivasan R, Yu F, Steele P, Li Q, Mitchell B, et al. Effect of acid, steam explosion, and size reduction pretreatments on bio-oil production from sweetgum, switchgrass, and corn stover. *Applied Biochemistry and Biotechnology* 2012;167:285–297. https://doi.org/10.1007/s12010-012-9678-8.

[122] Raveendran K, Ganesh A, Khilar KC. Influence of mineral matter on biomass pyrolysis characteristics. *Fuel* 1995;74:1812–1822. https://doi.org/10.1016/0016-2361(95)80013-8.

[123] Jae J, Tompsett GA, Lin Y-C, Carlson TR, Shen J, Zhang T, et al. Depolymerization of lignocellulosic biomass to fuel precursors: maximizing carbon efficiency by combining hydrolysis with pyrolysis. *Energy Environ Sci* 2010;3:358–365. https://doi.org/10.1039/B924621P.

[124] Misson M, Haron R, Kamaroddin MFA, Amin NAS. Pretreatment of empty palm fruit bunch for production of chemicals via catalytic pyrolysis. *Bioresource Technology* 2009;100:2867–2873. https://doi.org/10.1016/j.biortech.2008.12.060.

[125] Pittman CU, Mohan D, Eseyin A, Li Q, Ingram L, Hassan E-BM, et al. Characterization of bio-oils produced from fast pyrolysis of corn stalks in an auger reactor. *Energy Fuels* 2012;26:3816–3825. https://doi.org/10.1021/ef3003922.

Lignocellulose Biomass Pyrolysis for Bio-Oil Production

[126] Fahmi R, Bridgwater AV, Donnison I, Yates N, Jones JM. The effect of lignin and inorganic species in biomass on pyrolysis oil yields, quality and stability. *Fuel* 2008;87:1230–1240. https://doi.org/10.1016/j.fuel.2007.07.026.

[127] Das P, Ganesh A, Wangikar P. Influence of pretreatment for deashing of sugarcane bagasse on pyrolysis products. *Biomass and Bioenergy* 2004;27:445–457. https://doi.org/10.1016/j.biombioe.2004.04.002.

[128] Wigley T, Yip ACK, Pang S. Pretreating biomass via demineralisation and torrefaction to improve the quality of crude pyrolysis oil. *Energy* 2016;109:481–494. https://doi.org/10.1016/j.energy.2016.04.096.

[129] Chen D, Mei J, Li H, Li Y, Lu M, Ma T, et al. Combined pretreatment with torrefaction and washing using torrefaction liquid products to yield upgraded biomass and pyrolysis products. *Bioresource Technology* 2017;228:62–68. https://doi.org/10.1016/j.biortech.2016.12.088.

[130] Zhang S, Su Y, Xu D, Zhu S, Zhang H, Liu X. Effects of torrefaction and organic-acid leaching pretreatment on the pyrolysis behavior of rice husk. *Energy* 2018;149:804–813. https://doi.org/10.1016/j.energy.2018.02.110.

[131] Gong S-H, Im H-S, Um M, Lee H-W, Lee J-W. Enhancement of waste biomass fuel properties by sequential leaching and wet torrefaction. *Fuel* 2019;239:693–700. https://doi.org/10.1016/j.fuel.2018.11.069.

[132] Zhang D, Wang F, Zhang A, Yi W, Li Z, Shen X. Effect of pretreatment on chemical characteristic and thermal degradation behavior of corn stalk digestate: comparison of dry and wet torrefaction. *Bioresource Technology* 2019;275:239–246. https://doi.org/10.1016/j.biortech.2018.12.044.

[133] He C, Tang C, Li C, Yuan J, Tran K-Q, Bach Q-V, et al. Wet torrefaction of biomass for high quality solid fuel production: a review. *Renewable and Sustainable Energy Reviews* 2018;91:259–271. https://doi.org/10.1016/j.rser.2018.03.097.

[134] Hoekman SK, Broch A, Robbins C, Zielinska B, Felix L. Hydrothermal carbonization (HTC) of selected woody and herbaceous biomass feedstocks. *Biomass Conversion and Biorefinery* 2013;3:113–126. https://doi.org/10.1007/s13399-012-0066-y.

[135] Hoekman SK, Broch A, Robbins C. Hydrothermal carbonization (HTC) of lignocellulosic biomass. *Energy & Fuels* 2011;25:1802–1810. https://doi.org/10.1021/ef101745n.

[136] Chang S, Zhao Z, Zheng A, Li X, Wang X, Huang Z, et al. Effect of hydrothermal pretreatment on properties of bio-oil produced from fast pyrolysis of eucalyptus wood in a fluidized bed reactor. *Bioresource Technology* 2013;138:321–328. https://doi.org/10.1016/j.biortech.2013.03.170.

[137] Zhang S, Chen T, Xiong Y, Dong Q. Effects of wet torrefaction on the physicochemical properties and pyrolysis product properties of rice husk. *Energy Conversion and Management* 2017;141:403–409. https://doi.org/10.1016/j.enconman.2016.10.002.

[138] Tarves PC, Serapiglia MJ, Mullen CA, Boateng AA, Volk TA. Effects of hot water extraction pretreatment on pyrolysis of shrub willow. *Biomass and Bioenergy* 2017;107:299–304. https://doi.org/10.1016/j.biombioe.2017.10.024.

[139] Stephanidis S, Nitsos C, Kalogiannis K, Iliopoulou EF, Lappas AA, Triantafyllidis KS. Catalytic upgrading of lignocellulosic biomass pyrolysis vapours: effect of hydrothermal pre-treatment of biomass. *Catalysis Today* 2011;167:37–45. https://doi.org/10.1016/j.cattod.2010.12.049.

[140] Le Roux É, Chaouch M, Diouf PN, Stevanovic T. Impact of a pressurized hot water treatment on the quality of bio-oil produced from aspen. *Biomass and Bioenergy* 2015;81:202–209. https://doi.org/10.1016/j.biombioe.2015.07.005.

[141] Zheng A, Zhao Z, Chang S, Huang Z, Zhao K, Wei G, et al. Comparison of the effect of wet and dry torrefaction on chemical structure and pyrolysis behavior of corncobs. *Bioresource Technology* 2015;176:15–22. https://doi.org/10.1016/j.biortech.2014.10.157.

[142] Zeng K, He X, Yang H, Wang X, Chen H. The effect of combined pretreatments on the pyrolysis of corn stalk. *Bioresource Technology* 2019;281:309–317. https://doi.org/10.1016/j.biortech.2019.02.107.

[143] Su Y, Liu L, Dong Q, Xie Y, Wang P, Zhang S, et al. Investigation of molten salt in wet torrefaction and its effects on fast pyrolysis behaviors. *Energy Sources, Part A: Recovery, Utilization, and Environmental Effects* 2019;1–9. https://doi.org/10.1080/15567036.2019.1587104.

[144] Hu J, Jiang B, Wang J, Qiao Y, Zuo T, Sun Y, et al. Physicochemical characteristics and pyrolysis performance of corn stalk torrefied in aqueous ammonia by microwave heating. *Bioresource Technology* 2019;274:83–88. https://doi.org/10.1016/j.biortech.2018.11.076.

[145] Granados DA, Basu P, Nhuchhen DR, Chejne F. Investigation into torrefaction kinetics of biomass and combustion behaviors of raw, torrefied and char samples. *Biofuels* 2019;1–11. https://doi.org/10.1080/17597269.2018.1558837.

[146] Bach Q-V, Tran K-Q, Skreiberg Ø, Trinh TT. Effects of wet torrefaction on pyrolysis of woody biomass fuels. *Energy* 2015;88:443–456. https://doi.org/10.1016/j.energy.2015.05.062.

[147] Biswas AK, Umeki K, Yang W, Blasiak W. Change of pyrolysis characteristics and structure of woody biomass due to steam explosion pretreatment. *Fuel Processing Technology* 2011;92:1849–1854. https://doi.org/10.1016/j.fuproc.2011.04.038.

[148] Inagaki T, Siesler HW, Mitsui K, Tsuchikawa S. Difference of the crystal structure of cellulose in wood after hydrothermal and aging degradation: a NIR spectroscopy and XRD study. *Biomacromolecules* 2010;11:2300–2305. https://doi.org/10.1021/bm100403y.

[149] Li M-F, Shen Y, Sun J-K, Bian J, Chen C-Z, Sun R-C. Wet torrefaction of bamboo in hydrochloric acid solution by microwave heating. *ACS Sustainable Chemistry & Engineering* 2015;3:2022–2029. https://doi.org/10.1021/acssuschemeng.5b00296.

[150] Lynam JG, Coronella CJ, Yan W, Reza MT, Vasquez VR. Acetic acid and lithium chloride effects on hydrothermal carbonization of lignocellulosic biomass. *Bioresource Technology* 2011;102:6192–6199. https://doi.org/10.1016/j.biortech.2011.02.035.

[151] Xu X, Tu R, Sun Y, Wu Y, Jiang E, Zhen J. The influence of combined pretreatment with surfactant/ultrasonic and hydrothermal carbonization on fuel properties, pyrolysis and combustion behavior of corn stalk. *Bioresource Technology* 2019;271:427–438. https://doi.org/10.1016/j.biortech.2018.09.066.

[152] Kumar P, Barrett DM, Delwiche MJ, Stroeve P. Methods for pretreatment of lignocellulosic biomass for efficient hydrolysis and biofuel production. *Industrial & Engineering Chemistry Research* 2009;48:3713–3729. https://doi.org/10.1021/ie801542g.

[153] Balan V, Bals B, Chundawat SPS, Marshall D, Dale BE. Lignocellulosic biomass pretreatment using AFEX. In: Mielenz JR, editor. *Biofuels*, vol. 581, Totowa, NJ: Humana Press, 2009; pp. 61–77. https://doi.org/10.1007/978-1-60761-214-8_5.

[154] Chundawat SPS, Donohoe BS, da Costa Sousa L, Elder T, Agarwal UP, Lu F, et al. Multi-scale visualization and characterization of lignocellulosic plant cell wall deconstruction during thermochemical pretreatment. *Energy & Environmental Science* 2011;4:973. https://doi.org/10.1039/c0ee00574f.

[155] Jacquet N, Maniet G, Vanderghem C, Delvigne F, Richel A. Application of steam explosion as pretreatment on lignocellulosic material: a review. *Industrial & Engineering Chemistry Research* 2015;54:2593–2598. https://doi.org/10.1021/ie503151g.

[156] Deepa B, Abraham E, Cherian BM, Bismarck A, Blaker JJ, Pothan LA, et al. Structure, morphology and thermal characteristics of banana nano fibers obtained by steam explosion. *Bioresource Technology* 2011;102:1988–1997. https://doi.org/10.1016/j.biortech.2010.09.030.

[157] Shi W, Li S, Jia J, Zhao Y. Highly efficient conversion of cellulose to bio-oil in hot-compressed water with ultrasonic pretreatment. *Industrial & Engineering Chemistry Research* 2013;52:586–593. https://doi.org/10.1021/ie3024966.

[158] Tarves PC, Serapiglia MJ, Mullen CA, Boateng AA, Volk TA. Effects of hot water extraction pretreatment on pyrolysis of shrub willow. *Biomass and Bioenergy* 2017;107:299–304. https://doi.org/10.1016/j.biombioe.2017.10.024.

[159] Le Roux É, Diouf PN, Stevanovic T. Analytical pyrolysis of hot water pretreated forest biomass. *Journal of Analytical and Applied Pyrolysis* 2015;111:121–131. https://doi.org/10.1016/j.jaap.2014.11.023.

[160] Eisenbies MH, Volk TA, Amidon TE, Shi S. Influence of blending and hot water extraction on the quality of wood pellets. *Fuel* 2019;241:1058–1067. https://doi.org/10.1016/j.fuel.2018.12.120.

[161] Sindhu R, Binod P, Pandey A. Biological pretreatment of lignocellulosic biomass – an overview. *Bioresource Technology* 2016;199:76–82. https://doi.org/10.1016/j.biortech.2015.08.030.

[162] Vasco-Correa J, Ge X, Li Y. Biological pretreatment of lignocellulosic biomass. In: *Biomass Fractionation Technologies for a Lignocellulosic Feedstock Based Biorefinery*, Elsevier, 2016; pp. 561–585. https://doi.org/10.1016/B978-0-12-802323-5.00024-4.

[163] Yu Y, Zeng Y, Zuo J, Ma F, Yang X, Zhang X, et al. Improving the conversion of biomass in catalytic fast pyrolysis via white-rot fungal pretreatment. *Bioresource Technology* 2013;134:198–203. https://doi.org/10.1016/j.biortech.2013.01.167.

[164] Longe LF, Couvreur J, Leriche Grandchamp M, Garnier G, Allais F, Saito K. Importance of mediators for lignin degradation by fungal laccase. *ACS Sustainable Chemistry & Engineering* 2018;6:10097–10107. https://doi.org/10.1021/acssuschemeng.8b01426.

[165] Yang X, Ma F, Yu H, Zhang X, Chen S. Effects of biopretreatment of corn stover with white-rot fungus on low-temperature pyrolysis products. *Bioresource Technology* 2011;102:3498–3503. https://doi.org/10.1016/j.biortech.2010.11.021.

[166] You T, Li X, Wang R, Zhang X, Xu F. Effects of synergistic fungal pretreatment on structure and thermal properties of lignin from corncob. *Bioresource Technology* 2019;272:123–129. https://doi.org/10.1016/j.biortech.2018.09.145.

[167] Yan K, Liu F, Chen Q, Ke M, Huang X, Hu W, et al. Pyrolysis characteristics and kinetics of lignin derived from enzymatic hydrolysis residue of bamboo pretreated with white-rot fungus. *Biotechnology for Biofuels* 2016;9. https://doi.org/10.1186/s13068-016-0489-y.

[168] Agbor VB, Cicek N, Sparling R, Berlin A, Levin DB. Biomass pretreatment: fundamentals toward application. *Biotechnology Advances* 2011;29:675–685. https://doi.org/10.1016/j.biotechadv.2011.05.005.

[169] Adhikari S, Srinivasan V, Fasina O. Catalytic pyrolysis of raw and thermally treated lignin using different acidic zeolites. *Energy & Fuels* 2014;28:4532–4538. https://doi.org/10.1021/ef500902x.

[170] Ly HV, Choi JH, Woo HC, Kim S-S, Kim J. Upgrading bio-oil by catalytic fast pyrolysis of acid-washed Saccharina japonica alga in a fluidized-bed reactor. *Renewable Energy* 2019;133:11–22. https://doi.org/10.1016/j.renene.2018.09.103.

[171] Hoff TC, Gardner DW, Thilakaratne R, Wang K, Hansen TW, Brown RC, et al. Tailoring ZSM-5 zeolites for the fast pyrolysis of biomass to aromatic hydrocarbons. *ChemSusChem* 2016;9:1473–1482. https://doi.org/10.1002/cssc.201600186.

[172] Li X, Dong W, Zhang J, Shao S, Cai Y. Preparation of bio-oil derived from catalytic upgrading of biomass vacuum pyrolysis vapor over metal-loaded HZSM-5 zeolites. *Journal of the Energy Institute* 2019;S1743967119303599. https://doi.org/10.1016/j.joei.2019.06.005.

[173] Veses A, Puértolas B, López JM, Callén MS, Solsona B, García T. Promoting deoxygenation of bio-oil by metal-loaded hierarchical ZSM-5 zeolites. *ACS Sustainable Chemistry & Engineering* 2016;4:1653–1660. https://doi.org/10.1021/acssuschemeng.5b01606.

[174] Lee S, Lee M-G, Park J. Catalytic upgrading pyrolysis of pine sawdust for bio-oil with metal oxides. *J Mater Cycles Waste Manag* 2018;20:1553–1561. https://doi.org/10.1007/s10163-018-0716-7.

[175] Lin X, Zhang Z, Zhang Z, Sun J, Wang Q, Pittman CU. Catalytic fast pyrolysis of a wood-plastic composite with metal oxides as catalysts. *Waste Management* 2018;79:38–47. https://doi.org/10.1016/j.wasman.2018.07.021.

[176] Kumar R, Strezov V, Lovell E, Kan T, Weldekidan H, He J, et al. Enhanced bio-oil deoxygenation activity by Cu/zeolite and Ni/zeolite catalysts in combined in-situ and ex-situ biomass pyrolysis. *Journal of Analytical and Applied Pyrolysis* 2019. https://doi.org/10.1016/j.jaap.2019.03.008.

[177] Wang K, Johnston PA, Brown RC. Comparison of in-situ and ex-situ catalytic pyrolysis in a micro-reactor system. *Bioresource Technology* 2014;173:124–131. https://doi.org/10.1016/j.biortech.2014.09.097.

[178] Huang Y, Wei L, Crandall Z, Julson J, Gu Z. Combining Mo–Cu/HZSM-5 with a two-stage catalytic pyrolysis system for pine sawdust thermal conversion. *Fuel* 2015;150:656–663. https://doi.org/10.1016/j.fuel.2015.02.071.

[179] Hu C, Xiao R, Zhang H. Ex-situ catalytic fast pyrolysis of biomass over HZSM-5 in a two-stage fluidized-bed/fixed-bed combination reactor. *Bioresource Technology* 2017;243:1133–1140. https://doi.org/10.1016/j.biortech.2017.07.011.

[180] Adjaye JD, Bakhshi NN. Production of hydrocarbons by catalytic upgrading of a fast pyrolysis bio-oil. Part I: conversion over various catalysts. *Fuel Processing Technology* 1995;45:161–183. https://doi.org/10.1016/0378-3820(95)00034-5.

[181] Leung A, Boocock DGB, Konar SK. Pathway for the catalytic conversion of carboxylic acids to hydrocarbons over activated alumina. *Energy Fuels* 1995;9:913–920. https://doi.org/10.1021/ef00053a026.

[182] Shi Y, Xing E, Wu K, Wang J, Yang M, Wu Y. Recent progress on upgrading of bio-oil to hydrocarbons over metal/zeolite bifunctional catalysts. *Catalysis Science & Technology* 2017;7:2385–2415. https://doi.org/10.1039/C7CY00574A.

[183] Rahimi N, Karimzadeh R. Catalytic cracking of hydrocarbons over modified ZSM-5 zeolites to produce light olefins: a review. *Applied Catalysis A: General* 2011;398:1–17. https://doi.org/10.1016/j.apcata.2011.03.009.

[184] Hernando H, Hernández-Giménez AM, Ochoa-Hernández C, Bruijnincx PCA, Houben K, Baldus M, et al. Engineering the acidity and accessibility of the zeolite ZSM-5 for efficient bio-oil upgrading in catalytic pyrolysis of lignocellulose. *Green Chemistry* 2018. https://doi.org/10.1039/C8GC01722K.

[185] Puértolas B, Veses A, Callén MS, Mitchell S, García T, Pérez-Ramírez J. Porosity-acidity interplay in hierarchical ZSM-5 zeolites for pyrolysis oil valorization to aromatics. *ChemSusChem* 2015;8:3283–3293. https://doi.org/10.1002/cssc.201500685.

[186] Gou J, Wang Z, Li C, Qi X, Vattipalli V, Cheng Y-T, et al. The effects of ZSM-5 mesoporosity and morphology on the catalytic fast pyrolysis of furan. *Green Chemistry* 2017;19:3549–3557. https://doi.org/10.1039/C7GC01395G.

[187] Baloch HA, Nizamuddin S, Siddiqui MTH, Riaz S, Jatoi AS, Dumbre DK, et al. Recent advances in production and upgrading of bio-oil from biomass: a critical overview. *Journal of Environmental Chemical Engineering* 2018;6:5101–5118. https://doi.org/10.1016/j.jece.2018.07.050.

[188] Lian X, Xue Y, Zhao Z, Xu G, Han S, Yu H. Progress on upgrading methods of bio-oil: a review: upgrading progress of bio-oil. *International Journal of Energy Research* 2017;41:1798–1816. https://doi.org/10.1002/er.3726.

[189] Srinivasan V, Adhikari S, Chattanathan SA, Park S. Catalytic pyrolysis of torrefied biomass for hydrocarbons production. *Energy & Fuels* 2012;26:7347–7353. https://doi.org/10.1021/ef301469t.

[190] Neupane S, Adhikari S, Wang Z, Ragauskas AJ, Pu Y. Effect of torrefaction on biomass structure and hydrocarbon production from fast pyrolysis. *Green Chemistry* 2015;17:2406–2417. https://doi.org/10.1039/C4GC02383H.

Lignocellulose Biomass Pyrolysis for Bio-Oil Production

[191] Chen Z, Wang M, Jiang E, Wang D, Zhang K, Ren Y, et al. Pyrolysis of torrefied biomass. *Trends in Biotechnology* 2018;36:1287–1298. https://doi.org/10.1016/j.tibtech.2018.07.005.

[192] Zhang S, Zhang H, Liu X, Zhu S, Hu L, Zhang Q. Upgrading of bio-oil from catalytic pyrolysis of pretreated rice husk over Fe-modified ZSM-5 zeolite catalyst. *Fuel Processing Technology* 2018;175:17–25. https://doi.org/10.1016/j.fuproc.2018.03.002.

[193] Custodis VBF, Hemberger P, Ma Z, van Bokhoven JA. Mechanism of fast pyrolysis of lignin: studying model compounds. *The Journal of Physical Chemistry B* 2014;118:8524–8531. https://doi.org/10.1021/jp5036579.

[194] Bu Q, Lei H, Qian M, Yadavalli G. A thermal behavior and kinetics study of the catalytic pyrolysis of lignin. *RSC Advances* 2016;6:100700–100707. https://doi.org/10.1039/C6RA22967K.

[195] Arteaga-Pérez LE, Jiménez R, Grob N, Gómez O, Romero R, Ronsse F. Catalytic upgrading of biomass-derived vapors on carbon aerogel-supported Ni: effect of temperature, metal cluster size and catalyst-to-biomass ratio. *Fuel Processing Technology* 2018;178:251–261. https://doi.org/10.1016/j.fuproc.2018.05.036.

[196] Bach Q-V, Tran K-Q, Skreiberg Ø, Trinh TT. Effects of wet torrefaction on pyrolysis of woody biomass fuels. *Energy* 2015;88:443–456. https://doi.org/10.1016/j.energy.2015.05.062.

[197] Stephanidis S, Nitsos C, Kalogiannis K, Iliopoulou EF, Lappas AA, Triantafyllidis KS. Catalytic upgrading of lignocellulosic biomass pyrolysis vapours: effect of hydrothermal pre-treatment of biomass. *Catalysis Today* 2011;167:37–45. https://doi.org/10.1016/j.cattod.2010.12.049.

[198] Arteaga-Pérez LE, Gómez Cápiro O, Romero R, Delgado A, Olivera P, Ronsse F, et al. In situ catalytic fast pyrolysis of crude and torrefied Eucalyptus globulus using carbon aerogel-supported catalysts. *Energy* 2017;128:701–712. https://doi.org/10.1016/j.energy.2017.04.024.

[199] Mahadevan R, Adhikari S, Shakya R, Wang K, Dayton DC, Li M, et al. Effect of torrefaction temperature on lignin macromolecule and product distribution from HZSM-5 catalytic pyrolysis. *Journal of Analytical and Applied Pyrolysis* 2016;122:95–105. https://doi.org/10.1016/j.jaap.2016.10.011.

[200] Chen D, Li Y, Deng M, Wang J, Chen M, Yan B, et al. Effect of torrefaction pretreatment and catalytic pyrolysis on the pyrolysis poly-generation of pine wood. *Bioresource Technology* 2016;214:615–622. https://doi.org/10.1016/j.biortech.2016.04.058.

[201] Persson H, Yang W. Catalytic pyrolysis of demineralized lignocellulosic biomass. *Fuel* 2019;252:200–209. https://doi.org/10.1016/j.fuel.2019.04.087.

[202] Baral NR, Shah A. Comparative techno-economic analysis of steam explosion, dilute sulfuric acid, ammonia fiber explosion and biological pretreatments of corn stover. *Bioresource Technology* 2017;232:331–343. https://doi.org/10.1016/j.biortech.2017.02.068.

[203] Brown TR, Zhang Y, Hu G, Brown RC. Techno-economic analysis of biobased chemicals production via integrated catalytic processing. *Biofuels, Bioproducts and Biorefining* 2012;6:73–87. https://doi.org/10.1002/bbb.344.

[204] Shemfe M, Gu S, Fidalgo B. Techno-economic analysis of biofuel production via bio-oil zeolite upgrading: an evaluation of two catalyst regeneration systems. *Biomass and Bioenergy* 2017;98:182–193. https://doi.org/10.1016/j.biombioe.2017.01.020.

[205] Rogers JG, Brammer JG. Estimation of the production cost of fast pyrolysis bio-oil. *Biomass and Bioenergy* 2012;36:208–217. https://doi.org/10.1016/j.biombioe.2011.10.028.

[206] Chai L, Saffron CM, Yang Y, Zhang Z, Munro RW, Kriegel RM. Integration of decentralized torrefaction with centralized catalytic pyrolysis to produce green aromatics from coffee grounds. *Bioresource Technology* 2016;201:287–292. https://doi.org/10.1016/j.biortech.2015.11.065.

[207] Haberl H, Beringer T, Bhattacharya SC, Erb K-H, Hoogwijk M. The global technical potential of bio-energy in 2050 considering sustainability constraints. *Current Opinion in Environmental Sustainability* 2010;2:394–403. https://doi.org/10.1016/j.cosust.2010.10.007.

[208] He J, Strezov V, Kan T, Weldekidan H, Asumadu-Sarkodie S, Kumar R. Effect of temperature on heavy metal(loid) deportment during pyrolysis of Avicennia marina biomass obtained from phytoremediation. *Bioresource Technology* 2019;278:214–222. https://doi.org/10.1016/j.biortech.2019.01.101.

[209] Oasmaa A, Kyt M, Sipil K. Pyrolysis oil combustion tests in an industrial boiler. In: Bridgwater AV, editor. *Progress in Thermochemical Biomass Conversion*, Oxford, UK: Blackwell Science Ltd, 2001; pp. 1468–1481. https://doi.org/10.1002/9780470694954.ch121.

[210] Cataluña R, Kuamoto PM, Petzhold CL, Caramão EB, Machado ME, da Silva R. Using bio-oil produced by biomass pyrolysis as diesel fuel. *Energy & Fuels* 2013;27:6831–6838. https://doi.org/10.1021/ef401644v.

9 Thermochemical Production of Bio-Oil

Downstream Processing Technologies for Bio-Oil Upgrading, Production of Hydrogen, and High Value-Added Products

Kumar, R. and Strezov, V.[1]
1 School of Natural Sciences, Faculty of Science & Engineering, Macquarie University, Sydney, NSW, Australia

CONTENTS

9.1	Introduction	198
9.2	Biomass as a Renewable Feedstock for Bio-Oil Production	201
9.3	Methods for Downstream Bio-Oil Upgrading	205
	9.3.1 Solvent Addition	205
	9.3.2 Emulsification	212
	9.3.3 Filtration to Remove Solid Char Residue	216
	9.3.4 Electrochemical or Electrocatalytic Upgrading of Bio-Oil	220
	9.3.5 Hydrotreatment of Bio-Oil	222
9.4	Commercial Applications of Bio-Oils	235
9.5	Bio-Oil Upgrading to Hydrogen/Syngas *via* Steam Reforming	236
9.6	Trends and Future Perspectives	247
	9.6.1 Techno-economic Analysis	247
	9.6.2 Policy Analysis	250
	9.6.3 Challenges and Future Recommendations	250
9.7	Conclusions	252
9.8	Acknowledgments	253
	References	254

DOI: 10.1201/9781003265597-9

9.1 INTRODUCTION

The world economy continues to grow at a Gross Domestic Product (GDP) rate of 3.25% and has been estimated to grow at a faster rate in Asia, particularly in India and China [1]. Significant energy sources are also required to meet the desired economic development. The total energy demand is expected to increase worldwide by 28% by 2040 [1]. Among all the energy sectors, the transport sector, which mainly relies on liquid fuels, consumes the largest part of the energy and is predicted to reach nearly 3.3 billion tons worldwide by 2040 [1]. There are predictions of a significant increase in electric vehicles (cars and buses) or solar-assisted vehicles that may decrease the demand of liquid fuel; however, high-power transport vehicles, such as airplanes, long-haul trucks, and ships, will still require high-energy-density fuels. Therefore, potential alternatives to liquid fuels are required to meet the energy demand since conventional liquid fuels (petrol and diesel) are depleting. The most desirable alternatives could be renewable and sustainable fuels or fuels that can be produced from renewable feedstocks, and their combustion produces less greenhouse gas (GHG) emissions. In this regard, biomass has been considered the most suitable renewable energy source for the production of various second-generation liquid fuels. This is mainly because biomass is a dominant source of carbon and contains less nitrogenous and sulfur contents. Promising technologies can convert biomass into high-energy-density fuels [2–6]. In addition, it has also been reported that the combustion of fuels produced from biomass emits lower amounts of NO_x and SO_x compared to conventional liquid fuels, like bio-oil [7,8] or bio-based jet fuel [9], which consequently could help to reduce GHG emissions.

Pyrolysis and hydrothermal liquefaction (HTL) are the most widely used approaches to convert dry and wet lignocellulose biomass or organic wastes into liquid or other fuels and value-added chemicals [12–17]. Pyrolysis is a thermochemical process that degrades the various interlinkages between the biomass components as an effect of heating in an inert atmosphere where the main biomass components, such as cellulose, hemicellulose, and lignin, are further degraded into different organic compounds [18,19]. Figure 9.1 shows the major component of lignocellulose biomass. Biomass pyrolysis usually results in three products: bio-oil, bio-char, and pyrolytic gases. The yield of the products mainly depends on the composition of biomass and the pyrolysis temperature. Generally, at the temperature of 500–600 °C, the biomass with a higher proportion of cellulose results in a higher bio-oil yield, while the pyrolysis of biomass with a higher amount of hemicellulose and lignin may result in higher gas and char yield, respectively [20–22]. Other pyrolytic parameters, such as heating rate, the flow rate of carrier gas or residence time, holding time, and particle size of the feedstock, also influence the product yield or bio-oil composition [23]. On the other hand, HTL involves the decomposition of biomass (wet or dry biomass) in the presence of a solvent (water, methanol, ethanol, acetone, etc.) at the temperature of 250–550 °C and pressure of 5–25 MPa [24,25]. The process of biomass HTL firstly comprises the depolymerization of biomass into its individual components, followed by their decomposition via various reactions, such as dehydration, cleavage, decarboxylation, and deamination. In the last step, the reactive molecules are recombined or repolymerized to form high-molecular-weight compounds. Like pyrolysis,

Thermochemical Production of Bio-Oil

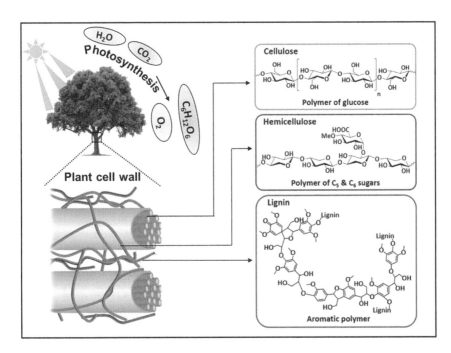

FIGURE 9.1 Structure of lignocellulosic biomass with cellulose, hemicellulose, and lignin.

Source: Reproduced with permission from [10,11].

the HTL process also generates three types of fuels, mainly bio-oil, bio-char, gases and a water phase that contains a high carbon content, and their yields depend on the type of feedstock and operating parameters of the process. For example, de Caprariis et al. [26] suggested that an increased bio-oil yield could be obtained with the biomass containing a higher content of lignin, while the minimum bio-oil yield was obtained with the biomass containing a higher content of cellulose. Generally, the temperature range of 250–330 °C is suitable for obtaining a higher bio-oil yield. The solvents with higher density and the ability to promote the solvolysis and hydration reactions are highly advantageous in the HTL process [27–29]. Other parameters, such as pressure, heating rate, and residence time, also play a critical role in obtaining quality bio-oil.

The bio-oil produced using either pyrolysis or HTL has been considered a clean and environmentally friendly energy fuel as its combustion generates lower GHG emissions compared to conventional fossil fuels [30,31]. For example, a study demonstrated the comparison of bio-oil combustion with heavy fuel oil in an industrial boiler. The results showed that the NO_x emissions for bio-oil were 88 mg/MJ, while the combustion of heavy fuel oil produced NO_x emissions of 193 mg/MJ [32]. However, the bio-oil properties, such as high acidity, low stability, low higher heating values (HHV), and the presence of solid char particles make it an unsuitable drop-in fuel [19,33,34]. Therefore, bio-oil upgrading is essential to produce bio-oil as a transport fuel or for its direct use in boilers and turbines for heat and power generation. There are different strategies to improve the properties of bio-oil, mainly based on the biomass pre-treatment, such as dry torrefaction [35,36], wet torrefaction [37,38], acid and alkali treatment [39–41], steam explosion, etc. [42], and downstream treatment of the bio-oil such as emulsification [43,44], solvent addition [45,46], filtration, etc. [47,48]. In terms of bio-oil upgrading, the biomass pre-treatment methods are usually advantageous to increase the conversion of oxygenated compounds into hydrocarbons and increase the bio-oil yield and HHV [28,29], while the downstream treatment methods generally help to increase the bio-oil stability and HHV, and decrease the viscosity and the amount of solid char particles. In addition, the bio-oil can also be upgraded using electrochemical hydrogenation, which generally converts the carbonyl-containing compounds into hydrocarbons or other value-added compounds [49,50]. Alternatively, the application of different catalysts during pyrolysis and HTL is a significant approach to improve the kinetics of the process and enhance the bio-oil properties and has been widely used for bio-oil upgrading in pyrolysis as well as in HTL [24,51,52]. Hydrotreatment is considered highly efficient for bio-oil upgrading as it removes oxygen in the form of H_2O, while in cracking, oxygen is removed in the form of CO_2 and CO, decreasing the total carbon yield [53,54]. Hydrotreatment of bio-oil obtained from pyrolysis and HTL process has been reported in several studies with various types of catalysts utilized for hydrotreatment of bio-oil to either convert it into a more valuable fuel with improved physicochemical properties or other value-added products. Biller et al. [55] studied the application of sulfided $NiMo/Al_2O_3$ and $CoMo/Al_2O_3$ for hydrotreatment of bio-oil obtained from HTL of *Chlorella*. The results reported a considerable increase in the conversion of oxygenated compounds into hydrocarbons with the application of sulfided catalysts, as a high number of hydrocarbons was observed in the upgraded bio-oil [55].

The bio-oil obtained from thermochemical techniques could also be a suitable feedstock for steam reforming (SR) for the production of H_2 or a mixture of CO and H_2, called syngas [56–61]. H_2 produced from SR of bio-oil can be further used as a clean fuel, while syngas can be further subjected to the Fischer-Tropsch process for the production of hydrocarbons. SR is a process involving the conversion of bio-oil containing oxygenated compounds or hydrocarbons into hydrogen in the presence of water at a temperature range of 350 to 1000 °C [62,63]. The technique also requires a highly active catalyst to enhance the conversion efficiency and hydrogen yield. Several studies have reported the application of various types of catalysts with promising results for hydrogen production [60,62].

Bio-oil is foreseen as a potential drop-in fuel; hence, bio-oil upgrading is highly important to make it competitive with conventional energy fuels. The methods used for bio-oil upgrading, such as catalytic cracking, hydrodeoxygenation [10,13,64], and biomass pre-treatments such as torrefaction and wet-torrefaction [37,65], have been comprehensively reviewed in previous publications. For example, Zacher et al. [66] critically reviewed the hydrotreatment process for bio-oil upgrading and discussed various parameters, techno-economic analysis, and challenges associated with the technique. Recently, Nishu et al. [67] published a review article focused on catalytic pyrolysis with ZSM-based catalysts for bio-oil upgrading. On the other hand, Bach and Skreiberg [65] published a review article on the effect of dry and wet torrefaction

Thermochemical Production of Bio-Oil

on bio-oil upgrading and other biofuel production. It was noticed that less attention had been paid to reviewing the methods applied for downstream bio-oil upgrading, and no review article has been published recently. In recent years, a number of research articles and reports have been published on various downstream techniques for bio-oil upgrading and production of other value-added fuels. Therefore, considering the significance of these methods for biofuel production, this article aims to provide the recent advances in the downstream upgrading of bio-oil produced either using the pyrolysis process or HTL. The article begins with critical insights into biomass's potential as a renewable resource and the conversion efficiency of pyrolysis and liquefaction for biofuel production. Later, it discusses the widely used methods for downstream bio-oil upgrading, such as solvent addition, emulsification, filtration, electrochemical hydrogenation, and hydrotreatment. Basic principles of the processes and effects of different parameters on bio-oil upgrading are thoroughly discussed, while key challenges and possible solutions are also provided. Bio-oil can be successfully converted to clean fuel like H_2 using the steam reforming technique (SR), which is critically discussed in the article. In addition, techno-economic analysis, policy analysis, challenges, and future recommendations related to downstream processes are provided in later sections of the article. Overall, this review article provides critical information about downstream bio-oil upgrading and other high-value-added fuel production.

9.2 BIOMASS AS A RENEWABLE FEEDSTOCK FOR BIO-OIL PRODUCTION

Biomass is a non-fossil, complex organic-inorganic solid product, mainly derived from plants and could also be obtained from animals, bacteria, fungi, etc. A recent study has estimated the amount of biomass among all the taxa (plants, bacteria, fungi, animals, viruses, archaea, protists) on Earth [68,69]. The study showed that approximately 550 Gt C is present on Earth, with 80%, or ~450 Gt C, covered by terrestrial plants, while the rest is dominated by bacteria and others [68]. Therefore, it could be suggested that out of the total biomass on earth, 80% of biomass could be estimated as the potential feedstock in different thermochemical technologies for biofuel production. Biomass is considered a renewable energy source since it does not contribute to the greenhouse effect because of CO_2-neutral conversion. The biomass plants store the energy in the primary products (monosaccharides) as a result of the photosynthesis process, which involves the uptake of water, CO_2, and solar energy by the plant pigments, which are converted into organic chemicals (monosaccharides like glucose) and oxygen, as shown in Eq. (9.1).

$$6H_2O + 6CO_2 + radiant\ energy \rightarrow C_6H_{12}O_6\left(glucose\right) + 6O_2 \qquad (9.1)$$

These primary products produced after photosynthesis act as precursors for the synthesis of all types of organic components of biomass and are further converted into secondary products, such as polysaccharides, proteins, lipids, and several other organic compounds. Generally, the higher the photosynthesis efficiency, the greater the biomass synthesis. It has been reported that the plants that fix CO_2 via C_3 pathway show higher photosynthesis efficiency at warm temperatures, while the plants fixing CO_2 via C_4 pathway exhibit higher rates of photosynthesis at cool temperatures [70]. Therefore, from a higher biomass production point of view, C3 or C4 plants can be cultured according to the preferred climate conditions in different parts of the world to enhance biomass production in a shorter span of time, which can be further utilized in various technologies for biofuel production.

The biomass's organic-inorganic composition and energy content are pivotal parameters for their utilization in conversion processes for the production of bio-oil or other biofuels. For example, the biomass that exhibits higher content of moisture could not be suitable for the pyrolysis process, while it could be a suitable feedstock for HTL as the excess water could be used as a reactant medium, or in anaerobic or fermentation processes for methane or bioethanol production. Similarly, the ash content is highly undesirable in the biomass as its higher content lowers the organic matter in the biomass and consequently decreases the HHV of the biomass. The ash content also contains certain metal oxides, such as calcium and potassium, which might affect the conversion processes due to their catalytic behavior, and their further presence in the bio-oil makes it highly unstable as these metal oxides may start the polymerization reactions. It is evident and well-known that different biomass exhibits varying compositions, chemical structures, and carbon contents. Generally, biomass with higher carbon content in reduced form shows a higher heating value, while the higher degree of oxygenation reduces the heating value of the biomass. For example, the monosaccharides contain carbon contents of nearly 40%, and their estimated HHV is 15.6 MJ/kg, while terpenes and lipids exhibit approximately 88% and 77% of carbon content and hence show higher HHV of 45.2 and 39.8 MJ/kg, respectively [71]. Table 9.1 shows the carbon content and HHV of specific biomass components.

TABLE 9.1
Typical Carbon Content and Heating Value of Selected Biomass Components.

Component	Carbon (wt%) on dry basis	HHV (MJ/kg)
Monosaccharides	40	15.6
Disaccharides	42	16.7
Polysaccharides	44	17.5
Crude proteins	53	24.0
Lignin	63	25.1
Lipids	76–77	39.8
Terpenes	88	45.2
Crude carbohydrates	41–44	16.7–17.7
Crude fibers	47–50	18.8–19.8
Crude triglycerides	74–78	36.5–40.0

Source: Reproduced with permission from [71].

Thermochemical Production of Bio-Oil

Extensive research has been carried out on both pyrolysis and HTL technologies for bio-oil production for optimization of process parameters and selection of biomass feedstock to obtain higher yield and quality of bio-oil. These parameters have been discussed in detail in several articles published already [20,21,92,93]. Therefore, they are not reviewed in this article. However, the key differences between pyrolysis and HTL in terms of bio-oil quality and energy conversion rate (ECR) are briefly discussed. ECR of the pyrolysis (or HTL) for a biomass feedstock at any temperature can be obtained using Eqs. (9.22) and (9.3).

$$\eta = \frac{Q_{recovered} - Q_{pyrolysis}}{Q_{biomass}} \times 100\% \quad (9.2)$$

where

$$Q_{recovered} = HHV_{gas} \times mass_{gas} + HHV_{liquid} \times mass_{liquid} + HHV_{char} \times mass_{char} \quad (9.3)$$

The comparative studies of pyrolysis and HTL suggest that HTL produces better bio-oil quality compared to pyrolysis [62,85,86]. For instance, Jena and Das [72] compared the quality of bio-oil produced from pyrolysis and HTL. They used *Spirulina platensis* as the feedstock and carried out the pyrolysis process at temperatures of 350 and 550 °C, with a heating rate of 3.5 °C/min and 7 °C/min, respectively, while the HTL process was carried out in a 1.8-L Parr reactor at 350 °C with the water pressure of 20.6 MPa and a heating rate of 3.3 °C/min, and the residence time of 60 min. The properties of the bio-oil that resulted from both processes are shown in Table 9.2, which suggests that the bio-oil from HTL showed better thermal stability and HHV than the pyrolytic oils [72]. However, the higher content of inorganic species was found in the bio-oil collected from the HTL process, which could be mainly because of the leaching of inorganic species from the char into the bio-oil, as the liquid and solid products are usually kept in the reactor until the reactor is cooled down and the bio-oil is separated from the solid char [94,95]. In terms of ECR, HTL also proved more efficient than the pyrolysis process. The study showed that HTL could convert approximately 67.9% of energy present in biomass into the bio-oil, while the ECR during pyrolysis was only 33.9% and 46.7% for the bio-oils obtained at the temperature of 350 and 500 °C, respectively. The lower ECR in pyrolysis could be attributed to more energy inputs required for the pyrolysis process, mainly for drying the biomass feedstock before pyrolysis. The conversion efficiency of the pyrolysis process could be further enhanced if the energy inputs are provided by the energy products generated during the pyrolysis or using solar thermal energy. In a recent study, Weldekidan et al. [96] showed that the pyrolysis process could be highly efficient if the heat required to carry out the pyrolysis process is supplied by the combustion of the evolved pyrolytic gas products. In this scenario, the ECR (for all pyrolytic products) calculated for the pyrolysis of rice husk biomass (at 500 °C and heating rate of 10 °C/min) was 89%, and if the solar thermal energy is used for the pyrolysis process, the ECR of 94% could also be achieved [96]. Overall, it can be suggested that pyrolysis could be an efficient and equivalent approach for bio-oil production when compared to HTL.

TABLE 9.2
Physical Properties, Ultimate Analysis, Inorganic Elements of Algal Bio-Oil Samples, and Energy and Mass Balance in HTL and Pyrolysis Processes.

Bio-oil properties	HTL[a] (350 °C)	Pyr[b] (350 °C)	Pyr[b] (550°C)
Color	black	reddish brown	reddish brown
Odor	smoky	acrid smoky	acrid smoky
pH	9.60	9.35	9.52
density, kg/L	0.97	1.20	1.05
viscosity, cP			
at 60 °C	51.20	34.30	23.10
at 40 °C	189.90	100.67	79.20
C, %	73.73	67.52	74.66
H, %	8.90	9.82	10.57
N, %	6.30	10.71	7.13
S, %	0.90	0.45	0.81
O, %	10.17	11.34	6.81
H/C ratio	1.44	1.73	1.68
O/C ratio	0.10	0.13	0.06
HHV, MJ/kg	34.20	29.30	33.62
Inorganics in ash, mg/kg			
Na	14.6	14.6	14.0
Mg	69.3	11.3	2.3
Al	60.1	58.8	10.7
Si	115	54.8	15.5
P	249	63.2	39.6
Ca	116	35.4	7.6
Fe	848	135	180
Ni	72.1	6.4	24.1
Energy and mass balance			
ER[c], %	67.9	33.9	46.7
ECR[d], net energy ratio	0.70	2.11	1.56
CHR[e], %	71.7	39.3	51.3

Source: Reproduced with permission from [72]. Copyright © 2011, American Chemical Society.
[a] HTL: Hydrothermal liquefaction, [b] Pyr: Pyrolysis, [c] ER: Energy recovery, [d] ECR: Net energy ratio, [e] CHR: Carbon and hydrogen recovery

Pyrolysis is a commercial process used for bio-oil production at a pilot scale. For example, KiOR and Envergent use a Circulating Fluid Bed configuration, while Dynamotive applies a Bubbling Fluidized Bed for biomass pyrolysis [97]. BTG-Bioliquids uses Rotating Cone Reactor fast pyrolysis technology for

Thermochemical Production of Bio-Oil

bio-oil production at a commercial level and claims to obtain 70% of bio-oil yield. However, the commercially produced bio-oil is still of low quality in terms of calorific value and H/C ratios. Hence, the companies have to use an upgrading approach to improve the bio-oil properties. On the other hand, HTL has not been used commercially, mainly because of the high capital cost of the system. Other key challenges of HTL are associated with reactor designs, high cost for solvent, catalyst, and purification of the bio-oil. A continuous reactor system is required to scale up the HTL process for bio-oil production as the batch reactors possess certain limitations regarding process parameters and a mixture of bio-oil and biochar in the reactor that further requires a purification step to separate [69]. However, continuous reactors have some challenges when operating under high pressures and temperature conditions. For example, they require the preparation of biomass slurries and pumping into the reactor, which is a challenging task to perform under high pressures. The requirement for pumping instrumentation and operation is also an economic challenge, increasing the total operating cost. The development of highly effective, cheaper, and simple purification techniques, the application of advanced, cost-effective, and versatile catalysts, and minimizing the use of solvents are major breakthroughs required for the successful application of HTL at a commercial level.

Tables 9.3 and summarize a few studies on the production of bio-oil using general pyrolysis and HTL (without any upgrading approach), respectively. It can be estimated that the bio-oil produced using either pyrolysis or HTL cannot be directly used as a drop-in fuel, and it is highly important to improve its properties and increase the energy content to make it a competitive fuel to the currently available conventional fuels. In this regard, several methods have been demonstrated for bio-oil upgrading, which can be applied during pyrolysis or HTL process that mainly comprises catalytic approaches, such as catalytic cracking, hydrodeoxygenation, and esterification, or pre-pyrolysis or pre-HTL approaches, which mainly involve biomass pre-treatment methods, such as torrefaction, acid and alkali treatments, or steam explosion. Alternatively, the bio-oil properties can be improved during post-pyrolysis or HTL process, such as with solvent addition, emulsification, filtration, electrochemical hydrogenation, and hydrotreatment, which are comprehensively discussed in the further sections of the article.

9.3 METHODS FOR DOWNSTREAM BIO-OIL UPGRADING

In this section, major downstream approaches for bio-oil upgrading have been comprehensively reviewed. Basic principles of the processes, the effect of key parameters on bio-oil properties, challenges, and feasibility have been thoroughly discussed.

9.3.1 SOLVENT ADDITION

The application of polar solvents has been shown to improve certain properties of the bio-oil. The main objective of using solvents is to increase the stability and decrease the viscosity of the bio-oil. The increase in viscosity during the storage is generally

TABLE 9.3

Properties of Bio-Oils Obtained from Biomass Pyrolysis without Using Any Upgrading Technique.

Biomass	Pyrolysis temp. (°C)	Pyrolysis reactor	Bio-oil yield (wt%)	Bio-oil properties							References
				HHV (MJ/kg)	Water content (wt%)	pH	Viscosity	TAN	Density (g/mL)	
Pine wood	500	/	/	19.5	/	/	175 cP	/	/	[44]
Saccharina japonica	300	Fluidized-bed	31.27	28.63	1.76	5.9	-	/	/	[73]
Pine wood	450	Auger reactor	/	22.49	16.9	3.08	55.2 cSt	69.5	1.18	[74]
Pine wood	450	Auger reactor	54.00	16.1	20.83	2.65	6.49 cSt	90.06	1.17	[75]
Sweetgum	450	Auger reactor	52.00	2.65	38.3	2.65	8.26 cSt	119.2	1.16	[76]
Switchgrass	450	Auger reactor	33.00	2.98	61.7	2.98	1.51 cSt	88.4	1.08	[76]
Corn stover	450	Auger reactor	35.00	2.66	54.7	2.66	1.60 cSt	85.8	1.08	[76]
Saccharina japonica	470	Fixed-bed	/	35.0	34.7	/	/	43	1.13	[77]
Eucalyptus bark	550	FFFP unit	52.79	12.77	29.89	2.38	/	/	1.14	[78]
Eucalyptus bark	500	FFFP unit	55.54	12.23	32.86	2.87	/	/	1.14	[78]
Eucalyptus bark	450	FFFP unit	64.99	13.89	27.98	2.76	/	/	1.15	[78]
Eucalyptus bark	400	FFFP unit	58.25	12.45	26.07	2.78	/	/	1.13	[78]
Walnut shell	550	Spouted bed	/	/	18.87	4.38	7.98 cSt	/	0.94	[79]
Walnut shell	550	Spouted bed	/	/	23.29	4.28	3.29 cSt	/	0.95	[34]
Prairie cord grass	400	Spouted bed	/	15.2	/	2.59	2.5 cP	/	1.25	[34]
Switchgrass	400	Spouted bed	/	14.9	/	2.77	2.1 cP	/	1.25	[34]
Napier grass	600	Fixed-bed	30.06	20.97	26.01	2.95	2.71 cP	/	1.05	[80]
Pine wood	500	/	/	14.46	29.78	/	18.49 cSt	40.7	/	[81]

TAN- Total acid number (mg of KOH/g), FFFP unit- Free-fall fast pyrolysis unit

TABLE 9.4
Properties of Bio-Oils Obtained from HTL Process without Using Any Upgrading Technique.

Feedstock	HTL process				Bio-oil fuel properties								References
	T (°C)	Pressure (MPa)	Reaction time (min)	Solvent	HHV (MJ/kg)	Water content (wt%)	pH	Viscosity	TAN	Density (g/mL)	H/C	O/C	
Spirulina platensis	350	20.6	60	water	34.21	/	9.60	51.20 cP	/	0.97	1.44	0.10	[72]
Aspen wood	400	32	/	/	37.4	1.4	/	2.10 X 10⁵ cP	/	1.07	1.25	0.10	[82]
Blackcurrant Pomace	300	1	60	Ethyl acetate	33.4	/	3.2	/	134	/	/	/	[83]
Blackcurrant Pomace	300	1	60	hexane	38.4	/	3.2	/	159	/	/	/	[83]
Blackcurrant Pomace	300	1	60	acetone	35.0	/	3.2	/	134	/	/	/	[83]
Blackcurrant Pomace	300	1	60	Isopropyl alcohol	34.6	/	3.2	/	137				[83]
Barley straw	500	35	15	water	17.19	/	/	/	/	/	0.95	0.56	[84]
Swine manure	340	6.8	15	water	36.05	2.37	/	843 cP	/	/	1.61	0.13	[85]
Chlorella pyrenoidosa	300	/	20	water	19.01	/	/	/	/	/	1.49	0.53	[86]
Barley straw	300	9	15	water	24.87	/	/	/	/	/	1.23	0.36	[87]
Nannochloropsis sp.	320	3.4	240	/	40.1	/	/	/	256.5	/	1.63	0.06	[88]
Nannochloropsis sp.	320		30	water	36.44	1.25	/	68.83 cSt	23.26	/	1.64	0.06	[89]
Sewage sludge	350	9.4–10.1	20	ethanol	36.14	/	/	818.3 cP	/	0.91	1.56	0.11	[90]
Rice straw	350	9.4–10.1	20	ethanol	33.90	/	/	1224 cP	/	1.03	1.38	0.17	[90]
Spirulina sp.	350	9.4–10.1	20	ethanol	34.33	/	/	962 cP	/	0.97	1.49	0.12	[90]
Litsea cubeba seed	290	/	60	water	40.8	8	/	/	100	/	1.9	0.10	[91]

linked with the formation of water, resulting in the separation of lignin-rich sludge at the bottom. The bio-oil, along with water, contains other oxygenated compounds and degraded lignin. Upon aging, the quantity of water-insoluble fraction increases, which further increases the bio-oil's average molecular mass and viscosity. The formation of water and water-insoluble fractions is usually due to the occurrence of condensation and polymerization reactions. The presence of impurities in the bio-oil, like char particles or heavy metals absorbed from the biomass during pyrolysis or HTL process, cancatalyze condensation and polymerization reactions. The addition of a solvent generally affects the viscosity of the bio-oil mainly by diluting the bio-oil without affecting the chemical reaction rate. In addition, the chemical reactions between the solvent and the bio-oil components also help to prevent polymerization reactions. The primary chemical reactions that occur between the alcohol solvent (such as ethanol and methanol) and the bio-oil components are esterification and acetalization. Table 9.5 shows some examples of solvents used to improve the physicochemical properties of bio-oil. Several solvents, such as ethanol, isopropanol, methanol, acetone, and N, N-dimethylformamide (DMF), have been successfully demonstrated for bio-oil upgrading. For example, Oasmaa et al. [98] investigated the effect of alcohol on the improvement of bio-oil properties. The results demonstrated that adding 5% of ethanol or isopropanol increased the solubility of hydrophobic components of the bio-oil and the amount of water content decreased by approximately 7 wt% in the top phase (that constitutes nearly 25% of the total liquid product) of the bio-oil, while no significant change in the water content was observed in the bottom phase. Moreover, the addition of solvent decreased the viscosity and density, whereas the heating value of the bio-oil increased proportionally with the concentration of the solvent, reaching a maximum of 17.5 MJ/kg with 10% of isopropanol [98]. A recent study demonstrated the use of different proportions of methanol from 3 to 15 wt% to improve the storage stability of bio-oil from pine wood pyrolysis [99]. The increasing concentration of methanol demonstrated a decrease in viscosity, which could be attributed to the change in the bio-oil microstructure, physical dilution, and prevention of chain reactions due to the interactions between methanol and bio-oil constituents [99,100]. In addition, the concentration above 6 wt% of methanol showed to increase the pH with the storage time, which could be ascribed to the fact that the neutral dilution effect of methanol or methanol could also inhibit the activity of H^+ in the bio-oil [99–101]. In a similar study, Liu et al. [102] investigated the influence of varying concentrations of acetone (3–15 wt%) on the physicochemical properties of bio-oil obtained from the pyrolysis of pinewood at 500 °C in a continuously fed bubbling fluidized bed reactor. The results indicated that acetone had a significant effect on improving the overall bio-oil properties. The increasing concentration of acetone increased the pH of bio-oil proportionally, while the formation of water content decreased with an increase in the concentration, obtaining approximately a 12% decrease with 15 wt% acetone. On the other hand, a maximum of 84.6% decrease was observed in the viscosity with the addition of 15 wt% of acetone in the bio-oil [102].

The previous studies discussed above utilized an individual solvent separately to analyze its effect on bio-oil upgrading. However, a compound additive comprising two or more solvents in varying proportions has also been tested to improve

TABLE 9.5
Solvents Used to Improve Physicochemical Properties of Bio-Oil.

Bio-oil properties				Solvents with bio-oil	Upgraded bio-oil properties				References
Viscosity (mm²/s)	Water content (wt%)	pH	HHV (MJ/kg)		Viscosity (mm²/s)	Water content (wt%)	pH	HHV (MJ/kg)	
1244.60	9.36	4.84	19.31	50% Ethyl acetate	6.16	8.12	4.43	26.48	[46]
1244.60	9.36	4.84	19.31	50% Acetone	6.50	7.31	5.48	29.03	[46]
1244.60	9.36	4.84	19.31	50% n-octanol	35.74	9.09	4.92	25.76	[46]
1244.60	9.36	4.84	19.31	50% PEG 400[a]	127.54	8.96	3.30	33.22	[46]
1244.60	9.36	4.84	19.31	50% Ethyl acetate + ultrasonication-150 W, 12 min	18.52	6.96	3.88	29.24	[46]
1244.60	9.36	4.84	19.31	50% Acetone + ultrasonication-150 W, 12 min	22.51	7.33	4.18	29.93	[46]
1244.60	9.36	4.84	19.31	50% n-octanol+ ultrasonication-150 W, 12 min	34.13	9.04	4.80	35.21	[46]
1244.60	9.36	4.84	19.31	50% PEG 400[a]+ ultrasonication-150 W, 12 min	127.29	8.93	5.42	34.77	[46]
560.77	16.64	3.36	22.55	10% Methanol	78.82	17.35	3.66	22.38	[103]
560.77	16.64	3.36	22.55	10% Acetone	76.04	17.04	3.49	23.06	[103]
560.77	16.64	3.36	22.55	10% Ethyl acetate	93.86	17.35	3.48	22.60	[103]
178.2	23.5	/	18.9	4.3% Glycerol, 1.9% methanol	130.1	/	/	18.90	[33]
178.2	23.5	/	18.9	22.8%, Glycerol, 13.4%methanol	40.3	/	/	19.08	[33]
178.2	23.5	/	18.9	10.8%, Glycerol, 51.1% methanol	22.5	/	/	19.48	[33]
12.14	21.77	4.14	/	2.42% n-butanol, 2.32% DMSO[b], 3.25% ethyl acetate	8.26	19.39	4.43	/	[79]
12.14	21.77	4.14	/	1.96% n-butanol, 5.03% DMSO[b], 1% ethyl acetate	9.34	19.50	4.40	/	[79]
/	32.86	2.87	12.23	2.5% Ethanol	/	32.61	2.50	12.23	[78]
/	32.86	2.87	12.23	5% Ethanol	/	32.76	2.53	13.65	[78]
/	32.86	2.87	12.23	10% Ethanol	/	31.25	2.55	15.62	[78]

(*Continued*)

TABLE 9.5 *(Continued)*

Bio-oil properties				Solvents with bio-oil	Upgraded bio-oil properties				References
Viscosity (mm²/s)	Water content (wt%)	pH	HHV (MJ/kg)		Viscosity (mm²/s)	Water content (wt%)	pH	HHV (MJ/kg)	
/	32.86	2.87	12.23	2.5% Methanol	/	32.31	2.47	12.46	[78]
/	32.86	2.87	12.23	5% Methanol	/	31.21	2.54	13.30	[78]
/	32.86	2.87	12.23	10% Methanol		27.48	2.57	14.63	[78]
6.43	28.03	4.04	/	8% Methanol	4.54	24.12	4.38	/	[34]
6.43	28.03	4.04	/	8% Acetone	4.95	24.30	4.36	/	[34]
6.43	28.03	4.04	/	8% DMF	4.67	23.97	4.42	/	[34]
6.43	28.03	4.04	/	1% Methanol, 1.94% acetone, 5.06% DMF	4.36	24.03	4.49	/	[34]

[a] polyethylene glycol (PEG); [b] dimethyl sulfoxide (DMSO)

[c] *N,N*-dimethylformamide (DMF)

T: Temperature

Thermochemical Production of Bio-Oil

the bio-oil quality, showing better bio-oil upgrading results compared to its single solvent counterparts. For example, a compound additive with 1 wt% methanol, 5.06 wt% DMF, and 1.94 wt% acetone proved the best combination to produce the most significant quality bio-oil as compared to either of the single solvents and increased the overall storage properties of the bio-oil [34]. The addition of compound additives was believed to prevent the polymerization of low-molecular compounds during aging. In a similar demonstration, Zhu et al. [79] examined the effect of a compound additive (2.42 wt% n-butanol, 2.32 wt% dimethyl sulfoxide, and 3.25 wt% ethyl acetate) on bio-oil properties during its storage at 80 °C for up to 48 h. It was reported that the compound additive showed noteworthy bio-oil stability as compared to the single solvent. For instance, the water content in the bio-oil with ethyl acetate was 8.18%, which decreased to 1.60% with the compound additive used in the study [79]. Moreover, Zhang et al. [103] also investigated the application of a mixed additive, containing methanol, acetone, and ethyl acetate in certain percentages, for bio-oil upgrading, and the results were satisfactory, showing substantial improvement in the viscosity and water content in the bio-oil. In comparison to single solvent, mixed additives proved more advantageous for bio-oil upgrading, which can be attributed to the chemical activity of the solvents in the compound additive that react with a greater number of constituents of the bio-oil and also prevent the polymerization reactions, consequently leading to a stable bio-oil.

The bio-oil upgrading with solvents can be further improved with physical treatments, such as ultrasonication, that could result in frequent particle movements and hence could allow the solvents molecules to interact better with the constituents of bio-oil. Noticeably, Xu et al. [46] successfully demonstrated the application of ultrasonication for bio-oil upgrading. They used n-octanol as the solvent mixed with the bio-oil in a ratio of 1:1, and the ultrasonic power of 150 W was applied for different exposure times from 2 to 20 minutes. The results revealed that increasing the exposure time of ultrasonication enhanced the bio-oil properties. For example, the bio-oil without ultrasonication showed lower pH of 4.92 and HHV of 25.76 MJ/kg, while the ultrasonication with an exposure time of 20 min increased the pH to 5.11 and HHV to 38.32 MJ/kg [46]. The increase in pH was attributed to the increase in alcoholysis of organic compounds of bio-oil upon ultrasonication. It was also suggested that ultrasonication promotes mechanical and cavitation effects at higher temperatures, which trigger the decomposition of large chain compounds into smaller compounds that can be evaporated as gas, consequently leading to a decrease in the moisture content of the bio-oil. A recent study also investigated the effect of ultrasonication power and exposure time on bio-oil properties, such as HHV, viscosity, and moisture content, using methanol and octanol blends [104]. Authors reported that bio-oil blends with solvents without ultrasonication treatment showed an HHV of 26 MJ/kg, viscosity of 316 mPa.s, and moisture content of 17%, while ultrasonication of the blends at the power of 55 W/L for 11 min increased the HHV to 34.2 MJ/kg and reduced the viscosity and moisture content to 260 mPa.s and 14.4%, respectively [104]. The enhanced properties of the blends were attributed to the breaking of larger compounds and forming free radicals upon ultrasonication, which reacted with other compounds in the bio-oil and formed stable compounds [104]. Ultrasonication was also believed to promote ring opening and hemiacetylation reactions by breaking the double bonds in ketones, alcohols, and polyaromatic hydrocarbons, leading to

212 Biowaste and Biomass in Biofuel Applications

the reduction in the content of ketones and alcohols and an increase in the content of alkanes and alkynes in the bio-oil [105].

The application of solvents is quite a simple and significant approach to enhancing the bio-oil properties, such as viscosity and calorific value. The solvents also react with the constituents of the bio-oil, such as organic compounds, minerals, and alkali metals, and prevent the polymerization reactions, thereby leading to a stable bio-oil. However, less information is available about the reaction mechanism between the solvent and bio-oil constituents due to the complexity and bio-oil composition. Therefore, more research should be conducted to understand the chemical reactions between the solvent and constituents of bio-oil.

9.3.2 Emulsification

Similar to solvent addition, emulsification can also be used to improve the bio-oil properties and increase the total energy content of the resultant bio-oil. Where the polar solvents are miscible in the bio-oil, emulsification involves two immiscible liquids in which the tiny particles of one liquid are suspended in the larger particles of the second liquid. The successful emulsion of the two liquids may result in different sizes of droplets, such as 1–10 µm, while the emulsion that results in droplets of the size 1–100 nm is termed as microemulsion [43]. Emulsion and microemulsions are formed almost in a similar way, but some key factors differentiate them from each other. It has been stated that microemulsions are thermodynamically more stable than emulsions and hence possess less probability of phase separation at a broad range of temperature. On the other hand, emulsions are comparatively less stable and require more energy to form [106]. Emulsification is a simple and effective approach for bio-oil upgrading as the resultant mixture can be directly used for heat or power generation [43]. Generally, the bio-oil is emulsified with other petroleum fuels, such as diesel or biodiesel. Since bio-oil and diesel are less miscible in nature, their emulsification could be carried out in the presence of a surfactant (such as Atlox 4914, Tween 80, and Span 80) and sometimes co-surfactants (for example, methanol, ethanol, and n-butanol) can also be used to improve the emulsion stability [107]. Generally, the surfactant molecules are made up of two parts, a polar hydrophilic 'head' and a nonpolar lipophilic "tail". During the emulsion of a polar liquid, such as bio-oil, and a nonpolar liquid, like diesel, the hydrophilic part of the surfactant adsorbs onto the droplet's surface, and the lipophilic part points outward into the nonpolar liquid. The surfactant molecules form a thin layer around the droplets and protect them from coalescing when they interact in the emulsion. This type of emulsion is known as water-in-oil (W/O) emulsion. Alternatively, when the droplets of a nonpolar liquid are dispersed in an aqueous liquid, they are termed as oil in water (O/W) emulsion, as shown in Figure 9.2A. In addition to this, other physical methods such as ultrasonication, stirring, and the selection of favorable parameters can be employed to obtain stable emulsions, which ultimately affect the physicochemical properties of the resultant bio-oil. Usually, the bio-oil upgrading through emulsification with diesel reduces the viscosity and enhances the calorific value and cetane number as the liquid fuel [106]. Table 9.6 compares the fuel properties of bio-oils and emulsions prepared using bio-oil and emulsifiers.

Thermochemical Production of Bio-Oil

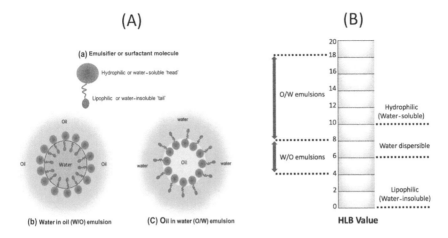

FIGURE 9.2 (A) Type of emulsions and (B) HLB values for different emulsions and mixture behaviors.

To obtain a stable emulsion, the volumetric ratios of bio-oil/diesel and the concentration of the emulsifier/surfactant are the important parameters, while other factors, like temperature, stirring intensity, and mixing time, are also critical to obtain a stable emulsion which subsequently would affect the bio-oil upgrading. In other words, a stable emulsion would result in a high-quality bio-oil having a longer stability duration, while an unstable emulsion would lead to a poor-quality bio-oil. Jiang and Ellis [108] investigated the emulsification of bio-oil with biodiesel optimization using octanol as the surfactant and studied the effect of various parameters on the stability of emulsion and their effect on the bio-oil properties. The study concluded that the mixing ratio of bio-oil/biodiesel of 40%/60% produced the most stable emulsion, while 4% octanol (surfactant) was optimum for obtaining a stable emulsion. They found that at the lower concentrations of octanol, the mixture was unstable due to the agglomeration of the oil droplets, whereas the emulsion was disrupted due to rapid coalescence at the higher concentrations of octanol [43,108,109]. Emulsification of the bio-oil with biodiesel decreased the viscosity to 4.66 mPa.s compared to 67.39 mPa.s of the sole bio-oil, while the HHV of the mixture significantly increased from 15.28 to 35.76 MJ/kg [108]. In a recent study, the bio-oil was emulsified with diesel using Span 80 and Tween 60 as surfactants. The resultant mixture showed an HHV value of 44.32 MJ/kg, which was close to the commercial diesel fuel (45.65 MJ/kg) [110]. Another important factor that plays a key role in obtaining a stable emulsion and thereby a high-quality bio-oil is the hydrophilic-lipophilic balance (HLB) number of the surfactant. HLB is a measure of the degree to which a surfactant is hydrophilic or lipophilic in nature. HLB generally varies between 0 and 18. Figure 9.2B shows the scale of HLB values, indicating that a surfactant having an HLB range of 4–8 would result in W/O emulsions, while a surfactant with an HLB range of 9–12 would lead to O/W emulsions. Bio-oil emulsification with diesel or biodiesel using surfactants of varying HLB values has been investigated to improve bio-oil stability and other properties. For instance, Martin et al. [111] demonstrated the effect of

TABLE 9.6
Comparative Analysis of Bio-Oil Fuel Properties and Emulsions Fuel Properties.

Bio-oil fuel properties					Emulsification			Emulsions fuel properties					References
C wt%	H wt%	O wt%	N wt%	HHV (MJ/kg)	Mixture	Emulsifier	HLB	C wt%	H wt%	O wt%	N wt%	HHV (MJ/kg)	
42.60	8.47	48.85	0.08	19.50	BO + 10% CG	/	/	42.11	8.54	49.27	0.08	19.40	[44]
42.60	8.47	48.85	0.08	19.50	BO + 20% CG	/	/	41.62	8.61	49.70	0.07	19.30	[44]
42.60	8.47	48.85	0.08	19.50	BO + 10% CG	0.5% Span 80	/	42.21	8.55	49.17	0.08	19.40	[44]
47.02	7.63	44.81	0.54	21.38	BO[a] + 90% D	5% (Span 80 and Tween 60)	7.3	82.47	13.56	0	3.97	44.32	[110]
47.02	7.63	44.81	0.54	21.38	BO[a] + 86% D	6.6% (Span 80 and Tween 60)	7.3	83.26	13.66	0.06	3.97	43.68	[110]
61.35	6.34	32.07	0.24	23.50	BO + 80% D	/	/	80.93	12.26	6.77	0.05	41.20	[114]
61.35	6.34	32.07	0.24	23.50	BO + 80% Et	/	/	53.98	11.77	34.20	0.05	28.60	[114]
75.65	5.20	18.97	0.17	28.90	BO + 80% D	/	/	84.11	12.06	3.79	0.03	42.30	[114]
42.64	7.55	49.59	0.22	18.90	BO + 4.35% G + 1.95% Mt	/	/	42.39	7.69	49.72	0.20	18.90	[33]
42.64	7.55	49.59	0.22	18.90	BO + 10.8% G + 5% Mt	/	/	42.0	7.92	49.90	0.18	18.95	[33]
42.64	7.55	49.59	0.22	18.90	BO + 22.8% G + 13.4% Mt	/	/	41.15	8.47	50.24	0.14	19.08	[33]
42.64	7.55	49.59	0.22	18.90	BO + 30.1% G + 23.1% Mt	/	/	40.40	9.03	50.47	0.10	19.24	[33]
42.64	7.55	49.59	0.22	18.90	BO + 42.7% G + 32.6% Mt	/	/	39.47	9.65	50.83	0.05	19.40	[33]
42.64	7.55	49.59	0.22	18.90	BO + 51.1% G + 38.1% Mt	/	/	38.89	10.02	51.07	0.02	19.48	[33]
39.96	7.74	52.19	0.11	15.27	BO + 60% D	4% octanol	/	77.54	11.75	9.71	1.00	41.43	[108]
/	/	/	/	13.8	BO + 90% D	10% Tween 80	/	/	/	/	/	41.38	[115]
/	/	/	/	13.8	BO + 90% D	10% Brij 58	/	/	/	/	/	41.18	[115]

BO: Bio-oil; CG: Crude glycerol; G: Glycerol; D: Diesel; Et: Ethanol; Mt: Methanol; HLB: Hydrophilic-lipophilic balance; [a] BO: Ether-extracted bio-oil was used in the study

Thermochemical Production of Bio-Oil

surfactant polyethylene glycol-dipolyhydroxystearate (PEG-DPHS) of varying HLB values on the stability of bio-oil emulsion with diesel fuel. The results revealed that the surfactant with an HLB of 4.75 produced the most stable emulsion with uniform size (~0.48 μm) of droplets when the diesel/bio-oil/surfactant ratio of 32:8:1 was used in the experiments. It was further reported that the droplets were quite stable until seven days, as no coalescence was observed. Such an emulsion showed greatly improved fuel properties, exhibiting the HHV value of 41.2 MJ/kg, which was approximately 75% higher than the raw bio-oil. A significant decrease in the viscosity and water content was also observed, which were 5.94 cP and 1.74 wt%, respectively [111]. In a separate study, Farooq et al. [110] investigated the emulsification of bio-oil with diesel using surfactant of varying HBL values. Firstly, they treated the raw bio-oil with ether and used the ether-extracted bio-oil for emulsification with diesel. Two surfactants, Tween 60 (HLB of 14.6) and Span 80 (4.3) were mixed to obtain the final surfactant with an HLB range of 4.3–8.8. An emulsion of bio-oil/surfactant/diesel was prepared with a ratio of 5/5/90 wt%, and the results showed that the surfactant with an HLB of 7.3 was optimal for obtaining the stable emulsion. The resultant emulsion showed a very high HHV value of 44.32 MJ/kg, which was nearly 107% higher than the raw bio-oil [110]. Based on the results from the previous two studies, it can be suggested that to obtain a stable emulsion, the optimal HLB value may differ on the type of surfactant and might vary depending on the composition of the bio-oil. For example, if the bio-oil contains a higher proportion of aromatic hydrocarbons, it would be miscible with diesel and may require a surfactant with a lower HLB value to produce a stable emulsion. On the hand, the bio-oil with no hydrocarbons and rich in oxygenated compounds may demand a surfactant with a higher HLB value to make a stable emulsion.

The emulsification of bio-oil with other than diesel or biodiesel fuel has also been investigated for bio-oil upgrading. For example, Zhang et al. [112] demonstrated bio-oil emulsification with crude glycerol using Span 80 as the surfactant. They studied the effect of various parameters to produce the stable emulsion with crude glycerol and found that the concentration of surfactant of 1% and temperature of below 45 °C was favorable for producing stable bio-oil/glycerol emulsions. However, they also reported the presence of some impurities in the crude glycerol, such as water, salt, and alkali metals, that significantly decreased the stability of emulsions [112]. The bio-oil emulsification can also be achieved without using any surfactant, which could make the process simpler and more cost-effective. It has been demonstrated that ultrasound emulsification with mechanical agitation is effective in breaking the droplets to produce stable emulsions. Therefore, it could prove highly advantageous over conventional emulsification and can also prevent the use of surfactants [44,113]. For instance, in their further study, Zhang et al. [44] demonstrated the emulsification of bio-oil with crude glycerol using ultrasound and mechanical agitation. To prepare a stable emulsion with bio-oil, the amount of glycerol was controlled so that it contained 1% of soap content to prevent the re-coalescence of droplets, while the ultrasound at 40% amplitude for four minutes and mechanical agitation for two minutes was applied to obtain a stable emulsion. The ultrasound treatment could help in the effective breakdown of droplets, while the mechanical agitation could prevent the re-coalescence of droplets. The results showed that the applied combined approach resulted in an emulsion that could be stable for a maximum of 15 h and improved the fuel properties compared to the raw bio-oil. For example, the produced emulsion showed a viscosity of 119.2 mPa.s, which was approximately 32% lower than the sole bio-oil [44].

Similar to solvent addition, emulsification could be a remarkable approach to improve the bio-oil properties, but it requires other physical techniques, such as stirring and ultrasonication, to produce a stable emulsion, and the use of additional surfactant that increases the cost of overall bio-oil upgrading.

9.3.3 Filtration to Remove Solid Char Residue

The crude bio-oil contains some solid char particles (1–10 μm) that also encompass metal ions, which are usually present in the biomass and are retained in the char particles during the pyrolysis process. The metal ions may act as a catalyst and promote the polymerization and condensation reactions during bio-oil storage, adversely affecting the chemical composition of the bio-oil and making it highly unstable to use as a drop-in fuel [116]. The char particles can also agglomerate and transform into larger particles, which can easily be deposited in engine valves and may block them, adversely affecting engine ignition. The char particles can also cause corrosion problems in the engines. Therefore, removing the char particles and metal ions is imperative to improve the bio-oil properties. In this regard, some successful attempts have been demonstrated using filtration techniques to remove the char particles from the bio-oil [47,48,117–122]. The filtration process can be divided mainly into liquid phase filtration and hot vapor filtration (HVF). Both modes of bio-oil filtration have shown positive results for the removal of char particles as well as improved bio-oil stability [66]. Figure 9.3a shows a schematic diagram of fast pyrolysis unit with HVF.

Liquid phase filtration is considered a post-pyrolysis treatment or a complete downstream bio-oil processing approach. It can be used to separate solid particles of 1–10 μm size [47,119]. Evidently, Javaid et al. [47] demonstrated the application of tubular ceramic membranes with a pore size of 0.5–0.8 μm for microfiltration of

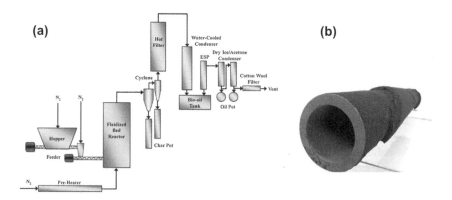

FIGURE 9.3 (a) Schematic diagram of fast pyrolysis unit with hot vapor filter [123]. (b) Filter candle with a cake layer [48].

Thermochemical Production of Bio-Oil

bio-oil at a temperature range of 38–45 °C and trans-membrane pressures of 1–3 bars. The authors reported a significant reduction in the char particles and overall ash content in the bio-oil, as confirmed by the microscopic analysis. However, insignificant changes were observed in the chemical composition of the bio-oil after the filtration process [47]. The most concerned problem of using membranes for bio-oil filtration is fouling of the membranes in long-run filtration, which can occur due to pore constriction, partial or complete blockage of pores, and the formation of a cake layer on its surface. Therefore, the regular washing of membranes with solvents, like methanol or acetic acid, is important to hamper the fouling.

On the other hand, HVF has proven more advantageous to remove char particles as well as to improve the bio-oil properties. It has been shown that char particles <10 µm can be removed using HVF. Unlike liquid filtration, which is a post-treatment method, HVF upgrades the bio-oil in mid pyrolysis process prior to the condensation. HVF can be further classified into two types based on the introduction of the filter, that is, *ex-situ* HVF and *in-situ* HVF. In *ex-situ* HVF, the filter can be placed downstream of the pyrolysis process before vapor condensation. Alternatively, in *in-situ* HVF, the filter is introduced in a continuous fluid bed pyrolysis system [66]. It has been observed that *ex-situ* HVF results in a significant decrease in bio-oil yield, while *in-situ* HVF could be advantageous to obtain higher bio-oil yields and lower cake formation on the filter [121]. Generally, an HVF unit is comprised of porous and permeable filter elements like filter candle, filter media, and membrane. Filters are usually made up of ceramic and metal elements applicable for high temperatures. Filter candles are cylindrical in shape and made up of ceramic monolith or other materials with 1 to 3 m in length, depending on the type of materials, and a diameter of 60–150 mm [124]. Filter media is made up of high or low-density ceramic-like silicon carbide alumina or cordierite or metal filter media which is made up of sintered metal or metal alloy. HVF units are coupled with a pyrolysis system for bio-oil filtration. During filtration, the pyrolytic vapors are passed through the filters, where the treated pyrolytic vapors leave the filter through an open end, while the untreated vapors enter the filter candles. Dust particles are also formed during the process, which aggregate on the surface of the candle and form a cake layer (shown in Figure 9.3b). The char particles or alkali and alkali earth metals are filtered in the HVF mainly by two mechanisms, surface filtration and depth filtration. In surface filtration, generally, the particles larger than the pore size of filters are filtered through a sieving mechanism where they attach to the surface of the filter. The cake on the filter is removed using jet pulsing techniques [124]. In depth filtration, particles are filtered on filter media where the particles are trapped through diffusion mechanism. The integration of HVF with the pyrolysis unit is challenging since the pyrolytic vapors form a sticky cake layer inside the filters which requires additional efforts to remove. Therefore, efficient techniques are required to remove the cake more easily and prevent the blocking of the filters.

Ex-situ HVF has been widely used for bio-oil upgrading. For example, Baldwin et al. [117] demonstrated the application of *ex-situ* HVF to remove the char particles from bio-oil produced from oak wood by employing the pyrolysis reactor, which was operated in the entrained-flow mode. The hot vapor filter comprised of either porous sintered stainless-steel metal powder or sintered ceramic powder was placed slipstream from the pyrolysis process development unit so that the filtered and unfiltered bio-oils could be separately collected for the comparison, while the bio-oil condensation and collection system was interfaced to the slipstream filter unit. The results demonstrated that the bio-oil obtained after the HVF using either of the filtration systems showed significantly less alkali metals than the unfiltered bio-oil. For example, the bio-oil obtained from the filtration system using porous sintered stainless-steel metal powder showed concentrations of sodium and potassium at 7 and 14 ppm, which were 49 and 50 ppm in the unfiltered bio-oil, respectively. Similarly, the sodium and potassium concentrations in the bio-oil obtained from the sintered ceramic powder filtration system were less than 5 ppm. Consequently, the bio-oil's significant effect on aging and viscosity reduction was noticed in the filtered bio-oil. However, stainless-steel filter was not found appropriate as a high concentration of iron was detected in the bio-oil filtered using a stainless-steel filter that was probably due to leaching from the filter, which indicates the importance of filter material for effective bio-oil upgrading. Another important observation in the study was the major decrease of 10–30% in the bio-oil yield, which was attributed to the catalytic activity of alkali metals and char present on the filter that probably reduced the activation energy of secondary cracking reactions for the pyrolytic vapors and increased the production of hydrogen and methane [117].

The temperature of the filter unit plays an important role in the removal of alkali metals, physical properties of the bio-oil, and the yields of pyrolytic products (bio-oil, bio-char, gases). Mei et al. [120] demonstrated the effect of the temperature of HVF on the removal of alkali metals and analyzed its effect on the bio-oil properties. They used a ceramic hot vapor filter to upgrade the bio-oil produced under fast pyrolysis of pine wood in a fluidized-bed reactor and varying HVF temperature from 350 to 500 °C. The results showed higher bio-oil yield obtained under HVF temperature of 400 °C when compared to 350 or 500 °C, while the concentrations of alkali metals and solid contents were also lower in the bio-oil obtained at this temperature. Consequently, the filtered bio-oil showed the HHV value of 23.29 MJ/kg, which was slightly lower than the bio-oil produced at 500 °C (25.88 MJ/kg), however, the viscosity of 26.9 mm^2/s was the lowest compared to either 350 or 500 °C, which were 28.6 and 37.6 mm^2/s, respectively [120]. Similarly, Chen et al. [119] investigated the effect of HVF to filter the char and solid particles in rice husk bio-oil and showed a noticeable decrease in the contents of char and alkali metals compared to unfiltered bio-oil. This study also reported a decrease of ~2.2% in the bio-oil with HVF process. Another study demonstrated the effect of filter temperature on yields of pyrolytic products with results shown in Figure 9.4, which suggests an increase in the bio-oil yield from 400 to 475 °C, while a decrease in the bio-oil yield was noticed as the temperatures increased to 550 °C [123]. Significant increase in char and gas yields was observed with HVF compared to non HVF fast pyrolysis [123]. The decrease in bio-oil yield is mainly attributed to the promotion of secondary cracking reactions catalyzed by char and metal particles present in the cake layer. A study revealed that during the filtration process major cracking reactions occur in the homogeneous gas phase, while some other reactions like dehydration and decarboxylation take place heterogeneously by char particles or metals present in the cake layer [48]. The physical characteristics of the cake, concentration of metals and

Thermochemical Production of Bio-Oil

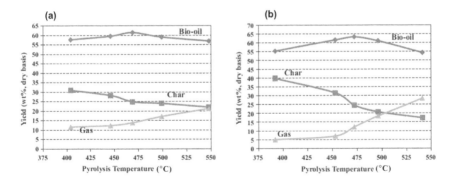

FIGURE 9.4 Effect of temperature on product yields from fast pyrolysis of cassava rhizome (a) without hot vapor filter and (b) with hot vapor filter.

Source: Reproduced with permission from [123].

porosity may have significant effect on bio-oil composition, which should be studied in the future. Hence, it can be suggested that *ex-situ* HVF could prove significant for the removal of char and metal particles but the bio-oil yield could decrease due to the catalytic activity of char and metal particles attached to the filter that promote the secondary cracking reactions [66,117,120]. However, these challenges encountered in *ex-situ* HVF can be overcome and the filter fouling can be diminished if the filter is used *in-situ* in a continuous fluidized bed pyrolysis system. Hoekstra et al. [121] successfully tested *in-situ* filtration of the char particles using wire mesh filters with a 5 μm pore size. The results revealed less filter fouling and efficient process stability achieved during the continuous run of 2 h, while a significant decrease in solid contents and alkali metals was noticed in the filtered bio-oil. Besides, the liquid yield of approximately 61–62% was achieved which was comparably higher than that of pyrolysis without HVF process [121].

This technique is highly advantageous to remove the solid char particles that, if present in the bio-oil, could initiate the polymerization and condensation reactions, making the bio-oil highly unstable, hence, filtration can increase the bio-oil stability and also decreases the viscosity. However, HVF may reduce bio-oil yield significantly. The presence of char and alkali metals promotes secondary cracking reactions of pyrolytic vapors and extra residence time in the filter might also boost the cracking reactions, thereby reducing the bio-oil yields and increasing gas and char yields. Cake formation on the filter also leads to pressure deviations in filter media, which can make the operation process of filtration quite challenging. Therefore, it is very important to maintain the cake removal or regeneration to prevent pressure deviations and make filtration process stable for bio-oil upgrading. In addition, the use of filtration may increase the cost of bio-oil upgrading as the membranes used in the process are highly expensive. Besides, they need regular washing with solvents which can further make the process costly. Therefore, cost-effective and more efficient membranes should be developed for bio-oil upgrading to make the process economical and more significant. Very little or nothing has been studied to estimate the cost of filtration for bio-oil upgrading. Hence, a techno-economic study is further proposed to determine the capital and operational costs of the process and estimate the cost of the upgraded bio-oil. Filtration process removes contaminants and improves certain bio-oil properties like viscosity but high oxygen and water content and low HHV make the bio-oil a poor drop-in fuel. Therefore, filtration technique should be further integrated with other bio-oil upgrading technique such as hydrotreatment to improve the calorific value.

9.3.4 Electrochemical or Electrocatalytic Upgrading of Bio-Oil

Electrochemical upgrading, widely known as electrocatalytic hydrogenation, is a well-known process of converting oxygenated or carbonyl-containing compounds into value-added organic compounds or hydrocarbons [125–127]. However, only recently, electrocatalytic upgrading of bio-oil has been reported, which is believed to be a noteworthy alternative for conventional hydrogenation process that occurs at high temperatures and hydrogen pressures of up to 2000 MPa. Electrocatalytic hydrogenation is generally carried out in an electrolytic membrane fuel cell. The fuel cell utilizes the protons for bio-oil hydrogenation that result from the oxidation of water, therefore, eliminating the use of high-pressure hydrogen and high temperature for bio-oil upgrading, which decreases the cost of bio-oil upgrading or other chemicals. Figure 9.5 shows an electrochemical cell used for bio-oil upgrading, made up of two compartments, the anode and the cathode, separated by a polymer membrane that could be either a cation exchange membrane (CEM) or anion exchange membrane (AEM). At the anode, the oxidation of H_2O takes place, releasing O_2 and H^+, while at the cathode, the oxygenated compounds (in this case, bio-oil containing oxygenated compounds) are hydrogenated by the addition of H^+ transferred through the membrane from the anode, evolving hydrogen during the process. At the cathode, a catalyst can be used to reduce the overpotential of hydrogen evolution reaction (HER) and increase the conversion efficiency of the compound

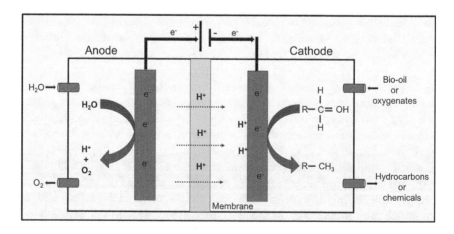

FIGURE 9.5 Electrochemical cell for bio-oil upgrading.

Thermochemical Production of Bio-Oil

to the desired product. Similarly, the anode can also be modified with catalysts to improve efficiency.

A number of studies have reported the electrocatalytic hydrogenation of bio-oil model compounds to stable or value-added compounds, however, only a few studies have demonstrated the application of electrochemical cells for real bio-oil upgrading. For example, Zhao et al. [128] demonstrated the electrocatalytic hydrogenation of furfural to furfuryl alcohol. Furfural is one of the main compounds formed during pyrolysis of hemicellulose, which can be hydrogenated to a high-value compounds, that is, furfuryl alcohol, which is widely used in chemical and polymer industries. Conventionally, furfuryl alcohol is prepared by vapor phase catalytic hydrogenation of furfural under high temperatures and high hydrogen pressures. Alternatively, electrocatalytic hydrogenation can be operated at mild temperatures and can eliminate the external supply of hydrogen, which otherwise uses the *in-situ* produced H_2 during the electrocatalytic hydrogenation. The study by Zhao et al. [129] used H-type electrochemical cell for hydrogenation of furfural with different metal and metal-activated carbon fiber catalysts at the cathode. The results showed that sole platinum cathode showed better selectivity of approximately 99% for furfuryl alcohol as compared to copper, lead and nickel cathodes. However, the conversion or hydrogenation efficiency was found lower (8%) for the platinum cathode due to low active surface area. Subsequently, the platinum cathode was modified with high surface area activated carbon fiber catalysts, which enhanced the conversion efficiency to 82% [128]. Similarly, electrocatalytic hydrogenation of some other bio-oil model compounds has been demonstrated. For instance, phenol, guaiacol, and syringol are the dominant compounds in the bio-oil composition, usually formed during the pyrolysis of the lignin content of the feedstock. Evidently, Li et al. [125] investigated the electrocatalytic hydrogenation of guaiacol in ruthenium/activated carbon cathode based two-chamber H-type electrochemical cell, Nafion-117 membrane and catholyte containing HCl, NaCl and NaOH. The major product of guaiacol hydrogenation was found to be cyclohexanol, while phenol was found to be the intermediate product. The study also suggested that during the electrochemical hydrogenation of guaiacol, demethoxygenation was the dominant deoxygenation reaction while in conventional catalytic upgrading of guaiacol, demethylation is one the major deoxygenation pathways, indicating that the former process retains more carbon in the liquid products than the latter and hence can prove more advantageous for enhanced bio-oil upgrading.

After the successful demonstration of electrocatalytic hydrogenation of bio-oil model compounds, this approach has been applied for real bio-oil upgrading in few studies that showed considerable positive results for bio-oil deoxygenation. For example, Elangovan et al. [126] demonstrated bio-oil deoxygenation using an oxygen ion conducting ceramic membrane-based electrochemical cells, operated at 550 °C, while a condenser was attached to the cell to condense the vapors and was kept at 10 °C. The results reported that approximately 24.5% oxygen reduction was observed in the bio-oil after electrochemical hydrogenation and approximately 16% increase in carbon content was achieved, which could be attributed to the conversion of oxygenated compounds into hydrocarbons. However, it was difficult to estimate the correct deoxygenation pathways due to the presence of numerous compounds in the bio-oil composition. In a recent study, bio-oil produced from the pine wood pyrolysis was upgraded in a dual membrane electrochemical cell, an AEM attached to the cathode and a CEM attached to the anode [127]. This demonstration showed improvements in few properties of the bio-oil, such as the pH increased from 2.6 to 4.5 and the total acid number decreased from 193 to 149 (mg of KOH/g, dry). This decrease in total acid number was attributed to the removal of carbonyl group-containing compounds, such as carboxylic acids and aldehydes, suggesting the successful hydrogenation of carbonyl moieties during the process [127].

Electrocatalytic upgrading could prove effective to convert the oxygenated compounds into hydrocarbons. However, the technique has not been used extensively for real bio-oil upgrading due to some major challenges. For example, the technique utilizes costly membranes and hydrogen, which makes the process highly expensive compared to the other techniques. Moreover, it requires supply of electricity to initiate the reactions. This electricity could also be provided from other renewable technology such as microbial fuel cells (MFCs) that can produce sufficient power for electrocatalytic hydrogenation. MFCs are also the electrochemical cells that use microorganisms to convert the chemical energy present in organic compounds into electricity [130,131]. Overall, it needs more development and research to make this technique more efficient and advanced to use for real bio-oil upgrading at a pilot-scale. Table 9.7 provides the main advantages and challenges of all methods for downstream bio-oil upgrading discussed in the previous sections. Besides making the bio-oil to a gasoline-like product, it can also be upgraded to produce other clean fuels, has been discussed in the following section.

9.3.5 Hydrotreatment of Bio-Oil

Hydrotreatment of bio-oil is the treatment with hydrogen in the presence of an active catalyst made up of metal or metal/support at temperatures between 200 and 500 °C and pressure in the range of 3–30 MPa [53–54]. It involves the removal of oxygen from oxygenated compounds of bio-oil through hydrodeoxygenation (HDO) reaction to produce hydrocarbons and water as the by-product. The main reactions involved in bio-oil upgrading under hydrotreatment are i) hydrogenation of $C - C$ and $C - O$ bonds, ii) breaking of $C - C$ bond by retro-aldol condensation and decarbonylation, iii) dehydration of $C - OH$ groups, and iv) hydrogenolysis of $C - O - C$ bonds. Hydrotreatment is considered highly efficient for bio-oil upgrading compared to cracking since it removes oxygen in the form of H_2O while in cracking oxygen is removed in the form of CO_2 and CO which decreases the total carbon yield [19,53,132]. More information on the reaction mechanisms involved in the conversion of oxygenated compounds to hydrocarbons can be found elsewhere [133–135]. Numerous studies have been conducted to examine the hydrotreatment of bio-oils and has proven most valuable approach among above discussed downstream technologies for bio-oil upgrading.

Hydrotreatment of bio-oils can be carried out in different reactors, such as batch, continuous and down flow reactors [136,137], are shown in Figure 9.6. Generally, the hydrotreatment is carried out in two steps. Firstly, the bio-oil is stabilized at lower temperature of between 100 and 300 °C in the presence of catalyst to convert the

Thermochemical Production of Bio-Oil

TABLE 9.7
Advantages and Challenges of Methods Used for Bio-Oil Upgrading.

No.	Method	Advantages	Challenges
1	Solvent addition	• A very simple approach for bio-oil upgrading • Decreases viscosity of bio-oil • Enhances stability of bio-oil • Increases heating value	• May increase water content • May decrease pH of bio-oil • Increases overall cost for bio-oil upgrading • Requires more research to understand the chemical reactions between the solvent and compounds of bio-oil
2	Emulsification	• A simple and effective approach for bio-oil upgrading • Reduces bio-oil viscosity • Enhances the calorific value and cetane number • Increases bio-oil stability	• The reaction mechanisms could be complex to understand • Requires other physical technique to produce a stable emulsion • Process parameters such as temperature and stirring are critical to obtain a stable emulsion • Requires an additional surfactant that increases the cost
3	Filtration	• An efficient approach to remove char particles and alkali metals • Filtered bio-oil exhibits lower viscosity and higher stability due to the removal of solid particles that can initiate the polymerization and condensation reactions. • Reduction in ageing reaction rate during storage • Removal of contaminants protects downstream equipment from corrosion and catalysts from poisoning	• Membranes are highly expensive • Membranes requires regular washing with solvents that can increase the cost • Some filter units require higher temperature • Cake formation causes pressure drops in the filter • Increases water content • Reduces HHV of bio-oil • Decreases bio-oil yield and increases char and gas yields by promoting secondary cracking reactions of vapors
4 5	Electrocatalytic Upgrading Hydrotreatment	• Increases the content of hydrocarbons in the bio-oil • Increases pH of bio-oil • Decreases acid number mainly due to the removal of carbonyl group-containing compounds • Can be used to convert bio-oil into high value-added compounds • Increases the content of hydrocarbons in the bio-oil • Other valuable products like phenols are also enhanced • Increases calorific value of bio-oil • Cost of upgraded bio-oil would be in range of $0.74–1.80/L	• An energy intensive process • Supply of hydrogen makes the process expensive • The use of membranes could be uneconomical • Needs more investigation to understand the chemical reactions during electrocatalytic bio-oil upgrading • Use of hydrogen makes the process highly expensive • Transportation and storage of hydrogen add the cost • Needs extra precautionary steps • Catalyst deactivation is a major challenge • Sulfur leaching from sulfided catalyst contaminates bio-oil that requires additional purification step

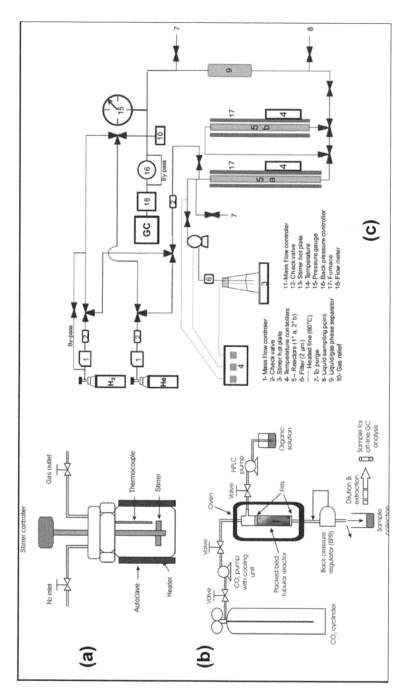

FIGURE 9.6 Schematic diagrams of batch reactor [136], continuous reactor [137], and down flow reactor [138] for hydrotreatment of bio-oils.

Source: Reproduced with permission from respective references.

Thermochemical Production of Bio-Oil

carboxyl and carbonyl functional groups to alcohol. Secondly, the stabilized bio-oil is treated at higher temperature around 350–400 °C where it undergoes HDO and cracking reactions in the presence of active catalysts [139,140]. The reactors can be operated at different optimized operating parameters such as temperature, pressure, relative flow rate and type of catalyst to obtain efficient bio-oil upgrading and less coke formation on the catalyst to prevent its early deactivation. For instance, temperature is one of the most important parameters to obtain the higher conversion of oxygenated compounds into hydrocarbons and hence decrease the oxygen content and increase the carbon and hydrogen content in the bio-oils. A number of studies suggest that in stabilization step of hydrotreatment, a temperature range of 100–300 °C, pressures between 29 and 290 bar and reaction time interval of 0.5–4 h are ideal to obtain the bio-oil yield in the range of 17–92 wt% and oxygen content of 1–16 wt% in the bio-oils [141,142]. However, for second step of hydrotreatment, higher temperatures of more than 300 °C are required to crack the larger molecules in the bio-oil but may vary depending on the type of catalyst used for the hydrotreatment. For example, Auersvald et al. [53] investigated the effect of temperature on bio-oil hydrotreatment in a continuous flow reactor in the presence of commercial sulfide $NiMo/Al_2O_3$ catalyst. The authors applied a range of temperatures of 240–360 °C and pressure of 2–8 MPa, while the hydrogen flow rate of 90 L h^{-1} was used in the experiments. Figure 9.7 shows the results for the effect of temperature on physicochemical properties of bio-oils. It can be clearly observed from the figure that undesirable properties of the bio-oils, such as acid number and content, significantly decreased with increase in temperature from 240 to 360 °C, while the desirable properties, such as heating value and degree of deoxygenation, considerably increased with increase in the reaction temperature. Therefore, it can be estimated that the higher temperatures enhanced the deoxygenation reactions like dehydration, decarboxylation, decarbonylation which were accompanied with hydrogenation reactions, leading to increase in H/C atomic ratio of bio-oils and decreasing O/C atomic ratio. The study also revealed that increase in hydrogen pressure from 2 to 8 MPa enhanced hydrogenation reactions, confirmed with the increase in H/C atomic ratio of bio-oils [53]. The selection of a temperature range is also essential to minimize the coke formation onto the catalyst surface during hydrotreatment of bio-oils. It is evident that temperature has a great influence on activation energies of the reactions that take place during hydrotreatment of bio-oils and it may promote the aromatization and polymerization reactions that usually favor coke formation and ultimately can lead to blockage of the reactor. Gholizadeh et al. [141] provided insightful information on the effect of temperature (370–470 °C) on coke formation and bio-oil properties during hydrotreatment of mallee wood pyrolysis oil in a continuous flow reactor using presulfided $NiMo/Al_2O_3$ catalyst. The results showed that increasing the temperature augmented the coke formation considerably. The study reported the formation of small and large aromatic ring structures that probably occupied the active sites of the catalyst and deactivated the catalyst. The study also revealed that the increase in temperature from 375 to 400 °C achieved the lowest oxygen content and highest carbon content in the bio-oils irrespective of varying bio-oil feed. However, further increase in temperature up to 450 °C marginally decreased the carbon content and increased the oxygen content in the bio-oils. The increase in oxygen content at

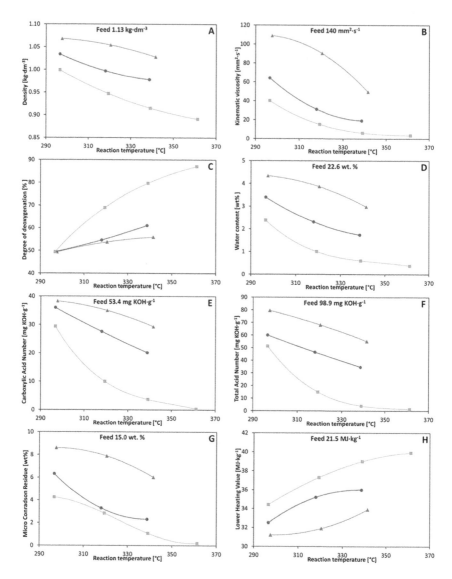

FIGURE 9.7 Effect of temperature and pressure on physicochemical properties of the organic phase of products: density (A), kinematic viscosity (B), degree of deoxygenation (DOD) (C), water content (D), carboxylic acid number (CAN) (E), total acid number (TAN) (F), micro Conradson carbonization residue (MCR) (G), lower heating value (H); blue triangle – 2 MPa, red circle – 4 MPa, green square – 8 MPa.

Source: Reproduced with permission from [53].

higher temperatures can be attributed to the reduced activity of the catalyst due to coke deposition [141]. The amount of coke formation on the catalyst surface can be reduced by heating the hydrogen at the inlet point of the reactor. Evidently, a study

Thermochemical Production of Bio-Oil

demonstrated the application of active hydrogen at the inlet point of bio-oil to heat and activate the catalyst [143]. The results showed decreased coke deposition and lesser reactor blockage during hydrotreatment of bio-oil. This is probably because the active hydrogen enhanced cracking activity and reduced polymerization of polycyclic aromatics of the bio-oils.

Similarly, other operating parameters such as hydrogen pressure, relative flow rate and catalyst to bio-oil feed ratio are also highly important to obtain the bio-oil with high carbon and less oxygen content and improved calorific values. It has been noticed that increasing the hydrogen pressure enhances hydrogenation and hydrodeoxygenation reactions, subsequently, increases deoxygenation activity and improves the conversion of oxygenated compounds to gasoline-like products and less heavy products, while the lower hydrogen pressure may favor condensation reactions and increases heavy products in the bio-oil. Figure 9.7 shows the results for the effect of hydrogen pressure on the physicochemical properties of bio-oil, investigated by Auersvald et al. [53]. It can be observed from the figure that the higher hydrogen pressure of 8 MPa showed a maximum deoxygenation activity of nearly 85% compared to the lower hydrogen pressure of 2 MPa. The study reported that high hydrogen pressure of 8 MPa enhanced the hydrogenation of oxygenated compounds and produced approximately 8% of heavy products, while a higher yield of nearly 12% of heavy products was obtained with 2 MPa, owing to the promotion of condensation reactions at the lower hydrogen pressure. In addition, the values for undesirable physicochemical properties such as density, acid number, viscosity, and water content decreased constantly with increase in hydrogen pressure [53]. On the other hand, the catalyst-to-bio-oil ratio in the case of batch reactor or liquid hourly space velocity (LHSV) in continuous bed reactor plays a significant role in the distribution of organic compounds in the bio-oil and coke formation on the catalyst, which ultimately affects the bio-oil quality and catalyst deactivation. LHSV is the rate at which bio-oil is fed into the hydrotreatment reactor and can be measured as h^{-1}. A number of studies reported the application of catalyst-to-bio-oil ratio of 1:20 and reaction time of 1–4 h in batch reactors and LHSV of 0.05–2 h^{-1} in continuous bed reactors. For instance, Gholizadeh et al. [142] investigated the influence of LHSV on product distribution during the hydrotreatment of bio-oil in a continuous bed reactor. They applied LHSV of 1, 2, and 3 h^{-1} with different amounts of bio-oil (100–900 mL) at a temperature of 375 °C and a hydrogen pressure of 7 MPa. The yields of organics from the hydrotreatment of bio-oil as a function of the volume of bio-oil fed into the reactor and LHSV are shown in Figure 9.8. They suggest that increasing the LHSV from 1 to 3 h^{-1} increased the yield of organics and reached plateau values when more than 500 mL of bio-oil was fed into the reactor. The study also revealed that a low LHSV of 1 h^{-1} produced less coke yield compared to the LHSV of 3 h^{-1}. This is probably because increasing LHSV offered less residence time, providing less time for hydrotreatment reactions. Moreover, the number of accessible active sites of hydrogen decreases as the concentration of heavy liquid increases in the reactor with an increase in LHSV. Consequently, in the absence of active hydrogen, hydrogenation and hydrocracking reactions are less favored, while polymerization reactions could be enhanced, which ultimately could result in the formation of heavy products and carbonaceous species.

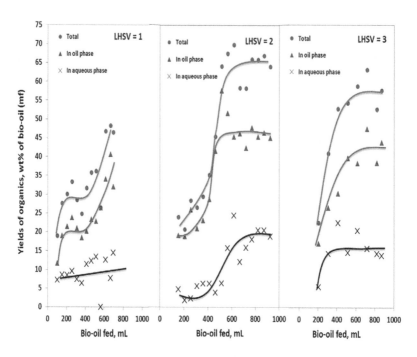

FIGURE 9.8 The yields of organics from the hydrotreatment of bio-oil as a function of the volume of bio-oil fed into the reactor and LHSV (h^{-1}).

Source: Reproduced with permission from [142].

Hydrotreatment of bio-oil obtained from pyrolysis and HTL process has been reported in several studies, and various types of catalysts have been utilized for hydrotreatment of bio-oil to either convert it into a more valuable fuel with improved physicochemical properties or other value-added products [139,156,157]. The major catalyst types used for HDO include the commercialized metal sulfides (MoS_2, $Ni-MoS_2$, and $Co-MoS_2$), efficient noble metals (Ru, Rh, Pd, Pt, and Re) and most commonly used transition metal-based catalysts (Cu, Fe, Mo, Co, and Ni) [138,158,159]. Noble metal-based catalysts are markedly favorable for bio-oil upgrading through the HDO pathway [159]. However, their high cost and high hydrogenation activity lead to excessive hydrogen consumption, which increases the overall cost of the process [136,138]. These catalysts are highly prone to the poisoning of sulfur content present in the bio-oils. On the other hand, transition metals are comparatively cheaper and possess competitive activity for bio-oil upgrading and therefore have been extensively studied for hydrotreatment of bio-oil as well as bio-oil model compounds. Table 9.8 presents the summary of catalysts used for the hydrotreatment of bio-oil and upgraded bio-oil properties.

Metal sulfide catalysts like $NiMoS/Al_2O_3$ and $CoMoS/Al_2O_3$ are commercialized catalysts used in petroleum refining and have been successfully utilized for the hydrotreatment of bio-oils [147,160,161]. In these catalysts, Mo and S act as active parts of the catalyst. The retention of sulfur content is highly important to keep the

TABLE 9.8

Catalysts Applied for Hydrotreatment of Bio-Oils and Properties of Upgraded Bio-Oils.

Catalyst	Hydrotreatment operating parameters						Upgraded bio-oil properties (wt%)					References
	Reactor type	Bio-oil source	Temp (°C)	Pressure (MPa)	Time (h) or LHSV (h⁻¹)	C/B	Bio-oil yield	C	H	O	H_2O	
$NiCu/TiO_2$	Batch	Pine wood	350	20.0	1 h	1:10	45.5	73.0	9.1	15.1	3.6	[144]
$NiCu/Al_2O_3$	Batch	Wheat straw	340	8.0	4 h	1:20	17.9	74.9	9.7	14.3	/	[145]
$NiMo/SiO_2\text{-}Al_2O_3$	Batch	Pine wood	350	14.0	4 h	1:20	42.4	77.2	9.6	13.2	2.9	[146]
$NiMoCe/\delta\text{-}Al_2O_3$	Batch	Cassava rhizome	300	1.0	1 h	1:6.7	/	67.8	7.1	22.2	/	[147]
$NiCu/CeO_2\text{-}ZrO_2$	Batch	Pine wood	350	20.0	1 h	1:10	40.6	78.3	8.5	13.2	8.1	[144]
$NiCu/ZrO_2$	Batch	Pine wood	350	20.0	1 h	1:10	38.9	72.1	8.7	16.1	4.1	[144]
NiCu/CRH	Batch	Pine wood	350	20.0	1 h	1:10	44.9	76.2	8.1	17.7	3.9	[144]
NiCu/Sibunite	Batch	Pine wood	350	20.0	1 h	1:10	35.9	87.6	6.8	5.4	12.5	[144]
$NiCu/\delta\text{-}Al_2O_3$	Batch	Pine wood	350	20.0	1 h	1:10	42.2	74.5	8.4	17.1	4.1	[144]
Ni/Cr_2O_3	Batch	Beech wood	225	8.0	2 h	1:20	42.86	58.3	8.0	33.7	10.5	[148]
$Ni\text{-}Cr/Cr_2O_3$	Batch	Beech wood	225	8.0	2 h	1:20	37.48	60.1	8.2	31.7	10.1	[148]
Ru/C	Batch	Beech wood	225	8.0	2 h	1:20	46.41	59.9	8.1	31.8	10.6	[148]
$NiCu/Al_2O_3$	Batch	Wheat straw	250	8.0	4 h	1:20	/	71.4	9.3	18.2	11.8	[145]
Ru/C	Batch	Pine wood	350	14.0	4 h	1:20	41.5	81.4	9.5	9.0	4.4	[146]
$Ni/SiO_2\text{-}Al_2O_3$	Batch	Pine wood	350	140	4 h	1:20	52.7	75.8	9.0	15.0	5.2	[146]
$NiCu/SiO_2\text{-}Al_2O_3$	Batch	Pine wood	350	14.0	4 h	1:20	49.5	76.0	9.1	14.8	4.6	[146]
$NiPd/SiO_2$	Batch	Pine wood	350	14.0	4 h	1:20	52.5	75.1	9.2	15.5	4.7	[146]
$NiPdCu/SiO_2$	Batch	Pine wood	350	14.0	4 h	1:20	53.1	75.8	9.2	14.9	5.6	[146]

(Continued)

TABLE 9.8 (Continued)

Catalyst	Reactor type	Bio-oil source	Temp (°C)	Pressure (MPa)	Time (h) or LHSV (h⁻¹)	C/B	Bio-oil yield	C	H	O	H₂O	References
							Upgraded bio-oil properties (wt%)					
NiMoCu/SiO₂-Al₂O₃	Batch	Pine wood	350	14.0	4 h	1:20	43.2	77.1	9.4	13.3	2.9	[146]
NiMo/δ-Al₂O₃	Batch	Cassava rhizome	300	1.0	1 h	1:6.7	/	59.2	6.8	31.3	/	[147]
NiMoCu/δ-Al₂O₃	Batch	Cassava rhizome	300	1.0	1 h	1:6.7	/	67.7	7.1	22.3	/	[147]
Ni/C	Batch	/	275	10.0	4 h	1:20	47.6	50.83	9.19	39.24	/	[149]
Ru/C	Packed bed	Pine wood	300	10.0	0.4 h⁻¹	/	49.0	75.0	12.2	10.2	0.44	[150]
Ru/C	Batch	Pine wood	350	20.0	4 h	1:31.5	17.5	79.1	9.3	11.6	/	[151]
Pt/C	Batch	Switchgrass	320	14.5	4 h	1:18	46.6	75.4	8.48	15.04	2.1	[152]
Ru/C	Batch	Corn stover	300	12.5	4 h	/	54.4	78.6	9.69	8.8	2.1	[140]
Pd/C	Batch	Corn stover	300	12.5	4 h	/	52.6	77.8	9.30	10.6	1.8	[140]
Ru/C	Batch	Hardwood	300	5.0	3 h	1:20	63.5	71.0	8.5	20.5	/	[153]
Ni/AC	Batch	Hardwood	300	5.0	3 h	1:20	60.0	72.8	8.3	18.8	/	[153]
NiP/AC	Batch	Hardwood	300	5.0	3 h	1:20	59.1	80.0	8.4	18.1	/	[153]
NiRu/AC	Batch	Hardwood	300	5.0	3 h	1:20	55.4	73.4	9.0	17.6	/	[153]
NiRuP/AC	Batch	Hardwood	300	5.0	3 h	1:20	58.7	73.0	8.5	18.3	/	[153]
Co/AC	Batch	Hardwood	300	5.0	3 h	1:20	58.4	72.6	8.2	19.2	/	[153]
CoP/AC	Batch	Hardwood	300	5.0	3 h	1:20	37.2	73.0	7.7	19.2	/	[153]
CoRu/AC	Batch	Hardwood	300	5.0	3 h	1:20	61.2	71.8	8.4	19.7	/	[153]
CoRuP/AC	Batch	Hardwood	300	5.0	3 h	1:20	63.5	73.2	8.4	18.4	/	[153]
Ni/SiO₂-Al₂O₃	Batch	PJ chips	350	7.0	1 h	1:5	55.7	69.2	10.4	20.1	/	[154]
Ni/SiO₂-Al₂O₃	Batch	PJ chips	400	7.0	1 h	1:5	49.4	75.1	12.5	12.2	/	[154]

Thermochemical Production of Bio-Oil

Ni/SiO$_2$-Al$_2$O$_3$	Batch	PJ chips	450	7.0	1 h	1:5	44.8	83.4	16.4	0.0	/	[154]
Ni/Al$_2$O$_3$	Batch	Wheat straw	340	8.0	1.6 h	1:20	76.2	73.5	9.5	15.9	4.7	[155]
NiCu/Al$_2$O$_3$	Batch	Wheat straw	340	8.0	1.6 h	1:20	78.0	69.8	9.8	19.4	6.8	[155]
Ni/SiO$_2$	Batch	Wheat straw	340	8.0	1.6 h	1:20	76.0	70.0	9.2	19.7	6.8	[155]
Ni/ZrO$_2$	Batch	Wheat straw	340	8.0	1.6 h	1:20	76.5	69.9	9.1	20.0	7.4	[155]
NiW/AC	Batch	Wheat straw	340	8.0	1.6 h	1:20	76.0	70.4	9.4	19.3	6.9	[155]
Ni/TiO$_2$	Batch	Wheat straw	340	8.0	1.6 h	1:20	76.8	73.0	9.1	16.8	4.9	[155]
Ru/C	Batch	Wheat straw	340	8.0	1.6 h	1:20	78.0	71.6	10.5	16.9	5.4	[155]

Note: PJ: Pinyon juniper; C/B: catalyst-to-bio-oil ratio

catalyst active during the hydrotreatment of bio-oils. Since the bio-oil contains very low amount of sulfur, sulfur-containing compounds like dimethyl sulfide, H_2S is required to add to the feed to overcome the loss of sulfur and avoid catalyst deactivation [160]. The presence of sulfur vacancies in the catalysts, mainly at the catalyst edges are thought to work as active sites in metal sulfide catalysts that catalyze the hydrodeoxygenation reactions [135], while the catalysts support like Al_2O_3 also contains acidic sites that catalyze various deoxygenation reactions like dehydration, decarboxylation, decarbonylation and convert acids, aldehydes, ketones into hydrocarbons [162]. The addition of transition metals Ni and Cu can be used as Mo promoters and are believed to enhance the number of sulfur vacancies [147,161]. These promoters can donate their valence electrons to Mo, subsequently can make Mo – S weaker, resulting in more active sulfur vacancies. During hydrodeoxygenation on metal sulfide catalysts, the oxygen atom of the functional groups of the reactant is attached to sulfur vacancies and promotes the breaking of $C - O$ [163]. In addition, activated hydrogen from $S - H$ groups is believed to saturate the oxygen atom released from the breaking of $C - O$ [163]. A number of studies have reported the successful application of metal sulfide catalysts for the hydrotreatment of bio-oils. For instance, Grilc et al. [164] investigated the influence of metal sulfide catalysts like $NiMo/Al_2O_3$ and MoS_2 for hydrotreatment of bio-oils produced from HTL of spruce and fir sawdust at a temperature of 300°C and a hydrogen pressure of 8 MPa and compared their activity with other catalysts like Pd/Al_2O_3, Pd/C, and Ni/Al_2O_3-SiO_2. The authors examined the comparative effect of different catalysts studied on various reactions (such as hydrodeoxygenation, decarbonylation, decarboxylation, and catalytic cracking) and yields of upgraded bio-oils. The results suggested that sulfide NiMo catalysts produced a higher yield of upgraded bio-oil compared to oxide and reduced form of NiMo catalysts but lower than Pd/Al_2O_3 and Pd/C. In addition, sulfide NiMo catalysts showed high hydrodeoxygenation, decarboxylation, and catalytic cracking activity. The reduced form of NiMo catalyst also showed high hydrodeoxygenation activity but could not favor decarbonylation, decarboxylation, and cracking much more efficiently compared to sulfide NiMo catalyst. On the other hand, Pd/Al_2O_3, Pd/C, and Ni/Al_2O_3-SiO_2 exhibited lower activity for all the reactions compared to either reduced or sulfide NiMo catalysts [164]. Biller et al. [55] studied the application of sulfided $NiMo/Al_2O_3$ and $CoMo/Al_2O_3$ for hydrotreatment of bio-oil obtained from HTL of *Chlorella*. The hydrotreatment of bio-oil using both catalysts was investigated in a batch reactor at two temperatures of 350 and 405 °C, 13.8 MPa hydrogen pressure, and a catalyst-to-bio-oil ratio of 0.2 [55]. The results reported that the application of sulfided catalysts considerably increased the conversion of oxygenated compounds into hydrocarbons, as a high number of hydrocarbons was observed in the upgraded bio-oil [55]. Although the application of metal sulfide catalysts is highly advantageous for hydrotreatment techniques to obtain the bio-oil with enhanced physicochemical properties and energy density, it may also lead to coke formation and, subsequently, undesirable blockage of the reactor. The use of additives like methanol has been shown to reduce coke formation. Methanol may also react with carboxylic or esters groups of the bio-oil and help to reduce its corrosivity [160]. The other drawback of using sulfided catalysts is the leaching of catalyst-bound sulfur into the upgraded bio-oil. Therefore, additional upgrading approach may require to remove the impurities, which ultimately can increase the overall cost of the bio-oil upgrading.

The other types of catalysts widely used for hydrotreatment of bio-oils are noble metals-based catalysts, such as Rh/C, Rh/ZrO$_2$, Ru/C, Pt/SiO$_2$, and Pd/C, Pd/Al$_2$O$_3$ [140,151,159]. These catalysts show a high reactivity for H$_2$ activation and thus can effectively saturate the oxygen atom of the functional groups of the oxygenated compounds in the bio-oil, making them highly favorable candidates for the hydrotreatment of bio-oils [139]. The other advantage of noble metal-based catalysts is that they are less prone to deactivation by water or sulfur contents present in the bio-oil [134]. Consequently, a number of studies deployed noble metals on different catalytic supports for the hydrotreatment of bio-oil and showed considerable improvement in the bio-oil properties and an increase in the H/C ratio, indicating the successful conversion of oxygenated compounds into hydrocarbons. For example, Wildschut et al. [151] demonstrated the hydrotreatment of fast pyrolysis oil at 250 and 350 °C and hydrogen pressures of 10 and 20 MPa using Ru and Pt on different supports like Ru/C, Pt/C, Pd/C, Ru/Al$_2$O$_3$, and Ru/TiO$_2$. The results revealed that Ru/C achieved the highest yield of upgraded bio-oil and deoxygenation activity which were 60 wt% and 90 wt%, respectively, while Ru/TiO$_2$ showed the least deoxygenation activity that can be attributed to the low surface area of TiO$_2$ [151]. Authors further suggested that other physicochemical properties of bio-oils, like viscosity, water content, and density, were significantly reduced, and a notable increase in HHV of bio-oils was observed. Evidently, the HHV of upgraded bio-oil obtained using Ru/C was 43 MJ/kg, which was approximately two times higher than the feed bio-oil of 20 MJ/kg [151]. A recent study reported the application of Ru/α-Al$_2$O$_3$ and Ru/γ-Al$_2$O$_3$ on hydrotreatment of rice husk pyrolysis oil at 240 °C and a hydrogen pressure of 4 MPa, with a reaction time of 24 hours. The results showed that Ru/α-Al$_2$O$_3$ achieved superior activity for hydrotreatment compared to Ru/γ-Al$_2$O$_3$. Markedly, Ru/α-Al$_2$O$_3$ showed a higher bio-oil yield of nearly 80 wt%, while Ru/γ-Al$_2$O$_3$ could achieve a maximum bio-oil yield of 58.4 wt%. Ru/α-Al$_2$O$_3$ showed less coke formation than Ru/γ-Al$_2$O$_3$, which was ascribed to the higher acidic character of the latter catalyst [151]. In addition, Ru/α-Al$_2$O$_3$ produced a 23.15% yield of hydrocarbons comprised of alkyl-substituted cyclohexane and alkyl-substituted benzene. The use of noble metal-based catalysts showed promising results of bio-oil upgrading through a hydrotreatment approach. However, noble metals are considered rare earth metals and are not present abundantly. Moreover, noble metal-based catalysts are highly expensive, restricting their industrial-scale application for bio-oil upgrading. Therefore, comparatively cheaper catalysts can make the hydrotreatment approach more economical for bio-oil upgrading.

Transition metal-based catalysts are considered highly cost-effective and substantially efficient for the hydrotreatment of bio-oils. Considering their low cost and lower hydrogen consumption, transition metals like Ni, Cu, Co, and Fe have been extensively used with and without different supports as potential catalysts for the hydrotreatment of bio-oils [134,147,158]. The presence of valence electrons in their d-orbitals allows them to interact with reactants. However, the electron density in the d-orbitals plays a key role in the determination of vacant coordination sites [134]. The mechanism of hydrodeoxygenation reactions over transition metal-based catalysts can be understood more clearly using model compounds of the bio-oil components [165–167]. Consequently, many attempts have been made to understand the reaction mechanisms using model compounds, such as guaiacol, anisole, phenol, and p-cresol [167–169].

Several studies have reported hydrotreatment of bio-oils using different monometallic and bimetallic catalysts. For instance, Yin et al. [146] investigated the effect of different transition metal-based catalysts, such as Ni/SiO_2-ZrO_2, $NiCu/SiO_2$-ZrO_2, $NiMo/SiO_2$, and $NiMoCu/SiO_2$ for hydrotreatment of pine wood bio-oil at 350 and 400 °C and hydrogen pressure of 14 MPa for 4 h. The results suggested that upgraded bio-oil showed a higher H/C ratio with $NiMo/SiO_2$ and $NiMoCu/SiO_2$ catalysts compared to Ni/SiO_2-ZrO_2, $NiCu/SiO_2$-ZrO_2. The noticeable point was that Mo-based catalysts yielded more CH_4 due to enhanced methanation reactions, which could be an undesirable product in order to retain more carbon in the bio-oil [146]. Similar to transition metals, the application of metal oxides [134,147], metal phosphides [149,153,166], carbides [138,152], and nitrides [133,134] have also shown promising results for the hydrotreatment of bio-oils.

Hydrotreatment of bio-oils has proven an advantageous approach. Nevertheless, the use of external hydrogen, arduous transport, and exorbitant storage makes the overall process highly expensive. Therefore, it is important to adopt cost-effective measurements to develop the technique more affordable at the industrial scale. In order to reduce the cost of external hydrogen supply, liquid hydrogen donors, such as formic acid, ethanol, and methanol, can be successfully converted into hydrogen through catalytic aqueous phase reforming process. Subsequently, the produced hydrogen can be utilized in the hydro-deoxygenation of bio-oils [170–172]. This approach is called *in-situ* hydrodeoxygenation, where hydrogen is not supplied from outside but rather provided by reforming reactions of hydrogen-donating chemicals. In a recent study, Mohammed et al. [171] demonstrated the application of methanol in *in-situ* hydrodeoxygenation of Napier pyrolytic oil in the presence of Pd/C and Pt/C catalysts. The process was carried out at 350 °C, with 2 wt% catalyst and 20 wt% methanol, and 1 h reaction time. The results showed that the oxygenated compounds in the bio-oil were successfully converted into hydrocarbons. As a result, the upgraded bio-oil showed enhanced physicochemical properties compared to feed bio-oil. For example, feed bio-oil showed H/C ratio of 1.44, while H/C ratios of bio-oil obtained with Pd/C and Pt/C were 1.68 and 1.66, respectively. In addition, HHV was increased from 29.18 MJ/kg of feed bio-oil to 39.32 with Pd/C and 38.07 with Pt/C [171]. Alternative to the application of liquid hydrogen donors, hydrogen can also be generated from water using suitable catalysts. For instance, zinc hydrolysis can lead to the generation of $H_2(Zn + H_2O = ZnO + H_2)$, which can be further utilized for hydrotreatment of bio-oil [173]. Bio-oils also contain approximately 15–30 wt% of water content which can be converted to hydrogen, and the *in-situ* produced hydrogen can be used for bio-oil upgrading making the whole process highly independent from an external source of hydrogen. However, the amount of water present in the bio-oil might not be enough to act as a solvent for all reactants to form a supercritical reaction system, hence, demanding the addition of water. A study attempted *in-situ* hydrodeoxygenation of bio-oil using the water content of bio-oil to produce hydrogen, but the authors also added water and methanol since the bio-oil contained

Thermochemical Production of Bio-Oil

14.5 wt% water only, which might not be adequate to generate the required amount of hydrogen for the treatment [136]. In a typical experiment, authors utilized 6 g zinc powder, 5 g Pd/C catalyst, 50 g bio-oil, 50 mL deionized water and 63 mL methanol as solvents, and loaded them in a 500 mL autoclave reactor. The experiments were carried out at 200–300 °C and 5 h reaction time. The results suggested significant production of hydrocarbons in the upgraded bio-oils, producing 12.47 wt% at 200 °C and 19.36 wt% at 300 °C, while 250 °C produced the maximum hydrocarbons of 24.09 wt%. The oxygenated compounds like phenols, acids, aldehydes, and ketones were reduced considerably, although esters were substantially increased. This was possibly because ketones and aldehydes were hydrogenated during the hydrotreatment process into alcohols that further underwent esterification reactions to yield esters [126,157]. Therefore, *in-situ* hydrodeoxygenation could be an advantageous approach economically as it reduces the cost of external hydrogen supply, but it also produces a low-quality bio-oil. Hence, a comparative techno-economic study considering the quality of bio-oils should be conducted to understand the impact of both types of hydro-deoxygenations.

9.4 COMMERCIAL APPLICATIONS OF BIO-OILS

The main goal of bio-oil upgrading is to make it a competitive fuel to replace heavy fuel oil or light fuel oil for heat generation or use it as a transport fuel. The early bio-oil combustion tests for heating applications at the industrial scale have indicated the bio-oil as a suitable fuel to replace heavy fuel oil. To date, few commercial-scale applications of bio-oil have been reported for combustion in boilers, turbines, and diesel engines. However, some specific modifications are required in the combustion equipment for bio-oil as compared to conventional fuels. In boilers, a variety of fuels can be used for heat generation, whereas bio-oil has also proved to be a suitable fuel for boilers for heat generation with acceptable emissions. For example, the combustion properties of bio-oils were tested in a test boiler on a 4 MW output level in Finland [32]. The study demonstrated the combustion of different bio-oils in the boiler, modified with a special type of front head to avoid heat loss and an extra cylinder inside the furnace to obtain higher temperature and faster volatilization. The bio-oil samples were added with 10% methanol to increase the homogeneity and enhance the combustibility and ignition. The combustion results suggested that the bio-oils were of high grade and the NO_x emissions were competitive to heavy fuel oil and extremely lower than the standard emission value (120 mg/MJ for 50–150 MW boiler) in Finland. Noticeably, the NO_x emissions were reported to be 88 mg/MJ for bio-oil, while the combustion of heavy fuel oil produced NO_x emissions of 88 mg/MJ [32]. Alternatively, bio-oil combustion has also been tested in a gas turbine for heat generation. Earlier, [174] carried out bio-oil combustion in small gas turbine type T216 with the capacity to generate 75kW electric power. The combustion chamber of the gas turbine was modified with inline fuel nozzles, that is, an ignition nozzle and second the main nozzle. The gas turbine was started using diesel oil, firstly, diesel oil was used to operate the ignition nozzle, and the bio-oil was supplied to the main nozzle using an external fuel pump. This gas turbine with dual fuel operation generated a power of 580 kWth, which was lower than the sole diesel fuel operation

(791kWth). However, the former mode resulted in lower NOx emissions as compared to the latter [174]. Recently, a study also reported the bio-oil combustion in a micro gas turbine [30]. The tests were performed using pure bio-oil and bio-oil/ethanol ratios of 20/80 and 50/50% (volume fractions), and the results were compared with the combustion of sole diesel fuel and ethanol. The results reported that pure bio-oil and the blend fuels with a higher fraction of bio-oil showed higher emissions of CO and NO_x than sole diesel fuel and ethanol. These increased emissions of CO and NO_x were attributed to the formation of larger droplets by the viscous bio-oil and fuel-bound nitrogen, respectively. However, the blend fuels showed better electrical efficiency compared to the diesel fuel, which was ascribed to the higher production of water vapor during the combustion process [30]. In addition to boilers and turbines, bio-oil combustion has been successfully demonstrated in diesel engines for power generation. Generally, diesel engines show higher power generation efficiency than boilers and turbines. Laesecke et al. [8] demonstrated bio-oil combustion in a diesel engine using a 0.45 L Ricardo single-cylinder direct injection diesel engine. The bio-oil showed approximately similar thermal efficiency to the diesel fuel. However, combustion air preheating of bio-oil (55 °C) was required for ignition. The longer ignition delay time with the bio-oil could be related to the chemical composition of the bio-oil. Recently, another demonstration showed the combustion behavior of bio-oil and its blends with biodiesel in a single-cylinder research engine [31]. The testing results indicated that pure bio-oil and the blend fuels with higher concentrations of bio-oil showed longer ignition delays than diesel fuel due to the reduction in cetane number and lower heating values.

The above discussion suggests that bio-oil has a great potential to serve as a potential fuel in turbines, boilers, and diesel engines for heat and power generation. However, some modifications are still required either in the combustion units or mixing the bio-oil with the solvents like ethanol, methanol, or diesel fuel to avoid ignition time delays. On the other hand, the application of bio-oil as a transport fuel needs more investigation. Currently, the lower heating values, chemical instability, and other poor physical properties restrict its use in internal combustion engines. The bio-oil upgrading to a suitable transport fuel needs the complete removal of oxygenated compounds, and the presence of naphthenes, paraffins, and aromatic hydrocarbons, and the other physical properties should also be improved to make it a realistic drop-in fuel. Besides, the production of bio-oil at a large scale, similar to the cost of conventional fuels, is one of the key challenges to overcome to make bio-oil economical and affordable to consumers.

9.5 BIO-OIL UPGRADING TO HYDROGEN/SYNGAS *VIA* STEAM REFORMING

The bio-oil generated from biomass pyrolysis or HTL process could also be a suitable feedstock for the steam reforming (SR) technique for the production of H_2 gas and synthesis gas (also termed as syngas; a mixture of CO and H_2). H_2 produced from SR of bio-oil can be further used as a clean fuel as its combustion produces water and no harmful gases are generated, or it can also be used in hydrodeoxygenation of bio-oil for the synthesis of gasoline-like products, while syngas can be further subjected

Thermochemical Production of Bio-Oil

to Fischer-Tropsch process for the production of hydrocarbons. SR is a process that involves the conversion of bio-oil containing oxygenated compounds or hydrocarbons into hydrogen in the presence of water at a temperature range of 350–1000 °C [62,63]. SR of an oxygenated compound of bio-oil is shown in Eq. 9.4.

$$C_n H_m O_k + (n-k) H_2 O \rightarrow n CO + \left(n + \frac{m}{2} - k\right) H_2 \tag{9.4}$$

The presence of a higher amount of steam in the process can lead to a water-gas shift reaction (WGSR) that involves the conversion of CO into CO_2 and H_2 gas, as shown in Eq. 3, while at low temperatures, H_2 produced in the process can combine with CO to generate methane, as given in Eq. 9.4.

$$CO + H_2 O \leftrightarrow CO_2 + H_2 \tag{9.5}$$

$$CO + 3H_2 \leftrightarrow CH_4 + H_2 O \tag{9.6}$$

It is also interesting to note that for a complete SR reaction, one mole of CO is lost for each mole of H_2 produced (Eq. 9.3), and in a methanation reaction (Eq. 9.4), three moles of hydrogen are lost for each mole of CH_4. From a thermodynamics point of view, the reforming reaction (Eq. 9.2) is an endothermic reaction and occurs at high temperatures and low pressures, while WGSR and methanation, shown in Eqs. 9.3 and 9.4, respectively, are exothermic reactions and take place at lower temperatures [175]. Therefore, the endothermic reforming reaction is usually performed in the high-temperature reactor, and the resultant products are transferred to another reactor of lower temperature to carry out the exothermic conversion reactions.

SR of bio-oil can be carried out in different types of reactors, such as combined two-stage pyrolysis-reforming reactor, separate fixed-bed reactor and fluidized bed reactor, tubular quartz micro-reactor, membrane reactor, spouted bed reactor, and nozzle-fed reactor [56]. Some reactors are shown in Figures 9.9, 9.10, and 9.11. Several studies have employed fixed-bed reactors for SR of bio-oil [56,175,176]. However, it is believed that fixed-bed reactor is convenient to reform only lighter model compounds of bio-oil such as acetic acid and ethanol, while the reforming of larger model compounds or crude bio-oil leaves a large amount of residue in the reactor and subsequent heating may lead to thermal degradation and formation of coke. Therefore, a fluidized bed reactor has been widely used to reduce the coke formation during SR of bio-oil or larger bio-oil model compounds. It is thought that the reforming process can be operated more efficiently than fixed-bed reactor [56,59,60]. Where in fixed-bed reactor, a layer of coke can be easily formed, in a fluidized bed reactor, the circulated catalyst particles are in direct contact with bio-oil components, and thus, less coke formation and more hydrogen yield can be obtained. Evidently, a study compared the activity of SR of bio-oil for hydrogen production in a fixed and fluidized bed reactor using Ni-based catalyst and also observed the coke formation in both reactors at similar reaction conditions [177]. The results revealed that carbon deposition was severe in fixed bed reactor compared to fluidized bed, suggesting quicker catalyst deactivation in the former. Since the fluidized bed showed lesser

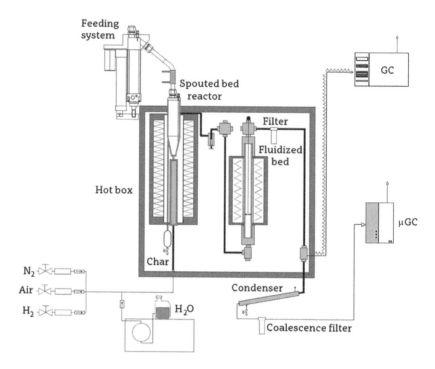

FIGURE 9.9 Scheme of the bench scale plant for continuous biomass pyrolysis-reforming. *Source*: Reproduced with permission from [182].

coke formation, it produced a higher yield of hydrogen, approximately 76%, which was 7% greater than the fixed bed [177]. However, coke deposition is still one of the limitations of fluidized beds. Other limitations associated with catalyst deactivation in fluidized beds are sintering and attrition. These processes result in the loss of active components of catalysts. More information on the mechanism of attrition of catalyst in fluidized bed can be found elsewhere [178]. Fluidized bed reactors could be made up of two beds, in which one bed is used for SR process, and the other is used to regenerate the catalyst by gasification or oxidation. Alternatively, combined fixed and fluidized bed reactor can also be used for SR of bio-oil, which allows the process to carry out at two different temperatures [56,179]. In this combined unit, a fluidized bed is used to evaporate the bio-oil at lower temperatures of 430–500 °C, while steam reforming is carried out in the fixed bed at a higher temperature of >700 °C in the presence of an active catalyst [179].

Another alternative to reduce the coke deposition on the catalyst is applying the two-stage catalytic reforming process, as shown in Figure 9.11 [180,181]. In the first stage, a less active catalyst is used at a temperature of 400–600 °C, while the second stage is operated with a more active catalyst at a temperature >700 °C. It is believed that in two-stage reactor systems, coke-generating precursors are reduced in the first stage, converting macromolecules of bio-oil into smaller compounds that lower coke

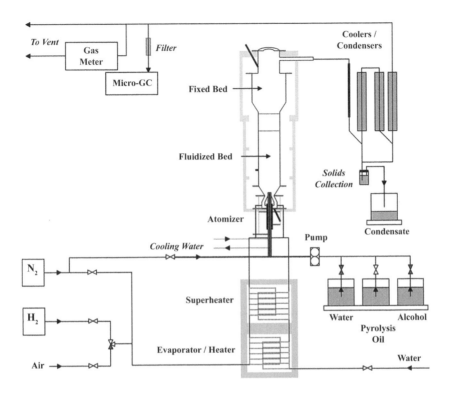

FIGURE 9.10 Schematic overview of the fluidized-bed setup for bio-oil reforming.

Source: Reproduced with permission from [179].

deposition in the second stage. Consequently, it produces an enhanced yield of syngas or H_2 and stabilizes the activity of a catalyst in long-term reaction. For example, Ren et al. [181] demonstrated the application of two-stage SR of bio-oil, using quartz sand in the first stage, fluidized bed reactor and Ni/dolomite for the second stage fixed-bed reactor, and compared the reforming results with single-stage fixed-bed SR at 800 °C. The results showed that two-stage SR produced a higher H_2 yield of 85.3% in 1 h of reaction time, while single-stage could produce 80% of H_2 yield. After 3 h of reaction time, H_2 yield decreased nearly 10% in the single-stage fixed reactor, but only 5.6% reduction in H_2 yield was observed in the two-stage system, owing to reduced coke formation in the system [179]. Another study by Liu et al. [180] performed two-stage catalytic SR of bio-oil using Fe/biochar in the first stage (or pre-reforming) at 350–600 °C and Ni-Ca/γ-Al_2O_3 in the second stage at 700 °C. The study suggested that Fe/biochar in the pre-reforming stage converted coke precursors like polycyclic aromatics, naphthalenes, and benzene into furans, phenols, and other non-aromatic compounds, which were successfully converted to H_2 and syngas in the second stage by Ni catalyst. The decrease in coke precursor compounds inhibits the polymerization of volatiles and hence the coke formation on the catalyst in the second stage [181]. As a result, an enhanced yield of H_2 was achieved, indicating that

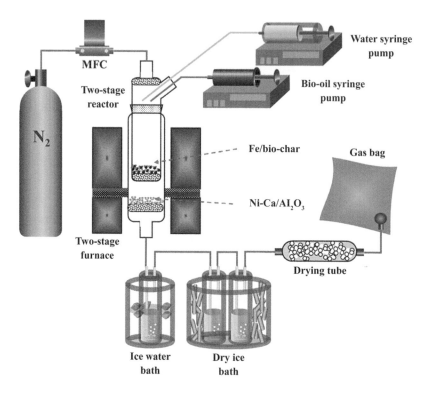

FIGURE 9.11 Schematic diagram of two-stage catalytic reforming system.

Source: Reproduced with permission from [180].

the two-stage catalytic reforming process is an advantageous and efficient approach to reduce the coke formation and obtain a higher yield of H_2.

SR of bio-oil can be performed in different reactors on the type or composition of bio-oil under varying operating parameters, such as temperature, steam/carbon (S/C) ratio, and weight hourly space velocity (WHSV) or space-time, which greatly influence the conversion rate of bio-oil, yield of H_2, and coke formation on the catalyst [62,175,183]. Generally, the smaller compounds like acetic acid require a low temperature of nearly 450 °C for their full conversion, while the larger compounds or polyaromatic compounds require a higher temperature of >750 °C for their complete conversion in the process. Therefore, SR of bio-oil is usually carried out between 400 and 1000 °C in a fixed or fluidized bed reactor. Valle et al. [184] investigated the effect of the temperature range of 550–700 °C on H_2 yield, bio-oil conversion, and coke formation during SR of pine wood bio-oil in a continuous two-step system using Ni/La_2O_3-αAl_2O_3 as the catalyst. It was found that H_2 yield and bio-oil conversion increased with an increase in temperature, showing the H_2 yield of nearly 30% at 550 °C which increased to above 70% at 700 °C with a space-time of >0.10$g_{catalyst}$ h/$g_{bio\text{-}oil}$ and S/C ratio of 1.5. However, the temperature increased the coke deposition on the Ni catalyst. For example, 14.8 wt% coke was observed at 600 °C, whereas 700 °C

Thermochemical Production of Bio-Oil

produced 21.4 wt% of coke with 0.04 $g_{catalyst}$ h/$g_{bio-oil}$ of space-time, S/C ratio of 1.5 and 5 h of reaction time [184]. It was further noticed that temperature of 550–650 °C produced a filamentous type of coke, which does not block the active sites of the catalyst and therefore has less impact on the catalyst deactivation [184]. Similarly, Remiro et al. [185] examined the effect of the temperature range of 500–800 °C on the aqueous fraction of bio-oil. The results revealed that a complete bio-oil conversion was achieved at 700 °C, and the highest H_2 yield of 95% was obtained with 5 h of reaction time [185].

Another key parameter for SR is the S/C ratio to achieve a higher yield of H_2 [183,186]. Generally, water is added to the bio-oil to obtain the desirable S/C ratio. Studies have shown that a higher S/C ratio (>3) is advantageous to change the thermodynamic equilibrium of reforming and WGSR toward H_2 production, consequently leading to a higher yield of H_2. For instance, a study showed approximately 93% H_2 yield with an S/C ratio of 6, while an S/C ratio of 1.5 could achieve a maximum H_2 yield of nearly 78% [183]. Moreover, the higher amount of steam can also help to gasify some amount of carbonaceous species, thus, minimizing the risk of catalyst deactivation. However, the higher amount of steam can reduce the energy efficiency of SR process since it requires a higher amount of energy to evaporate water at the required temperature [187]. Therefore, a suitable S/C ratio is pivotal to achieving the maximum H_2 yield. In addition to the S/C ratio, the selection of space-time or WHSV is highly important to obtain an optimum yield of H_2 and bio-oil conversion in reforming reaction. Higher the space-time or WHSV, longer the time catalyst can react with bio-oil components, and therefore, it could be favorable to produce a high H_2 yield. Valle et al. [184] applied different space-time (0.04, 0.10, 0.19 and 0.38 $g_{catalyst}$ h/$g_{bio-oil}$) for SR of bio-oil and examined its effect on hydrogen production. The results of the study are shown in Figure 9.12, which suggested that space-time of 0.19 $g_{catalyst}$ h/$g_{bio-oil}$ was favorable to convert the bio-oil into H_2, obtaining the maximum H_2 yield of nearly 93% with an S/C ratio of 6 and temperature of 700 °C. In addition, these operating conditions were also ideal to form undesirable by-products, such as CH_4 and C_2-C_4 hydrocarbons, a negligible amount of CH_4 and nearly no C_2-C_4 hydrocarbons were found with a space-time of 0.19 $g_{catalyst}$ h/$g_{bio-oil}$ [184]. On the other hand, an increase in the space-time from 0.04 to 0.38 $g_{catalyst}$ h/$g_{bio-oil}$ showed a constant decrease in coke formation, 0.04 $g_{catalyst}$ h/$g_{bio-oil}$ producing the largest amount of coke of 17.3 wt% which reduced significantly to 6.7 wt% with 0.38 $g_{catalyst}$ h/$g_{bio-oil}$ [184].

A highly active and stable catalyst is usually required to enhance the rate of SR reaction and increase the yield of H_2 [188]. A desirable catalyst should be able to promote WGSR and favor the breaking of C—C, C—H, and O=H bonds and be less prone to deactivation due to coke formation [189]. In this regard, noble metals like Pt and Rh or non-noble metals such as Ni, Co, Ce, and Fe dispersed on different supports like Al_2O_3, ZrO_2, CeO_3-Al_2O_3, HZSM-5 and carbon nanotubes (CNT) have been widely explored in various modes of SR of bio-oil [62,182,188]. For instance, a study compared the activity of the noble metals Pt and Rh supported on Al_2O_3 and $CeZrO_2$ for SR for beech wood bio-oil [190]. The results of the study are shown in Figure 9.13. It can be predicted from the results that Al_2O_3-based catalysts were less active for hydrogen production compared to $CeZrO_2$ catalysts. This is probably because $CeZrO_2$ exhibits redox properties and may carry out an additional set of

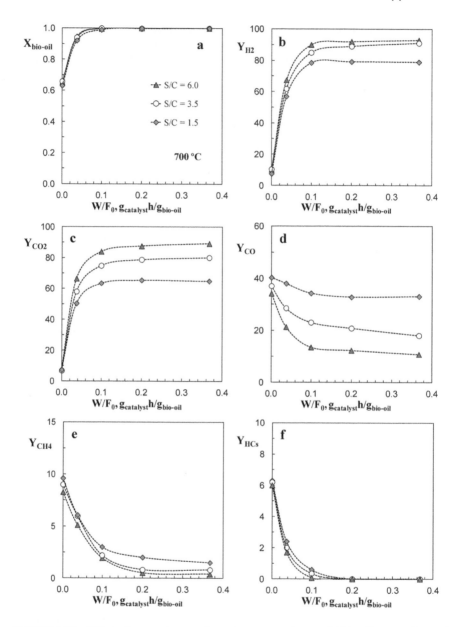

FIGURE 9.12 Effect of space-time on the values at zero time on (a) bio-oil conversion and yields of (b) H_2, (c) CO_2, (d) CO, (e) CH_4, and (f) C_2-C_4 hydrocarbons at 700 °C and for different values of S/C ratio.

Source: Reproduced with permission from [184].

reactions compared to Al_2O_3-based catalysts. It was further noticed that Rh/CeZrO$_2$ and Pt/CeZrO$_2$ catalysts showed almost similar yields of H_2 but Pt/CeZrO$_2$ catalyst was found to maintain the reforming activity for a long-term reaction, producing more

Thermochemical Production of Bio-Oil

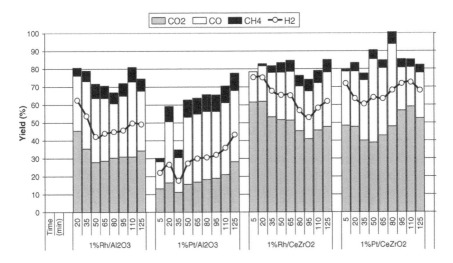

FIGURE 9.13 Activity of various catalysts for steam reforming of bio-oil as a function of time on stream. Experimental conditions: 200 catalyst + 1000 mg cordierite; T = 860 °C ± 30 °C; liquid flow rate: bio-oil = 14.0 μL min^{-1}, H$_2$O = 96.8 μL min^{-1}; S/C = 10.8; GeHSV = 3090 h^{-1}.

Source: Reproduced with permission from [190].

than 50% of H$_2$ over 9 h, which can be attributed to better WGSR activity of Pt [190]. On the other hand, among non-noble metals, Ni-based catalysts have shown promising activity for WGSR and bond breaking, and hence different Ni-based monometallic and bimetallic catalysts have been widely used for SR of bio-oil for enhanced H$_2$ production. For example, Santamaria et al. [182] demonstrated the application of Ni/ZrO$_2$ for SR of the bio-oil (produced from pyrolysis of pine wood at 500 °C) in a fluidized bed reactor at 600 °C and achieved a maximum H$_2$ yield of 92.4%. In a separate study, Bizkarra et al. [58] carried out SR of bio-oil in a continuous fixed bed reactor using different Ni-based monometallic and bimetallic catalysts. The SR reactions were operated using an S/C ratio of 5 and at atmospheric pressure. The results showed that the monometallic catalyst Ni/Al$_2$O$_3$ showed a maximum H$_2$ yield of 90%, which continuously decreased and reached 35% after 3 h of operating time, attributing to the faster deactivation of the catalyst due to coke formation. However, Ni/CeO$_3$-Al$_2$O$_3$ showed more resistance to the coke formation and maintained high activity for H$_2$ production for a longer period, which was attributed to the higher oxygen mobility by the ceria particles as compared to the sole Al$_2$O$_3$ [58]. Noticeably, compared to the monometallic catalysts, the bimetallic catalyst, Rh-Ni/CeO$_3$-Al$_2$O$_3$ showed better activity and stability for H$_2$ for a longer period of time. The catalyst showed an H$_2$ yield of nearly 60% from the start to the end of the reaction, which was ascribed to the significant activity of the catalyst for oxidation of carbon instead of favoring carbon deposition, consequently resulting in the higher resistance to catalyst deactivation and better catalytic activity toward H$_2$ production [58]. Several other catalysts using different metals and supports have been utilized for SR of bio-oil. Some examples are given in Table 9.9.

TABLE 9.9

Catalytic Steam Reforming of Bio-Oil for Hydrogen Production.

Bio-oil source	Catalyst	SR operating parameters					Maximum H_2 yield	References
		Reactor	Temperature (°C)	Pressure	S/C molar ratio	Space-time/WHSV[a]		
Pine wood sawdust	Ni/ZrO$_2$	Fluidized bed	600	/	7.7	20 g$_{cat}$ min/g$_{bio-oil}$	92.4 wt%	[182]
Pine wood sawdust	Ni/Al$_2$O$_3$	Fixed bed	800	1 atm	5	1.45 g$_{cat}$ h/g$_{bio-oil}$	~90 wt%	[58]
Pine wood sawdust	Ni/CeO$_2$-Al$_2$O$_3$	Fixed bed	800	1 atm	5	1.45 g$_{cat}$ h/g$_{bio-oil}$	~88 wt%	[58]
Pine wood sawdust	Ni/La$_2$O$_3$-Al$_2$O$_3$	Fixed bed	800	1 atm	5	1.45 g$_{cat}$ h/g$_{bio-oil}$	~73 wt%	[58]
Pine wood sawdust	Pd-Ni/CeO$_2$-Al$_2$O$_3$	Fixed bed	800	1 atm	5	1.45 g$_{cat}$ h/g$_{bio-oil}$	~70 wt%	[58]
Pine wood sawdust	Pt-Ni/CeO$_2$-Al$_2$O$_3$	Fixed bed	800	1 atm	5	1.45 g$_{cat}$ h/g$_{bio-oil}$	~72 wt%	[58]
Pine wood sawdust	Rh-Ni/CeO$_2$-Al$_2$O$_3$	Fixed bed	800	1 atm	5	1.45 g$_{cat}$ h/g$_{bio-oil}$	~61 wt%	[58]
Pine wood sawdust	Ni/La$_2$O$_3$-αAl$_2$O$_3$	Fluidized bed	700	/	6	0.38 g$_{cat}$ h/g$_{bio-oil}$	93% wt%	[183]
Coconut shell	Ni/Al$_2$O$_3$	Fixed bed	750	/	/	/	58.21 wt%	[57]
Cotton stalk	Ni/Al$_2$O$_3$	Fixed bed	750	/	/	/	57.95 wt%	[57]
Palm kernel shell	Ni/Al$_2$O$_3$	Fixed bed	750	/	/	/	57.36 wt%	[57]
Rice Husk	Ni/Al$_2$O$_3$	Fixed bed	750	/	/	/	57.63 wt%	[57]
Sugarcane	Ni/Al$_2$O$_3$	Fixed bed	750	/	/	/	59.23 wt%	[57]
Wheat straw	Ni/Al$_2$O$_3$	Fixed bed	750	/	/	/	54.06 wt%	[57]
Pine wood sawdust	Rh/CeO$_2$- ZrO$_2$	Fluidized bed	700	/	6	0.15 g$_{cat}$ h/g$_{bio-oil}$	0.95[c]	[63]
Pine wood sawdust	Ni/Al$_2$O$_3$	Fluidized bed	600	/	7.7	20 g$_{cat}$ min/g$_{bio-oil}$	~90 wt%	[195]
Pine wood sawdust	Ni/MgO	Fluidized bed	600	/	7.7	20 g$_{cat}$ min/g$_{bio-oil}$	~88 wt%	[195]
Pine wood sawdust	Ni/SiO$_2$	Fluidized bed	600	/	7.7	20 g$_{cat}$ min/g$_{bio-oil}$	~12 wt%	[195]

Pine wood sawdust	Ni/TiO$_2$	Fluidized bed	600	/	7.7	20 g$_{cat}$ min/g$_{bio-oil}$	~65 wt%	[195]
Commercial bio-oil	Ni-MgO/Al$_2$O$_3$	Fixed bed	850	/	1[b]	30 h^{-1}	61 wt%	[176]
Pine wood	Ni/Al	Fixed bed	600	1 atm	5.58	1.67 g$_{cat}$ min/g$_{bio-oil}$	0.064 g/g$_{org}$	[187]
Pine wood	Ni/Al	Fixed bed	700	1 atm	5.58	1.67 g$_{cat}$ min/g$_{bio-oil}$	0.097 g/g$_{org}$	[187]
Pine wood	Ni/Al	Fixed bed	800	1 atm	5.58	1.67 g$_{cat}$ min/g$_{bio-oil}$	0.087 g/g$_{org}$	[187]
Pine wood sawdust	Ni-Co/Al-Mg	Fixed bed	650	1 atm	7.6	4 g$_{cat}$ min/g$_{bio-oil}$	0.17 g/g$_{org}$	[196]
Pine wood sawdust	Ni-Co/Al-Mg	Fluidized bed	650	1 atm	7.6	4 g$_{cat}$ min/g$_{bio-oil}$	0.07 g/g$_{org}$	[196]
Maize stalk	Ni-Ce/Al$_2$O$_3$	Fixed bed	900	/	6	12 h^{-1}	71.4 wt%	[59]
Pine wood sawdust	NiO/MgO	Fluidized bed	800	/	10	1.0 h^{-1}	77.6%	[197]

[a] WHSV– Weight hourly space velocity

[b] Bio-oil/water ratio

[c] H$_2$ yield was calculated as: $Y_{H2}=F_{H2}/F^o_{H2}$, where F_{H2} is the H$_2$ molar flow rate in the product stream and F^o_{H2} is the stoichiometric molar flow rate.

The kinetics of SR process for bio-oil has been less explored so far. Although several studies have been conducted to understand the SR reactions using model compounds like butanol and ethanol [191–193]. For instance, Vaidya and Rodrigues [193] examined the kinetics of ethanol reforming for hydrogen production in the presence of Ru/Al_2O_3 catalyst at 600 and 700 °C. The authors concluded that SR of ethanol over Ru/Al_2O_3 catalyst involves three reactions in which the first reaction is irreversible, and the latter two are reversible:

1. $C_2H_5OH + H_2O \rightarrow CO_2 + CH_4 + 2H_2$ (9.7)

2. $CH_4 + H_2O \leftrightarrow CO + 3H_2$ (9.8)

4. $CO + H_2O \leftrightarrow CO_2 + H_2$ (9.9)

The study suggests that the increase in temperature enhances ethanol conversion, and above 700 °C, intermediate products like CH_4, C_2H_4, C_2H_6, and CH_2CHO are also formed that are steam reformed to produce CO_2 and H_2 [193]. A total of 6 mol of H_2 and 2 mol of CO_2 could be produced. It was further noticed that ethanol reforming follows first-order kinetics and requires activation energy of 96 kJ mol^{-1} [193]. However, the kinetics of ethanol reforming to hydrogen production under similar conditions over different catalysts can vary, and different activation energy values can be obtained [192,194]. Similarly, the kinetics of other oxygenated compounds, like acetic acid, have been widely studied on different types of catalysts.

Overall, SR of bio-oil is a promising approach to generate clean fuel like H_2, and studies have shown that significant conversion rates of bio-oil to H_2 or a higher H_2 yield of more than 90% can be obtained using catalytic SR. The main concern of catalytic SR is catalyst deactivation. As the reaction is usually carried out at higher temperatures, the metals such as Ni in the catalyst can be sintered, which consequently affects the catalytic activity during the SR reaction. The formation of carbonaceous species during the reaction could occupy or block the active sites on the catalyst surface, initiating the prompt deactivation of the catalyst and leading to decreased catalytic activity. In addition, Ni is believed to be less active for WGSR and more active for methanation, which may result in lower H_2 yields. Therefore, the performance of Ni-based catalysts can be further improved by its modification with the addition of Cu and Co metals that are highly active WGSR and less active for methanation. The addition of metal oxides, such as CeO_2 and MgO can also increase the adsorption and activation of water, thereby increasing WGSR. Metal oxides can also enhance the oxygen storage capacity, which can help to gasify carbonaceous species and minimize catalyst deactivation. Therefore, the development of versatile catalysts with multiple functions that are highly efficient and less prone to deactivation is necessary for the successful conversion of different compounds in SR process.

Thermochemical Production of Bio-Oil

9.6 TRENDS AND FUTURE PERSPECTIVES

9.6.1 TECHNO-ECONOMIC ANALYSIS

Thermochemical technologies, like fast pyrolysis and HTL, are used for bio-oil production, and subsequently, upgrading techniques are applied to enhance the bio-oil properties to make a competitive fuel for real applications. In addition to the quality of bio-oil, it is also important to examine the cost involved in different steps of these processes and estimate the price of upgraded bio-oil. Additionally, a comparative techno-economic analysis between different approaches can help to adopt the appropriate technique that suggests the highest energy conversion efficiency and maximum bio-oil production with minimum investment. In this regard, several techno-economic studies have been conducted for bio-oil production from fast pyrolysis, HTL, and combined upgrading techniques [199–201]. The major cost involved in pyrolysis bio-oil production is from buying, transporting, and drying feedstocks, and electrical consumption during the pyrolysis process. The total cost for electrical consumption can be reduced if the bio-oil produced from the pyrolysis process is used in a diesel engine for power generation. In this case, approximately 18% of bio-oil would be consumed. The cost of bio-oil production could be further reduced to 18% by selling the biochar that is also produced during the pyrolysis process [202]. The estimated cost for bio-oil production from fast pyrolysis of energy crops like willow and miscanthus is $12–$26/GJ [202]. A comparative techno-economic study between pyrolysis and HTL using a similar feedstock can provide better insights into economic bio-oil production. To confirm this, a recent study conducted a comparative techno-economic analysis for biofuel production through HTL and pyrolysis using sugarcane bagasse as the feedstock [198]. The estimated costs involved in different steps of pyrolysis and HTL of sugarcane bagasse have been outlined in Table 9.10 [198]. The study suggested that the pyrolysis technique is more profitable for biofuel production than HTL. The results showed that the liquefaction of biomass requires more energy inputs, mainly to pump liquefaction slurry at a high flow rate and liquefaction pressure. Besides, the use of ethanol also increases the operating cost in the liquefaction process, which is not required in pyrolysis. The total operating costs were estimated at $14.57 million/year for liquefaction and $6.16 million/year for the pyrolysis process using a similar amount of feedstock. On the other hand, the revenue obtained from the unit price for HTL was higher compared to the pyrolysis, which could be attributed to the generation of different annual volumes of the products. Since the operating costs are higher than the revenue, unit margin (US$/L) is more suitable to compare the profits or losses of the process, which can be calculated with the following formula:

$$Unit\,margin\left(\frac{US\$}{L}\right) = \frac{Annual\,revenue - Annual\,opearational\,costs}{Annual\,production\,volume}$$

The authors further suggested that the lower negative value of the unit margin indicates the cost-effectiveness or profitability of the process. In this regard, the unit

TABLE 9.10
Economic Results of Modeling of Liquefaction and Pyrolysis.

Quantity	Liquefaction	Pyrolysis
Plant capacity, tonnes/year feed as received	84000	84000
Capital cost estimates, million US$		
Total installed cost	17.87	23.20
Location-adjusted direct cost	44.46	38.42
Total indirect costs	16.20	4.95
Working capital	12.13	8.67
Total capital cost	72.79	52.05
Operating costs, million US$/year		
Feedstock cost	2.04	2.04
Electricity	0.30	<0.01
Heating	1.01	—
Ethanol or Amine make-up	3.37	—
Catalyst replacements	0.12	0.31
Hydrogen	1.77	1.17
Steam supply	2.07	—
Trade waste handling	0.06	<0.01
Water	1.46	0.60
Labor	1.17	1.17
Maintenance (2% FCI)	1.21	0.87
Total operating costs	14.57	6.16
Total products, million liters/year	25.78	11.58
Revenue, million US$/year	8.44	3.79
Base economic indicators		
Annual cash flow, million US$	−6.13	−2.37
Net present value, million US$	−113.7	−65.7

Source: Reproduced with permission from [198].

margin for pyrolysis was estimated to be $−0.21/L, while it was $−0.24/L for liquefaction [198]. Therefore, it can be suggested that the pyrolysis technique is more favorable or economical for bio-oil production than the liquefaction process. Various techno-economic studies of fast biomass pyrolysis estimated the cost of produced bio-oil to be in the range of $0.11–$0.65/L [200,203].

Integrating bio-oil production from either pyrolysis or liquefaction process with any upgrading approach, such as solvent addition or hydrotreatment, further increases bio-oil cost. Techno-economic analysis of an integrated process has been widely studied for hydrotreatment but has been rarely reported for other approaches, like emulsification, solvent addition, and electrochemical treatment. For example, Wright et al. [203] estimated the cost of bio-oil produced from fast pyrolysis of corn stover and upgraded with hydrotreatment, assuming two scenarios, one of which

Thermochemical Production of Bio-Oil

includes hydrogen production from a fraction of the bio-oil produced during the pyrolysis process and the other relies on purchasing hydrogen. Initial economic results showed that purchasing hydrogen for bio-oil upgrading would be more economical than producing the hydrogen as hydrogen production requires higher capital investment, which would be approximately $287 million compared to merchant hydrogen of $200 million. The study further suggested that the upgraded bio-oil would cost nearly $1.73 and $0.90 per liter for hydrogen production and merchant hydrogen scenarios, respectively [203]. Sensitivity results indicated that process variables such as biomass cost and electricity supply in both scenarios had a great influence on the final cost of the bio-oil, while the low fuel conversion yield could also be achieved due to reduced performance of the pyrolysis reactor, losses occurred during bio-oil collection and storage, and poor bio-oil upgrading yields [203]. On the other hand, Zhu et al. [204] conducted a techno-economic analysis of bio-oil production through HTL and its further upgrading via hydrotreatment. Two scenarios were applied to evaluate the bio-oil production cost. The first scenario was based on using the currently available parameters, and the second was on advanced technologies in a commercial system. The annual production rates for upgraded bio-oil for the first and second scenarios were $42.9 million and $69.9 million GGE (gallon gasoline equivalent), respectively. The second scenario assumes the utilization of advanced technology that could reduce the organic loss and enhance the bio-oil yield compared to the first scenario, showing approximately 40.5% bio-oil yield estimated to be 29.4% for the first scenario. The minimum fuel selling price for the upgraded bio-oil was estimated to be $0.74/liter for the second and $1.29/liter for the first scenario [204]. The major factors affecting the bio-oil production cost were found to be feedstock cost, product yield, and cost of upgrading equipment [204]. Furthermore, it has been inferred that the production of upgraded bio-oil, which is equivalent to gasoline- or diesel-like liquid fuel, could be economically attractive if the bio-oil is available at the cost of $0.11/L and should be sold at the cost of more than $0.31/L [97]. However, previous studies suggest that upgraded bio-oil production costs are still higher than the desired cost to make it a commercial liquid fuel. Therefore, more efforts are required to reduce the operating cost of the processes to obtain the bio-oil at lower prices.

The economic feasibility of hydrogen production through bio-oil SR has also been investigated [201,205,206]. Sarkar and Kumar [205] carried out fast pyrolysis of forest (whole-tree biomass and forest residue) and agricultural biomass (wheat and barley straw) for bio-oil production at a plant capacity of 2000 dry tonnes/day and its further SR for hydrogen production at a plant that has a capacity of processing 1198 tonnes bio-oil/day. The results showed that hydrogen production from forest biomass is economically more feasible compared to agricultural biomass, suggesting the cost of hydrogen production is around $2.40/kg of H_2 from whole-tree biomass, $3.00/kg of H_2 for forest residue and $4.55/kg of H_2 for agricultural biomass. Costs for feedstock transport and capital cost for bio-oil production were major contributions to the production of H_2 cost, contributing almost 34% of the total cost. In a separate study, Zhang et al. [201] estimated the cost of hydrogen production via SR of bio-oil and suggested that a total capital investment of $333 million would be required at a 2000

250   Biowaste and Biomass in Biofuel Applications

t/day capacity plant, which could produce hydrogen around 160 t/day, indicating the cost of H_2 in a range of \$2.33 to\$4.33/kg of H_2.

9.6.2 POLICY ANALYSIS

The Renewable Energy Directive of the European Commission has set the target to have 32% renewable fuels in the energy mix by 2030, which was nearly 17.5% in 2017. Pyrolysis and HTL technologies have shown promising potential to produce a low-cost liquid fuel that is bio-oil, which is foreseen to compete with conventional fossil fuels in the near future. However, the bio-oil's poor physicochemical properties, mainly due to the high oxygen content, is a great challenge to make it a drop-in fuel. Although several approaches can be employed to improve poor physicochemical properties and convert oxygen-containing compounds into high-energy-density hydrocarbons, the bio-oil is still not regarded as a drop-in fuel. This is mainly associated with the production cost of bio-oil regardless of the production technology and the integration with bio-oil upgrading technique that influences bio-oil commercialization. Different techno-economic studies estimate high costs for feedstock sourcing, capital, and operating expenses, and lower process yields that ultimately contribute to the high cost of produced bio-oil. Moreover, the degree of sensitivity for these parameters could vary for different bio-oil upgrading approaches. Therefore, there is a high need for dedicated policies to reduce the capital and operating costs to promote the development and commercialization of bio-oil. To reduce the cost of feedstock transportation, establishing facilities for bio-oil production near the feedstock source could be a feasible option. Sustainable management of land use is required for growing desirable crops that result in a higher yield of bio-oil that could be advantageous for economic bio-oil production at a largescale. On the other hand, the capital investment for bio-oil upgrading can be minimized by integrating the bio-oil production unit with the existing oil refining industry. This way, the already built infrastructure can be used for bio-oil upgrading facilities and minimize the capital cost. It has been estimated that oil refineries around the world would be used less for gasoline production and more for diesel and jet fuels, projecting the change in petroleum feed from fluid catalytic cracking units to hydrocracking units [97]. Therefore, oil refineries can be employed for the hydrotreatment of bio-oils. Overall, effective policies are essentially required to reduce the capital cost for bio-oil production and commercialization of bio-oil to achieve the desired target of renewable fuel generation.

9.6.3 CHALLENGES AND FUTURE RECOMMENDATIONS

The downstream approaches employed for bio-oil upgrading have shown promising results to improve certain physicochemical properties of the bio-oil. There are also certain challenges associated with the techniques, which can be seen as possible research opportunities in the near future. For example, solvent addition and emulsification approaches are highly advantageous to increase bio-oil's stability and calorific value. However, solvent addition can also increase the bio-oil's water content and decrease the pH. To obtain a stable emulsion, additional physical techniques

Thermochemical Production of Bio-Oil

like ultrasonication and stirring are required. The necessity of surfactants in emulsification further increases the cost of bio-oil upgrading. Very less is known about the reaction mechanisms between solvents and bio-oil components. Therefore, more research studies can be conducted using bio-oil model compounds to understand the reaction chemistry during solvent addition and emulsification techniques. On the other hand, filtration removes the solid char particles from the bio-oil, which otherwise could be detrimental to bio-oil stability as they can promote polymerization and condensation reactions. However, the use of filtration may increase the cost of bio-oil upgrading as the membranes used in the process are highly expensive. In addition, membranes need regular washing with solvents which can further make the process costly. Therefore, cost-effective and more efficient membranes should be developed for bio-oil upgrading to make the process economical.

The electrocatalytic hydrogenation approach is still in its infancy for real bio-oil upgrading, although it has been widely used for processing model compounds. The major challenge associated with the technique is the utilization of high-priced membranes and hydrogen. Thus, developing a cost-effective and high-performance ion exchange membrane is required to make the technique economical. To decrease the hydrogen cost, electrochemical cells can be integrated with other systems, such as steam reforming, that can utilize bio-oil for hydrogen production, although converting it into a reality would require extensive research work since it requires significant capital investment and operational costs. Another main challenge in electrochemical hydrogenation is the supply of electricity to initiate the reactions. To minimize the cost of electricity and make the technique more sustainable, it can be integrated with other renewable technologies, such as microbial fuel cells that can produce the required electricity that can be supplied to electrocatalytic hydrogenation of bio-oil. Furthermore, techno-economic analysis should be carried out to examine the extent of deoxygenation of bio-oil in electrochemical cells to optimize operating costs, use of external hydrogen, and greenhouse gas emissions.

Hydrotreatment of bio-oil is considered the most promising approach to obtain hydrocarbon-rich bio-oil and has shown almost 100% of conversion of oxygenated compounds to hydrocarbons and other high-value-added products. Nevertheless, the technique faces critical challenges which should be addressed to make the process feasible at the commercial scale. The major challenge is associated with the cost of external hydrogen storage and transportation. To reduce the cost of external hydrogen supply, some liquid hydrogen donors such as ethanol can be used for *in-situ* hydrogen production, and the produced hydrogen can be utilized in hydrodeoxygenation of bio-oil. However, the feasibility of producing affordable bio-oil has not been examined so far. Therefore, a techno-economic study should be conducted to determine the operating cost and degree of bio-oil upgrading. Other challenges in hydrotreatment process are associated with the application of catalysts. For example, metal sulfide catalysts are highly prone to coke formation, which may lead to unfavorable blockage of the reactor. The other disadvantage of using sulfided catalysts is the leaching of catalyst-bound sulfur into the upgraded bio-oil, which demands an additional upgrading approach to remove the impurities, which ultimately can increase the overall cost of the bio-oil upgrading. Noble metal-based catalysts are highly expensive, restricting their industrial-scale application for bio-oil upgrading.

252   Biowaste and Biomass in Biofuel Applications

On the other hand, transition metal-based catalysts are also sensitive to coke deposition at high temperature and pressure conditions, which leads to their early deactivation. The acidic nature of catalyst supports like Al_2O_3, zeolite is also unfavorable as the water content present in the bio-oils adsorbs onto active sites, resulting in catalyst deactivation [139]. The formation of aromatic hydrocarbons is suitable up to certain concentrations. For instance, 40% in gasoline as aromatics act as precursors for coke formation, and thus, their high concentrations are prone to coking reactions and, ultimately, reactor plugging. Hydrogenation of aromatic rings is quite challenging because it requires highly active catalysts and stringent reaction conditions like high temperatures and hydrogen pressures of up to 8 MPa [159]. To produce more stable bio-oil and less coke deposition, two-stage hydrotreatment can be carried out. In the first stage, lower temperatures up to 250 °C can be applied in the presence of a less active catalyst that converts large molecular compounds (which are thought to contribute to coke formation) into smaller compounds, the resultant bio-oil with intermediate compounds is considered stabilized. In the second stage, higher temperatures >350 °C can be applied in the presence of a more active catalyst to successfully convert the oxygenated compounds into high-energy-density hydrocarbons.

SR of bio-oil is a promising approach to generate H_2 or syngas. The main concern of catalytic SR is catalyst deactivation. The metals such as Ni in the catalyst can be sintered at higher temperatures, which consequently affect the catalytic activity during the SR reaction. In addition, coke formation blocks the active sites on the catalyst surface, initiating the prompt deactivation of the catalyst and leading to reduced catalytic activity. Therefore, the development of advanced catalysts that are highly efficient and less prone to deactivation is necessary for the SR process. The catalysts can be promoted with metal oxides like CeO_2 and MgO that increase adsorption and water activation, which helps enhance WGSR. Oxygen storage capacity of metal oxides can also help to gasify carbonaceous species and minimize catalyst deactivation.

9.7 CONCLUSIONS

This review article comprehensively critically reviewed predominantly applied downstream processing techniques, such as solvent addition, emulsification, filtration, hydrotreatment, electrochemical hydrogenation for bio-oil upgrading, and steam reforming of bio-oil for hydrogen production. Significant improvement in bio-oil properties can be achieved using these techniques. It has been shown that in the downstream bio-oil upgrading, certain bio-oil properties, such as viscosity, pH, HHV, and bio-oil stability, can be considerably improved with polar solvents, like ethanol and methanol, and by preparing emulsions with diesel using surfactants, like Span 80 and Tween 60. However, the addition of solvents may increase the water content and decrease the pH of the bio-oils. In addition, less is known about the reaction mechanisms between solvents and bio-oil components. Therefore, more research studies can be conducted to understand the mechanisms, which can help to make the process more feasible for enhanced bio-oil upgrading. Microfiltration and hot vapor filtration methods are highly beneficial to separate char particles and inorganic species present in the bio-oil but at the expense of a decrease in bio-oil yield due to

Thermochemical Production of Bio-Oil

enhanced secondary cracking reactions promoted by char particles and metals. Since filtration removes contaminants from the bio-oil, it protects downstream equipment from corrosion and catalysts from poisoning. Formation of the cake layer on the filter is another challenge with hot vapor filtration associated with fast pyrolysis. Therefore, it is very important to maintain the cake removal or regeneration to make the filtration process stable for bio-oil upgrading.

Hydrotreatment has proven an advantageous approach to obtain bio-oil rich in hydrocarbons and high energy density. Nevertheless, the use of external hydrogen, transport and storage makes the overall process highly expensive. The cost of upgraded bio-oil obtained from hydrotreatment has been estimated between $0.74 and $1.80/L, which is still higher than the desired cost to make it a commercial liquid fuel. Therefore, more efforts are required to reduce the operating cost of the processes to obtain the bio-oil at lower prices. Electrocatalytic hydrogenation has recently emerged as a novel approach for bio-oil upgrading and is effective in removing carbonyl-containing compounds in the bio-oil. It also improves the bio-oil properties, such as increasing the pH and decreasing the acid values. However, the technique requires an external supply of electricity and utilizes costly membranes and hydrogen, making the process more expensive than the other techniques. Extensive research is required to make this technique more efficient and advanced to use for real bio-oil upgrading at a pilot scale.

Alternatively, the bio-oil could also be subjected to steam reforming to generate H_2 and syngas, where H_2 can be directly used as a clean fuel, while syngas can be further subjected to Fischer-Tropsch process for the production of hydrocarbons. The main concern of catalytic steam reforming is catalyst deactivation. As the reaction is usually carried out at higher temperatures, the metals such as Ni in the catalyst can be sintered, which consequently affects the catalytic activity during the SR reaction. The addition of metals like Cu, Co, and metal oxides, such as CeO_2 and MgO, increase the adsorption and activation of water, thereby increasing water gas shift reaction and hydrogen production. Coke formation is a major challenge for steam reforming of bio-oil. Thus, the development of versatile catalysts with multiple functions that are highly efficient and less prone to deactivation is necessary for the successful conversion of different compounds in SR process.

To sum up, bio-oil is still not regarded as a drop-in fuel. This is mainly associated with the production cost of bio-oil regardless of the production technology and the integration with the bio-oil upgrading technique. Therefore, there is a high need for dedicated policies to reduce the capital and operating costs to promote the development and commercialization of bio-oil.

9.8 ACKNOWLEDGMENTS

This article is reproduced from "R. Kumar and V. Strezov, Thermochemical production of bio-oil: a review of downstream processing technologies for bio-oil upgrading, production of hydrogen and high value-added products, Renewable and Sustainable Energy Reviews, 135, 110152, 2021", with copyright license permission from Elsevier, license number 5336900658219.

254   Biowaste and Biomass in Biofuel Applications

REFERENCES

[1] Capuano DL. International Energy Outlook 2018 (IEO2018) 2000:21.

[2] He J, Strezov V, Kan T, Weldekidan H, Asumadu-Sarkodie S, Kumar R. Effect of temperature on heavy metal(loid) deportment during pyrolysis of Avicennia marina biomass obtained from phytoremediation. *Bioresource Technology* 2019. https://doi.org/10.1016/j.biortech.2019.01.101.

[3] Hognon C, Delrue F, Texier J, Grateau M, Thiery S, Miller H, et al. Comparison of pyrolysis and hydrothermal liquefaction of Chlamydomonas reinhardtii. Growth studies on the recovered hydrothermal aqueous phase. *Biomass and Bioenergy* 2015;73:23–31. https://doi.org/10.1016/j.biombioe.2014.11.025.

[4] Kumar R, Strezov V, Lovell E, Kan T, Weldekidan H, He J, et al. Enhanced bio-oil deoxygenation activity by Cu/zeolite and Ni/zeolite catalysts in combined in-situ and ex-situ biomass pyrolysis. *Journal of Analytical and Applied Pyrolysis* 2019. https://doi.org/10.1016/j.jaap.2019.03.008.

[5] Kumar R, Kumar P. Future microbial applications for bioenergy production: A perspective. *Frontiers in Microbiology* 2017;8. https://doi.org/10.3389/fmicb.2017.00450.

[6] Zhou YJ, Kerkhoven EJ, Nielsen J. Barriers and opportunities in bio-based production of hydrocarbons. *Nature Energy* 2018;3:925–935. https://doi.org/10.1038/s41560-018-0197-x.

[7] Khodier A, Kilgallon P, Legrave N, Simms N, Oakey J, Bridgwater T. Pilot-scale combustion of fast-pyrolysis bio-oil: Ash deposition and gaseous emissions. *Environmental Progress & Sustainable Energy* 2009;28:397–403. https://doi.org/10.1002/ep.10379.

[8] Shihadeh A, Hochgreb S. Diesel engine combustion of biomass pyrolysis oils. *Energy & Fuels* 2000;14:260–274. https://doi.org/10.1021/ef990044x.

[9] Moore RH, Thornhill KL, Weinzierl B, Sauer D, D'Ascoli E, Kim J, et al. Biofuel blending reduces particle emissions from aircraft engines at cruise conditions. *Nature* 2017;543:411–415. https://doi.org/10.1038/nature21420.

[10] Alonso DM, Wettstein SG, Dumesic JA. Bimetallic catalysts for upgrading of biomass to fuels and chemicals. *Chemical Society Reviews* 2012;41:8075. https://doi.org/10.1039/c2cs35188a.

[11] Sudarsanam P, Peeters E, Makshina EV, Parvulescu VI, Sels BF. Advances in porous and nanoscale catalysts for viable biomass conversion. *Chemical Society Reviews* 2019;48:2366–2421. https://doi.org/10.1039/C8CS00452H.

[12] Araújo A, Queiroz G, Maia D, Gondim A, Souza L, Fernandes V, et al. Fast pyrolysis of sunflower oil in the presence of microporous and mesoporous materials for production of bio-oil. *Catalysts* 2018;8:261. https://doi.org/10.3390/catal8070261.

[13] Baloch HA, Nizamuddin S, Siddiqui MTH, Riaz S, Jatoi AS, Dumbre DK, et al. Recent advances in production and upgrading of bio-oil from biomass: A critical overview. *Journal of Environmental Chemical Engineering* 2018;6:5101–5118. https://doi.org/10.1016/j.jece.2018.07.050.

[14] Li R, Xie Y, Yang T, Li B, Wang W, Kai X. Effects of chemical–biological pretreatment of corn stalks on the bio-oils produced by hydrothermal liquefaction. *Energy Conversion and Management* 2015;93:23–30. https://doi.org/10.1016/j.enconman.2014.12.089.

[15] Lian X, Xue Y, Zhao Z, Xu G, Han S, Yu H. Progress on upgrading methods of bio-oil: A review: Upgrading progress of bio-oil. *International Journal of Energy Research* 2017;41:1798–1816. https://doi.org/10.1002/er.3726.

[16] Weldekidan H, Strezov V, Kan T, Kumar R, He J, Town G. Solar assisted catalytic pyrolysis of chicken-litter waste with in-situ and ex-situ loading of CaO and char. *Fuel* 2019;246:408–416. https://doi.org/10.1016/j.fuel.2019.02.135.

[17] Weldekidan H, Strezov V, Town G. Review of solar energy for biofuel extraction. *Renewable and Sustainable Energy Reviews* 2018;88:184–192. https://doi.org/10.1016/j.rser.2018.02.027.

[18] Dhyani V, Bhaskar T. A comprehensive review on the pyrolysis of lignocellulosic biomass. *Renewable Energy* 2018;129:695–716. https://doi.org/10.1016/j.renene.2017.04.035.

[19] Mohan D, Pittman, CU, Steele PH. Pyrolysis of wood/biomass for bio-oil: A critical review. *Energy & Fuels* 2006;20:848–889. https://doi.org/10.1021/ef0502397.

[20] Fan L, Zhang Y, Liu S, Zhou N, Chen P, Cheng Y, et al. Bio-oil from fast pyrolysis of lignin: Effects of process and upgrading parameters. *Bioresource Technology* 2017;241:1118–1126. https://doi.org/10.1016/j.biortech.2017.05.129.

[21] Guedes RE, Luna AS, Torres AR. Operating parameters for bio-oil production in biomass pyrolysis: A review. *Journal of Analytical and Applied Pyrolysis* 2018;129:134–149. https://doi.org/10.1016/j.jaap.2017.11.019.

[22] Zhao S, Liu M, Zhao L, Zhu L. Influence of interactions among three biomass components on the pyrolysis behavior. *Industrial & Engineering Chemistry Research* 2018;57:5241–5249. https://doi.org/10.1021/acs.iecr.8b00593.

[23] Sharma A, Pareek V, Zhang D. Biomass pyrolysis—A review of modelling, process parameters and catalytic studies. *Renewable and Sustainable Energy Reviews* 2015;50:1081–1096. https://doi.org/10.1016/j.rser.2015.04.193.

[24] Gollakota ARK, Kishore N, Gu S. A review on hydrothermal liquefaction of biomass. *Renewable and Sustainable Energy Reviews* 2018;81:1378–1392. https://doi.org/10.1016/j.rser.2017.05.178.

[25] Toor SS, Rosendahl L, Rudolf A. Hydrothermal liquefaction of biomass: A review of subcritical water technologies. *Energy* 2011;36:2328–2342. https://doi.org/10.1016/j.energy.2011.03.013.

[26] de Caprariis B, De Filippis P, Petrullo A, Scarsella M. Hydrothermal liquefaction of biomass: Influence of temperature and biomass composition on the bio-oil production. *Fuel* 2017;208:618–625. https://doi.org/10.1016/j.fuel.2017.07.054.

[27] Akhtar J, Amin NAS. A review on process conditions for optimum bio-oil yield in hydrothermal liquefaction of biomass. *Renewable and Sustainable Energy Reviews* 2011;15:1615–1624. https://doi.org/10.1016/j.rser.2010.11.054.

[28] Kumar R, Strezov V, Kan T, Weldekidan H, He J, Jahan S. Investigating the effect of mono- and bimetallic/zeolite catalysts on hydrocarbon production during bio-oil upgrading from *Ex Situ* pyrolysis of biomass. *Energy Fuels* 2019. https://doi.org/10.1021/acs.energyfuels.9b02724.

[29] Kumar R, Strezov V, Weldekidan H, He J, Singh S, Kan T, et al. Lignocellulose biomass pyrolysis for bio-oil production: A review of biomass pre-treatment methods for production of drop-in fuels. *Renewable and Sustainable Energy Reviews* 2020;123:109763. https://doi.org/10.1016/j.rser.2020.109763.

[30] Buffi M, Cappelletti A, Rizzo AM, Martelli F, Chiaramonti D. Combustion of fast pyrolysis bio-oil and blends in a micro gas turbine. *Biomass and Bioenergy* 2018;115:174–185. https://doi.org/10.1016/j.biombioe.2018.04.020.

[31] Laesecke J, Ellis N, Kirchen P. Production, analysis and combustion characterization of biomass fast pyrolysis oil – Biodiesel blends for use in diesel engines. *Fuel* 2017;199:346–357. https://doi.org/10.1016/j.fuel.2017.01.093.

[32] Oasmaa A, Kyt M, Sipil K. Pyrolysis oil combustion tests in an industrial boiler. In: Bridgwater AV, editor. *Progress in Thermochemical Biomass Conversion*, Oxford, UK: Blackwell Science Ltd, 2001; pp. 1468–1481. https://doi.org/10.1002/9780470694954.ch121.

[33] Zhang M, Wu H. Phase behavior and fuel properties of bio-oil/glycerol/methanol blends. *Energy & Fuels* 2014;28:4650–4656. https://doi.org/10.1021/ef501176z.

[34] Zhu L, Li K, Zhang Y, Zhu X. Upgrading the storage properties of bio-oil by adding a compound additive. *Energy & Fuels* 2017;31:6221–6227. https://doi.org/10.1021/acs.energyfuels.7b00864.

[35] Bert V, Allemon J, Sajet P, Dieu S, Papin A, Collet S, et al. Torrefaction and pyrolysis of metal-enriched poplars from phytotechnologies: Effect of temperature and biomass chlorine content on metal distribution in end-products and valorization options. *Biomass and Bioenergy* 2017;96:1–11. https://doi.org/10.1016/j.biombioe.2016.11.003.

[36] Chen W-H, Wang C-W, Kumar G, Rousset P, Hsieh T-H. Effect of torrefaction pretreatment on the pyrolysis of rubber wood sawdust analyzed by Py-GC/MS. *Bioresource Technology* 2018;259:469–473. https://doi.org/10.1016/j.biortech.2018.03.033.

[37] He C, Tang C, Li C, Yuan J, Tran K-Q, Bach Q-V, et al. Wet torrefaction of biomass for high quality solid fuel production: A review. *Renewable and Sustainable Energy Reviews* 2018;91:259–271. https://doi.org/10.1016/j.rser.2018.03.097.

[38] Zhang D, Wang F, Zhang A, Yi W, Li Z, Shen X. Effect of pretreatment on chemical characteristic and thermal degradation behavior of corn stalk digestate: Comparison of dry and wet torrefaction. *Bioresource Technology* 2019;275:239–246. https://doi.org/10.1016/j.biortech.2018.12.044.

[39] Cao B, Wang S, Hu Y, Abomohra AE-F, Qian L, He Z, et al. Effect of washing with diluted acids on Enteromorpha clathrata pyrolysis products: Towards enhanced bio-oil from seaweeds. *Renewable Energy* 2019;138:29–38. https://doi.org/10.1016/j.renene.2019.01.084.

[40] Chen H, Cheng H, Zhou F, Chen K, Qiao K, Lu X, et al. Catalytic fast pyrolysis of rice straw to aromatic compounds over hierarchical HZSM-5 produced by alkali treatment and metal-modification. *Journal of Analytical and Applied Pyrolysis* 2018;131:76–84. https://doi.org/10.1016/j.jaap.2018.02.009.

[41] Liu G, Mba Wright M, Zhao Q, Brown RC. Hydrocarbon and ammonia production from catalytic pyrolysis of sewage sludge with acid pretreatment. *ACS Sustainable Chemistry & Engineering* 2016;4:1819–1826. https://doi.org/10.1021/acssuschemeng.6b00016.

[42] Wang H, Srinivasan R, Yu F, Steele P, Li Q, Mitchell B. Effect of acid, alkali, and steam explosion pretreatments on characteristics of bio-oil produced from pinewood. *Energy & Fuels* 2011;25:3758–3764. https://doi.org/10.1021/ef2004909.

[43] Leng L, Li H, Yuan X, Zhou W, Huang H. Bio-oil upgrading by emulsification/ microemulsification: A review. *Energy* 2018;161:214–232. https://doi.org/10.1016/j.energy.2018.07.117.

[44] Zhang M, Yewe-Siang Lee Shee We M, Wu H. Direct emulsification of crude glycerol and bio-oil without addition of surfactant via ultrasound and mechanical agitation. *Fuel* 2018;227:183–189. https://doi.org/10.1016/j.fuel.2018.04.099.

[45] Li H, Xia S, Ma P. Upgrading fast pyrolysis oil: Solvent–anti-solvent extraction and blending with diesel. *Energy Conversion and Management* 2016;110:378–385. https://doi.org/10.1016/j.enconman.2015.11.043.

[46] Xu X, Li Z, Sun Y, Jiang E, Huang L. High-quality fuel from the upgrading of heavy bio-oil by the combination of ultrasonic treatment and mutual solvent. *Energy & Fuels* 2018;32:3477–3487. https://doi.org/10.1021/acs.energyfuels.7b03483.

[47] Javaid A, Ryan T, Berg G, Pan X, Vispute T, Bhatia SR, et al. Removal of char particles from fast pyrolysis bio-oil by microfiltration. *Journal of Membrane Science* 2010;363:120–127. https://doi.org/10.1016/j.memsci.2010.07.021.

[48] Ruiz M, Martin E, Blin J, Van de Steene L, Broust F. Understanding the secondary reactions of flash pyrolysis vapors inside a hot gas filtration unit. *Energy & Fuels* 2017;31:13785–13795. https://doi.org/10.1021/acs.energyfuels.7b02923.

[49] Carroll KJ, Burger T, Langenegger L, Chavez S, Hunt ST, Román-Leshkov Y, et al. Electrocatalytic hydrogenation of oxygenates using earth-abundant transition-metal nanoparticles under mild conditions. *ChemSusChem* 2016;9:1904–1910. https://doi.org/10.1002/cssc.201600290.

[50] Elangovan S, Larsen D, Bay I, Mitchell E, Hartvigsen J, Millett B, et al. Electrochemical upgrading of bio-oil. *ECS Transactions* 2017;78:3149–3158. https://doi.org/10.1149/07801.3149ecst.

[51] Ding K, Zhong Z, Wang J, Zhang B, Fan L, Liu S, et al. Improving hydrocarbon yield from catalytic fast co-pyrolysis of hemicellulose and plastic in the dual-catalyst bed of CaO and HZSM-5. *Bioresource Technology* 2018;261:86–92. https://doi.org/10.1016/j.biortech.2018.03.138.

Thermochemical Production of Bio-Oil

[52] Iisa K, French RJ, Orton KA, Yung MM, Johnson DK, ten Dam J, et al. In situ and ex situ catalytic pyrolysis of pine in a bench-scale fluidized bed reactor system. *Energy & Fuels* 2016;30:2144–2157. https://doi.org/10.1021/acs.energyfuels.5b02165.

[53] Auersvald M, Shumeiko B, Vrtiška D, Straka P, Staš M, Šimáček P, et al. Hydrotreatment of straw bio-oil from ablative fast pyrolysis to produce suitable refinery intermediates. *Fuel* 2019;238:98–110. https://doi.org/10.1016/j.fuel.2018.10.090.

[54] Zhang X, Wang T, Ma L, Zhang Q, Jiang T. Hydrotreatment of bio-oil over Ni-based catalyst. *Bioresource Technology* 2013;127:306–311. https://doi.org/10.1016/j.biortech.2012.07.119.

[55] Biller P, Sharma BK, Kunwar B, Ross AB. Hydroprocessing of bio-crude from continuous hydrothermal liquefaction of microalgae. *Fuel* 2015;159:197–205. https://doi.org/10.1016/j.fuel.2015.06.077.

[56] Adeniyi AG, Otoikhian KS, Ighalo JO. Steam reforming of biomass pyrolysis oil: A review. *International Journal of Chemical Reactor Engineering* 2019;17. https://doi.org/10.1515/ijcre-2018-0328.

[57] Akubo K, Nahil MA, Williams PT. Pyrolysis-catalytic steam reforming of agricultural biomass wastes and biomass components for production of hydrogen/syngas. *Journal of the Energy Institute* 2018;S1743967118308742. https://doi.org/10.1016/j.joei.2018.10.013.

[58] Bizkarra K, Bermudez JM, Arcelus-Arrillaga P, Barrio VL, Cambra JF, Millan M. Nickel based monometallic and bimetallic catalysts for synthetic and real bio-oil steam reforming. *International Journal of Hydrogen Energy* 2018;43:11706–11718. https://doi.org/10.1016/j.ijhydene.2018.03.049.

[59] Fu P, Yi W, Li Z, Bai X, Zhang A, Li Y, et al. Investigation on hydrogen production by catalytic steam reforming of maize stalk fast pyrolysis bio-oil. *International Journal of Hydrogen Energy* 2014;39:13962–13971. https://doi.org/10.1016/j.ijhydene.2014.06.165.

[60] Santamaria L, Arregi A, Alvarez J, Artetxe M, Amutio M, Lopez G, et al. Performance of a Ni/ZrO_2 catalyst in the steam reforming of the volatiles derived from biomass pyrolysis. *Journal of Analytical and Applied Pyrolysis* 2018;136:222–231. https://doi.org/10.1016/j.jaap.2018.09.025.

[61] Singh S, Kumar R, Setiabudi HD, Nanda S, Vo D-VN. Advanced synthesis strategies of mesoporous SBA-15 supported catalysts for catalytic reforming applications: A state-of-the-art review. *Applied Catalysis A: General* 2018;559:57–74. https://doi.org/10.1016/j.apcata.2018.04.015.

[62] Choi I-H, Hwang K-R, Lee K-Y, Lee I-G. Catalytic steam reforming of biomass-derived acetic acid over modified $Ni/\gamma-Al_2O_3$ for sustainable hydrogen production. *International Journal of Hydrogen Energy* 2019;44:180–190. https://doi.org/10.1016/j.ijhydene.2018.04.192.

[63] Remiro A, Ochoa A, Arandia A, Castaño P, Bilbao J, Gayubo AG. On the dynamics and reversibility of the deactivation of a Rh/CeO_2ZrO_2 catalyst in raw bio-oil steam reforming. *International Journal of Hydrogen Energy* 2019;44:2620–2632. https://doi.org/10.1016/j.ijhydene.2018.12.073.

[64] Dabros TMH, Stummann MZ, Høj M, Jensen PA, Grunwaldt J-D, Gabrielsen J, et al. Transportation fuels from biomass fast pyrolysis, catalytic hydrodeoxygenation, and catalytic fast hydropyrolysis. *Progress in Energy and Combustion Science* 2018;68:268–309. https://doi.org/10.1016/j.pecs.2018.05.002.

[65] Bach Q-V, Skreiberg Ø. Upgrading biomass fuels via wet torrefaction: A review and comparison with dry torrefaction. *Renewable and Sustainable Energy Reviews* 2016;54:665–677. https://doi.org/10.1016/j.rser.2015.10.014.

[66] Zacher AH, Olarte MV, Santosa DM, Elliott DC, Jones SB. A review and perspective of recent bio-oil hydrotreating research. *Green Chemistry* 2014;16:491–515. https://doi.org/10.1039/C3GC41382A.

[67] Nishu, Liu R, Rahman MdM, Sarker M, Chai M, Li C, et al. A review on the catalytic pyrolysis of biomass for the bio-oil production with ZSM-5: Focus on structure. *Fuel Processing Technology* 2020;199:106301. https://doi.org/10.1016/j.fuproc.2019.106301.

[68] Bar-On YM, Phillips R, Milo R. The biomass distribution on earth. *Proceedings of the National Academy of Sciences* 2018;115:6506–6511. https://doi.org/10.1073/pnas.1711842115.

[69] Beims RF, Hu Y, Shui H, Xu C (Charles). Hydrothermal liquefaction of biomass to fuels and value-added chemicals: Products applications and challenges to develop large-scale operations. *Biomass and Bioenergy* 2020;135:105510. https://doi.org/10.1016/j.biombioe.2020.105510.

[70] Pearcy RW, Ehleringer J. Comparative ecophysiology of C3 and C4 plants. *Plant Cell & Environment* 1984;7:1–13. https://doi.org/10.1111/j.1365-3040.1984.tb01194.x.

[71] Klass DL. *Biomass For Renewable Energy, Fuels, and Chemicals*. San Diego: Academic Press, 1998.

[72] Jena U, Das KC. Comparative evaluation of thermochemical liquefaction and pyrolysis for bio-oil production from microalgae. *Energy & Fuels* 2011;25:5472–5482. https://doi.org/10.1021/ef201373m.

[73] Choi JH, Kim S-S, Ly HV, Kim J, Woo HC. Effects of water-washing Saccharina japonica on fast pyrolysis in a bubbling fluidized-bed reactor. *Biomass and Bioenergy* 2017;98:112–123. https://doi.org/10.1016/j.biombioe.2017.01.006.

[74] Hassan EM, Steele PH, Ingram L. Characterization of fast pyrolysis bio-oils produced from pretreated pine wood. *Applied Biochemistry and Biotechnology* 2009;154:3–13. https://doi.org/10.1007/s12010-008-8445-3.

[75] Wang H, Srinivasan R, Yu F, Steele P, Li Q, Mitchell B. Effect of acid, alkali, and steam explosion pretreatments on characteristics of bio-oil produced from pinewood. *Energy & Fuels* 2011;25:3758–3764. https://doi.org/10.1021/ef2004909.

[76] Wang H, Srinivasan R, Yu F, Steele P, Li Q, Mitchell B, et al. Effect of acid, steam explosion, and size reduction pretreatments on bio-oil production from sweetgum, switchgrass, and corn stover. *Applied Biochemistry and Biotechnology* 2012;167:285–297. https://doi.org/10.1007/s12010-012-9678-8.

[77] Choi J, Choi J-W, Suh DJ, Ha J-M, Hwang JW, Jung HW, et al. Production of brown algae pyrolysis oils for liquid biofuels depending on the chemical pretreatment methods. *Energy Conversion and Management* 2014;86:371–378. https://doi.org/10.1016/j.enconman.2014.04.094.

[78] Pidtasang B, Udomsap P, Sukkasi S, Chollacoop N, Pattiya A. Influence of alcohol addition on properties of bio-oil produced from fast pyrolysis of eucalyptus bark in a free-fall reactor. *Journal of Industrial and Engineering Chemistry* 2013;19:1851–1857. https://doi.org/10.1016/j.jiec.2013.02.031.

[79] Zhu L, Li K, Ding H, Zhu X. Studying on properties of bio-oil by adding blended additive during aging. *Fuel* 2018;211:704–711. https://doi.org/10.1016/j.fuel.2017.09.106.

[80] Mohammed IY, Abakr YA, Kazi FK, Yusuf S. Effects of pretreatments of Napier grass with deionized water, sulfuric acid and sodium hydroxide on pyrolysis oil characteristics. *Waste and Biomass Valorization* 2017;8:755–773. https://doi.org/10.1007/s12649-016-9594-1.

[81] Ye J, Jiang J, Xu J. Effect of alcohols on simultaneous bio-oil upgrading and separation of high value-added chemicals. *Waste and Biomass Valorization* 2018;9:1779–1785. https://doi.org/10.1007/s12649-017-9934-9.

[82] Yu J, Biller P, Mamahkel A, Klemmer M, Becker J, Glasius M, et al. Catalytic hydrotreatment of bio-crude produced from the hydrothermal liquefaction of aspen wood: A catalyst screening and parameter optimization study. *Sustainable Energy Fuels* 2017;1:832–841. https://doi.org/10.1039/C7SE00090A.

Thermochemical Production of Bio-Oil

[83] Anouti S, Haarlemmer G, Déniel M, Roubaud A. Analysis of physicochemical properties of bio-oil from hydrothermal liquefaction of blackcurrant pomace. *Energy Fuels* 2016;30:398–406. https://doi.org/10.1021/acs.energyfuels.5b02264.

[84] Zhu Z, Rosendahl L, Toor SS, Yu D, Chen G. Hydrothermal liquefaction of barley straw to bio-crude oil: Effects of reaction temperature and aqueous phase recirculation. *Applied Energy* 2015;137:183–192. https://doi.org/10.1016/j.apenergy.2014.10.005.

[85] Xiu S, Shahbazi A, Shirley V, Cheng D. Hydrothermal pyrolysis of swine manure to bio-oil: Effects of operating parameters on products yield and characterization of bio-oil. *Journal of Analytical and Applied Pyrolysis* 2010;88:73–79. https://doi.org/10.1016/j.jaap.2010.02.011.

[86] Xu Y, Zheng X, Yu H, Hu X. Hydrothermal liquefaction of Chlorella pyrenoidosa for bio-oil production over Ce/HZSM-5. *Bioresource Technology* 2014;156:1–5. https://doi.org/10.1016/j.biortech.2014.01.010.

[87] Zhu Z, Toor SS, Rosendahl L, Yu D, Chen G. Influence of alkali catalyst on product yield and properties via hydrothermal liquefaction of barley straw. *Energy* 2015;80:284–292. https://doi.org/10.1016/j.energy.2014.11.071.

[88] Duan P, Savage PE. Upgrading of crude algal bio-oil in supercritical water. *Bioresource Technology* 2011;102:1899–1906. https://doi.org/10.1016/j.biortech.2010.08.013.

[89] Shakya R, Adhikari S, Mahadevan R, Hassan EB, Dempster TA. Catalytic upgrading of bio-oil produced from hydrothermal liquefaction of Nannochloropsis sp. *Bioresource Technology* 2018;252:28–36. https://doi.org/10.1016/j.biortech.2017.12.067.

[90] Huang H, Yuan X, Zhu H, Li H, Liu Y, Wang X, et al. Comparative studies of thermochemical liquefaction characteristics of microalgae, lignocellulosic biomass and sewage sludge. *Energy* 2013;56:52–60. https://doi.org/10.1016/j.energy.2013.04.065.

[91] Wang F, Chang Z, Duan P, Yan W, Xu Y, Zhang L, et al. Hydrothermal liquefaction of Litsea cubeba seed to produce bio-oils. *Bioresource Technology* 2013;149:509–515. https://doi.org/10.1016/j.biortech.2013.09.108.

[92] Chan YH, Yusup S, Quitain AT, Tan RR, Sasaki M, Lam HL, et al. Effect of process parameters on hydrothermal liquefaction of oil palm biomass for bio-oil production and its life cycle assessment. *Energy Conversion and Management* 2015;104:180–188. https://doi.org/10.1016/j.enconman.2015.03.075.

[93] Kan T, Strezov V, Evans TJ. Lignocellulosic biomass pyrolysis: A review of product properties and effects of pyrolysis parameters. *Renewable and Sustainable Energy Reviews* 2016;57:1126–1140. https://doi.org/10.1016/j.rser.2015.12.185.

[94] Doassans-Carrère N, Ferrasse J-H, Boutin O, Mauviel G, Lédé J. Comparative study of biomass fast pyrolysis and direct liquefaction for bio-oils production: Products yield and characterizations. *Energy & Fuels* 2014;28:5103–5111. https://doi.org/10.1021/ef500641c.

[95] Vardon DR, Sharma BK, Blazina GV, Rajagopalan K, Strathmann TJ. Thermochemical conversion of raw and defatted algal biomass via hydrothermal liquefaction and slow pyrolysis. *Bioresource Technology* 2012;109:178–187. https://doi.org/10.1016/j.biortech.2012.01.008.

[96] Weldekidan H, Strezov V, He J, Kumar R, Sarkodie SA, Doyi I, et al. Energy conversion efficiency of pyrolysis of chicken litter and rice husk biomass. *Energy & Fuels* 2019:acs.energyfuels.9b01264. https://doi.org/10.1021/acs.energyfuels.9b01264.

[97] Karatzos S, McMillan JD, Saddler JN. The potential and challenges of drop-in biofuels: A report by IEA. *Bioenergy Task*2014;39.

[98] Oasmaa A, Kuoppala E, Selin J-F, Gust S, Solantausta Y. Fast pyrolysis of forestry residue and pine. 4. Improvement of the product quality by solvent addition. *Energy & Fuels* 2004;18:1578–1583. https://doi.org/10.1021/ef040038n.

[99] Mei Y, Chai M, Shen C, Liu B, Liu R. Effect of methanol addition on properties and aging reaction mechanism of bio-oil during storage. *Fuel* 2019;244:499–507. https://doi.org/10.1016/j.fuel.2019.02.012.

[100] Chen D, Zhou J, Zhang Q, Zhu X. Evaluation methods and research progresses in bio-oil storage stability. *Renewable and Sustainable Energy Reviews* 2014;40:69–79. https://doi.org/10.1016/j.rser.2014.07.159.

[101] Kim T-S, Kim J-Y, Kim K-H, Lee S, Choi D, Choi I-G, et al. The effect of storage duration on bio-oil properties. *Journal of Analytical and Applied Pyrolysis* 2012;95:118–125. https://doi.org/10.1016/j.jaap.2012.01.015.

[102] Liu R, Fei W, Shen C. Influence of acetone addition on the physicochemical properties of bio-oils. *Journal of the Energy Institute* 2014;87:127–133. https://doi.org/10.1016/j.joei.2013.08.001.

[103] Zhang L, Liu R, Yin R, Mei Y, Cai J. Optimization of a mixed additive and its effect on physicochemical properties of bio-oil. *Chemical Engineering & Technology* 2014;37:1181–1190. https://doi.org/10.1002/ceat.201300786.

[104] Qin L, Shao Y, Hou Z, Jia Y, Jiang E. Ultrasonic-assisted upgrading of the heavy bio-oil obtained from pyrolysis of pine nut shells with methanol and octanol solvents. *Energy Fuels* 2019;33:8640–8648. https://doi.org/10.1021/acs.energyfuels.9b01248.

[105] Mohapatra H, Kleiman M, Esser-Kahn AP. Mechanically controlled radical polymerization initiated by ultrasound. *Nature Chemistry* 2017;9:135–139. https://doi.org/10.1038/nchem.2633.

[106] Jiang X, Ellis N. Upgrading bio-oil through emulsification with biodiesel: Thermal stability. *Energy & Fuels* 2010;24:2699–2706. https://doi.org/10.1021/ef901517k.

[107] de Luna MDG, Cruz LAD, Chen W-H, Lin B-J, Hsieh T-H. Improving the stability of diesel emulsions with high pyrolysis bio-oil content by alcohol co-surfactants and high shear mixing strategies. *Energy* 2017;141:1416–1428. https://doi.org/10.1016/j.energy.2017.11.055.

[108] Jiang X, Ellis N. Upgrading bio-oil through Emulsification with biodiesel: Mixture production. *Energy & Fuels* 2010;24:1358–1364. https://doi.org/10.1021/ef9010669.

[109] Guo Z, Wang S, Wang X. Stability mechanism investigation of emulsion fuels from biomass pyrolysis oil and diesel. *Energy* 2014;66:250–255. https://doi.org/10.1016/j.energy.2014.01.010.

[110] Farooq A, Shafaghat H, Jae J, Jung S-C, Park Y-K. Enhanced stability of bio-oil and diesel fuel emulsion using Span 80 and Tween 60 emulsifiers. *Journal of Environmental Management* 2019;231:694–700. https://doi.org/10.1016/j.jenvman.2018.10.098.

[111] Martin JA, Mullen CA, Boateng AA. Maximizing the stability of pyrolysis oil/diesel fuel emulsions. *Energy & Fuels* 2014;28:5918–5929. https://doi.org/10.1021/ef5015583.

[112] Zhang M, Wu H. Stability of emulsion fuels prepared from fast pyrolysis bio-oil and glycerol. *Fuel* 2017;206:230–238. https://doi.org/10.1016/j.fuel.2017.06.010.

[113] Abismaïl B, Canselier JP, Wilhelm AM, Delmas H, Gourdon C. Emulsification by ultrasound: Drop size distribution and stability. *Ultrasonics Sonochemistry* 1999;6:75–83. https://doi.org/10.1016/S1350-4177(98)00027-3.

[114] Martin JA, Mullen CA, Boateng AA. Maximizing the stability of pyrolysis oil/diesel fuel emulsions. *Energy & Fuels* 2014;28:5918–5929. https://doi.org/10.1021/ef5015583.

[115] Chong YY, Thangalazhy-Gopakumar S., Ng HK, Ganesan PB, Gan S., Lee LY, et al. Emulsification of bio-oil and diesel. *Chemical Engineering Transactions* 2017;56:1801–1806. https://doi.org/10.3303/CET1756301.

[116] Yang Z, Kumar A, Huhnke RL. Review of recent developments to improve storage and transportation stability of bio-oil. *Renewable and Sustainable Energy Reviews* 2015;50:859–870. https://doi.org/10.1016/j.rser.2015.05.025.

[117] Baldwin RM, Feik CJ. Bio-oil stabilization and upgrading by hot gas filtration. *Energy & Fuels* 2013;27:3224–3238. https://doi.org/10.1021/ef400177t.

[118] Case PA, Wheeler MC, De Sisto WJ. Effect of residence time and hot gas filtration on the physical and chemical properties of pyrolysis oil. *Energy & Fuels* 2014;28:3964–3969. https://doi.org/10.1021/ef500850y.

Thermochemical Production of Bio-Oil

[119] Chen T, Wu C, Liu R, Fei W, Liu S. Effect of hot vapor filtration on the characterization of bio-oil from rice husks with fast pyrolysis in a fluidized-bed reactor. *Bioresource Technology* 2011;102:6178–6185. https://doi.org/10.1016/j.biortech.2011.02.023.

[120] Mei Y, Liu R, Wu W, Zhang L. Effect of hot vapor filter temperature on mass yield, energy balance, and properties of products of the fast pyrolysis of pine sawdust. *Energy & Fuels* 2016;30:10458–10469. https://doi.org/10.1021/acs.energyfuels.6b01877.

[121] Hoekstra E, Hogendoorn KJA, Wang X, Westerhof RJM, Kersten SRA, van Swaaij WPM, et al. Fast pyrolysis of biomass in a fluidized bed reactor: In situ filtering of the vapors. *Industrial & Engineering Chemistry Research* 2009;48:4744–4756. https://doi.org/10.1021/ie8017274.

[122] Elliott DC, Wang H, French R, Deutch S, Iisa K. Hydrocarbon liquid production from biomass via hot-vapor-filtered fast pyrolysis and catalytic hydroprocessing of the bio-oil. *Energy & Fuels* 2014;28:5909–5917. https://doi.org/10.1021/ef501536j.

[123] Pattiya A, Suttibak S. Production of bio-oil via fast pyrolysis of agricultural residues from cassava plantations in a fluidised-bed reactor with a hot vapour filtration unit. *Journal of Analytical and Applied Pyrolysis* 2012;95:227–235. https://doi.org/10.1016/j.jaap.2012.02.010.

[124] Heidenreich S. Hot gas filtration – A review. *Fuel* 2013;104:83–94. https://doi.org/10.1016/j.fuel.2012.07.059.

[125] Li Z, Garedew M, Lam CH, Jackson JE, Miller DJ, Saffron CM. Mild electrocatalytic hydrogenation and hydrodeoxygenation of bio-oil derived phenolic compounds using ruthenium supported on activated carbon cloth. *Green Chemistry* 2012;14:2540. https://doi.org/10.1039/c2gc35552c.

[126] Elangovan S, Larsen D, Bay I, Mitchell E, Hartvigsen J, Millett B, et al. Electrochemical upgrading of bio-oil. *ECS Transactions* 2017;78:3149–3158. https://doi.org/10.1149/07801.3149ecst.

[127] Lister TE, Diaz LA, Lilga MA, Padmaperuma AB, Lin Y, Palakkal VM, et al. Low-temperature electrochemical upgrading of bio-oils using polymer electrolyte membranes. *Energy & Fuels* 2018;32:5944–5950. https://doi.org/10.1021/acs.energyfuels.8b00134.

[128] Zhao B, Chen M, Guo Q, Fu Y. Electrocatalytic hydrogenation of furfural to furfuryl alcohol using platinum supported on activated carbon fibers. *Electrochimica Acta* 2014;135:139–146. https://doi.org/10.1016/j.electacta.2014.04.164.

[129] Hilten R, Weber J, Kastner JR. Continuous upgrading of fast pyrolysis oil by simultaneous esterification and hydrogenation. *Energy & Fuels* 2016;30:8357–8368. https://doi.org/10.1021/acs.energyfuels.6b01906.

[130] Kumar R, Singh L, Zularisam AW, Hai FI. Microbial fuel cell is emerging as a versatile technology: A review on its possible applications, challenges and strategies to improve the performances: Microbial fuel cell is emerging as a versatile technology. *International Journal of Energy Research* 2018;42:369–394. https://doi.org/10.1002/er.3780.

[131] Kumar R, Singh L, Zularisam AW. Exoelectrogens: Recent advances in molecular drivers involved in extracellular electron transfer and strategies used to improve it for microbial fuel cell applications. *Renewable and Sustainable Energy Reviews* 2016;56:1322–1336. https://doi.org/10.1016/j.rser.2015.12.029.

[132] Chen B, Shi Z, Jiang S, Tian H. Catalytic cracking mechanisms of tar model compounds. *Journal of Central South University* 2016;23:3100–3107. https://doi.org/10.1007/s11771-016-3375-7.

[133] Si Z, Zhang X, Wang C, Ma L, Dong R. An overview on catalytic hydrodeoxygenation of pyrolysis oil and its model compounds. *Catalysts* 2017;7:169. https://doi.org/10.3390/catal7060169.

[134] Kim S, Kwon EE, Kim YT, Jung S, Kim HJ, Huber GW, et al. Recent advances in hydrodeoxygenation of biomass-derived oxygenates over heterogeneous catalysts. *Green Chemistry* 2019:10.1039.C9GC01210A. https://doi.org/10.1039/C9GC01210A.

[135] Ruddy DA, Schaidle JA, Ferrell III JR, Wang J, Moens L, Hensley JE. Recent advances in heterogeneous catalysts for bio-oil upgrading via "ex situ catalytic fast pyrolysis": Catalyst development through the study of model compounds. *Green Chemistry* 2014;16:454–490. https://doi.org/10.1039/C3GC41354C.

[136] Cheng S, Wei L, Alsowij MR, Corbin F, Julson J, Boakye E, et al. In situ hydrodeoxygenation upgrading of pine sawdust bio-oil to hydrocarbon biofuel using Pd/C catalyst. *Journal of the Energy Institute* 2018;91:163–171. https://doi.org/10.1016/j.joei.2017.01.004.

[137] Lau PL, Allen RWK, Styring P. Continuous-flow Heck synthesis of 4-methoxybiphenyl and methyl 4-methoxycinnamate in supercritical carbon dioxide expanded solvent solutions. *Beilstein Journal of Organic Chemistry* 2013;9:2886–2897. https://doi.org/10.3762/bjoc.9.325.

[138] Sanna A, Vispute TP, Huber GW. Hydrodeoxygenation of the aqueous fraction of bio-oil with Ru/C and Pt/C catalysts. *Applied Catalysis B: Environmental* 2015;165:446–456. https://doi.org/10.1016/j.apcatb.2014.10.013.

[139] Han Y, Gholizadeh M, Tran C-C, Kaliaguine S, Li C-Z, Olarte M, et al. Hydrotreatment of pyrolysis bio-oil: A review. *Fuel Processing Technology* 2019;195:106140. https://doi.org/10.1016/j.fuproc.2019.106140.

[140] Capunitan JA, Capareda SC. Hydrotreatment of corn stover bio-oil using noble metal catalysts. *Fuel Processing Technology* 2014;125:190–199. https://doi.org/10.1016/j.fuproc.2014.03.029.

[141] Gholizadeh M, Gunawan R, Hu X, de Miguel Mercader F, Westerhof R, Chaitwat W, et al. Effects of temperature on the hydrotreatment behaviour of pyrolysis bio-oil and coke formation in a continuous hydrotreatment reactor. *Fuel Processing Technology* 2016;148:175–183. https://doi.org/10.1016/j.fuproc.2016.03.002.

[142] Gholizadeh M, Gunawan R, Hu X, Hasan MM, Kersten S, Westerhof R, et al. Different reaction behaviours of the light and heavy components of bio-oil during the hydrotreatment in a continuous pack-bed reactor. *Fuel Processing Technology* 2016;146:76–84. https://doi.org/10.1016/j.fuproc.2016.01.026.

[143] Gholizadeh M, Gunawan R, Hu X, Kadarwati S, Westerhof R, Chaiwat W, et al. Importance of hydrogen and bio-oil inlet temperature during the hydrotreatment of bio-oil. *Fuel Processing Technology* 2016;150:132–140. https://doi.org/10.1016/j.fuproc.2016.05.014.

[144] Ardiyanti AR, Khromova SA, Venderbosch RH, Yakovlev VA, Melián-Cabrera IV, Heeres HJ. Catalytic hydrotreatment of fast pyrolysis oil using bimetallic Ni–Cu catalysts on various supports. *Applied Catalysis A: General* 2012;449:121–130. https://doi.org/10.1016/j.apcata.2012.09.016.

[145] Boscagli C, Yang C, Welle A, Wang W, Behrens S, Raffelt K, et al. Effect of pyrolysis oil components on the activity and selectivity of nickel-based catalysts during hydrotreatment. *Applied Catalysis A: General* 2017;544:161–172. https://doi.org/10.1016/j.apcata.2017.07.025.

[146] Yin W, Venderbosch RH, He S, Bykova MV, Khromova SA, Yakovlev VA, et al. Mono-, bi-, and tri-metallic Ni-based catalysts for the catalytic hydrotreatment of pyrolysis liquids. *Biomass Conversion and Biorefinery* 2017;7:361–376. https://doi.org/10.1007/s13399-017-0267-5.

[147] Sangnikul P, Phanpa C, Xiao R, Zhang H, Reubroycharoen P, Kuchonthara P, et al. Role of copper- or cerium-promoters on NiMo/γ-Al$_2$O$_3$ catalysts in hydrodeoxygenation of guaiacol and bio-oil. *Applied Catalysis A: General* 2019;574:151–160. https://doi.org/10.1016/j.apcata.2019.02.004.

[148] Carriel Schmitt C, Zimina A, Fam Y, Raffelt K, Grunwaldt J-D, Dahmen N. Evaluation of high-loaded Ni-based catalysts for upgrading fast pyrolysis bio-oil. *Catalysts* 2019;9:784. https://doi.org/10.3390/catal9090784.

Thermochemical Production of Bio-Oil

[149] Schmitt CC, Raffelt K, Zimina A, Krause B, Otto T, Rapp M, et al. Hydrotreatment of fast pyrolysis bio-oil fractions over nickel-based catalyst. *Topics in Catalysis* 2018;61:1769–1782. https://doi.org/10.1007/s11244-018-1009-z.

[150] Kim G, Seo J, Choi J-W, Jae J, Ha J-M, Suh DJ, et al. Two-step continuous upgrading of sawdust pyrolysis oil to deoxygenated hydrocarbons using hydrotreating and hydrodeoxygenating catalysts. *Catalysis Today* 2018;303:130–135. https://doi.org/10.1016/j.cattod.2017.09.027.

[151] Wildschut J, Mahfud FH, Venderbosch RH, Heeres HJ. Hydrotreatment of fast pyrolysis oil using heterogeneous noble-metal catalysts. *Industrial & Engineering Chemistry Research* 2009;48:10324–10334. https://doi.org/10.1021/ie9006003.

[152] Elkasabi Y, Mullen CA, Pighinelli ALMT, Boateng AA. Hydrodeoxygenation of fast-pyrolysis bio-oils from various feedstocks using carbon-supported catalysts. *Fuel Processing Technology* 2014;123:11–18. https://doi.org/10.1016/j.fuproc.2014.01.039.

[153] Guo C, Rao KTV, Yuan Z, He S (Quan), Rohani S, Xu C (Charles). Hydrodeoxygenation of fast pyrolysis oil with novel activated carbon-supported NiP and CoP catalysts. *Chemical Engineering Science* 2018;178:248–259. https://doi.org/10.1016/j.ces.2017.12.048.

[154] Jahromi H, Agblevor FA. Upgrading of pinyon-juniper catalytic pyrolysis oil via hydrodeoxygenation. *Energy* 2017;141:2186–2195. https://doi.org/10.1016/j.energy.2017.11.149.

[155] Boscagli C, Raffelt K, Grunwaldt J-D. Reactivity of platform molecules in pyrolysis oil and in water during hydrotreatment over nickel and ruthenium catalysts. *Biomass and Bioenergy* 2017;106:63–73. https://doi.org/10.1016/j.biombioe.2017.08.013.

[156] Ardiyanti AR, Bykova MV, Khromova SA, Yin W, Venderbosch RH, Yakovlev VA, et al. Ni-Based Catalysts for the Hydrotreatment of Fast Pyrolysis Oil. *Energy & Fuels* 2016;30:1544–1554. https://doi.org/10.1021/acs.energyfuels.5b02223.

[157] Reyhanitash E, Tymchyshyn M, Yuan Z, Albion K, van Rossum G, (Charles) Xu C. Hydrotreatment of fast pyrolysis oil: Effects of esterification pre-treatment of the oil using alcohol at a small loading. *Fuel* 2016;179:45–51. https://doi.org/10.1016/j.fuel.2016.03.074.

[158] Jahromi H, Agblevor FA. Hydrodeoxygenation of aqueous-phase catalytic pyrolysis oil to liquid hydrocarbons using multifunctional Nickel catalyst. *Industrial & Engineering Chemistry Research* 2018;57:13257–13268. https://doi.org/10.1021/acs.iecr.8b02807.

[159] Mu W, Ben H, Du X, Zhang X, Hu F, Liu W, et al. Noble metal catalyzed aqueous phase hydrogenation and hydrodeoxygenation of lignin-derived pyrolysis oil and related model compounds. *Bioresource Technology* 2014;173:6–10. https://doi.org/10.1016/j.biortech.2014.09.067.

[160] Horáček J, Kubička D. Bio-oil hydrotreating over conventional CoMo & NiMo catalysts: The role of reaction conditions and additives. *Fuel* 2017;198:49–57. https://doi.org/10.1016/j.fuel.2016.10.003.

[161] Kadarwati S, Hu X, Gunawan R, Westerhof R, Gholizadeh M, Hasan MDM, et al. Coke formation during the hydrotreatment of bio-oil using NiMo and CoMo catalysts. *Fuel Processing Technology* 2017;155:261–268. https://doi.org/10.1016/j.fuproc.2016.08.021.

[162] Eschenbacher A, Saraeian A, Jensen PA, Shanks BH, Li C, Duus JØ, et al. Deoxygenation of wheat straw fast pyrolysis vapors over Na-Al$_2$O$_3$ catalyst for production of bio-oil with low acidity. *Chemical Engineering Journal* 2020;394:124878. https://doi.org/10.1016/j.cej.2020.124878.

[163] Romero Y, Richard F, Brunet S. Hydrodeoxygenation of 2-ethylphenol as a model compound of bio-crude over sulfided Mo-based catalysts: Promoting effect and reaction mechanism. *Applied Catalysis B: Environmental* 2010;98:213–223. https://doi.org/10.1016/j.apcatb.2010.05.031.

[164] Grilc M, Likozar B, Levec J. Hydrodeoxygenation and hydrocracking of solvolysed lignocellulosic biomass by oxide, reduced and sulphide form of NiMo, Ni, Mo and Pd catalysts. *Applied Catalysis B: Environmental* 2014;150–151:275–287. https://doi.org/10.1016/j.apcatb.2013.12.030.

[165] Jin W, Pastor-Pérez L, Villora-Picó JJ, Sepúlveda-Escribano A, Gu S, Reina TR. Investigating new routes for biomass upgrading: "H_2-Free" hydrodeoxygenation using Ni-based catalysts. *ACS Sustainable Chemistry & Engineering* 2019;7:16041–16049. https://doi.org/10.1021/acssuschemeng.9b02712.

[166] Li K, Wang R, Chen J. Hydrodeoxygenation of Anisole over Silica-Supported Ni_2P, MoP, and NiMoP Catalysts. *Energy Fuels* 2011;25:854–863. https://doi.org/10.1021/ef101258j.

[167] Tu C, Chen J, Li W, Wang H, Deng K, Vinokurov VA, et al. Hydrodeoxygenation of bio-derived anisole to cyclohexane over bi-functional IM-5 zeolite supported Ni catalysts. *Sustainable Energy Fuels* 2019;3:3462–3472. https://doi.org/10.1039/C9SE00554D.

[168] Dongil AB, Ghampson IT, García R, Fierro JLG, Escalona N. Hydrodeoxygenation of guaiacol over Ni/carbon catalysts: Effect of the support and Ni loading. *RSC Advances* 2016;6:2611–2623. https://doi.org/10.1039/C5RA22540J.

[169] Zhang J, Fidalgo B, Kolios A, Shen D, Gu S. Mechanism of deoxygenation in anisole decomposition over single-metal loaded HZSM-5: Experimental study. *Chemical Engineering Journal* 2018;336:211–222. https://doi.org/10.1016/j.cej.2017.11.128.

[170] Wang Z, Zeng Y, Lin W, Song W. In-situ hydrodeoxygenation of phenol by supported Ni catalyst – explanation for catalyst performance. *International Journal of Hydrogen Energy* 2017;42:21040–21047. https://doi.org/10.1016/j.ijhydene.2017.07.053.

[171] Mohammed IY, Abakr YA, Mokaya R. Catalytic upgrading of pyrolytic oil via in-situ hydrodeoxygenation. *Waste Biomass Valor* 2020;11:2935–2947. https://doi.org/10.1007/s12649-019-00613-0.

[172] Wang L, Ye P, Yuan F, Li S, Ye Z. Liquid phase in-situ hydrodeoxygenation of bio-derived phenol over Raney Ni and Nafion/SiO_2. *International Journal of Hydrogen Energy* 2015;40:14790–14797. https://doi.org/10.1016/j.ijhydene.2015.09.014.

[173] Lv M, Zhou J, Yang W, Cen K. Thermogravimetric analysis of the hydrolysis of zinc particles. *International Journal of Hydrogen Energy* 2010;35:2617–2621. https://doi.org/10.1016/j.ijhydene.2009.04.017.

[174] Strenziok R, Hansen U, Knstner H. Combustion of bio-oil in a gas turbine. In: Bridgwater AV, editor. *Progress in Thermochemical Biomass Conversion*, Oxford, UK: Blackwell Science Ltd, 2001; pp. 1452–1458. https://doi.org/10.1002/9780470694954.ch119.

[175] Trane R, Dahl S, Skjøth-Rasmussen MS, Jensen AD. Catalytic steam reforming of bio-oil. *International Journal of Hydrogen Energy* 2012;37:6447–6472. https://doi.org/10.1016/j.ijhydene.2012.01.023.

[176] Seyedeyn-Azad F, Abedi J, Sampouri S. Catalytic steam reforming of aqueous phase of bio-oil over Ni-based alumina-supported catalysts. *Industrial & Engineering Chemistry Research* 2014;53:17937–17944. https://doi.org/10.1021/ie5034705.

[177] Lan P, Xu Q, Zhou M, Lan L, Zhang S, Yan Y. Catalytic steam reforming of fast pyrolysis bio-oil in fixed bed and fluidized bed reactors. *Chemical Engineering & Technology* 2010;33:2021–2028. https://doi.org/10.1002/ceat.201000169.

[178] Werther J, Reppenhagen J. Catalyst attrition in fluidized-bed systems. *AIChE Journal* 1999;45:2001–2010. https://doi.org/10.1002/aic.690450916.

[179] van Rossum G, Kersten SRA, van Swaaij WPM. Staged catalytic gasification/steam reforming of pyrolysis oil. *Industrial & Engineering Chemistry Research* 2009;48:5857–5866. https://doi.org/10.1021/ie900194j.

[180] Liu Q, Xiong Z, Syed-Hassan SSA, Deng Z, Zhao X, Su S, et al. Effect of the pre-reforming by Fe/bio-char catalyst on a two-stage catalytic steam reforming of bio-oil. *Fuel* 2019;239:282–289. https://doi.org/10.1016/j.fuel.2018.11.029.

[181] Ren Z-Z, Lan P, Ma H-R, Wang T, Shi X-H, Zhang S-P, et al. Hydrogen production via catalytic steam reforming of bio-oil model compound in a two-stage reaction system. *Energy Sources, Part A: Recovery, Utilization, and Environmental Effects* 2014;36:1921–1930. https://doi.org/10.1080/15567036.2011.582615.

Thermochemical Production of Bio-Oil

265

[182] Santamaria L, Lopez G, Arregi A, Amutio M, Artetxe M, Bilbao J, et al. Influence of the support on Ni catalysts performance in the in-line steam reforming of biomass fast pyrolysis derived volatiles. *Applied Catalysis B: Environmental* 2018;229:105–113. https://doi.org/10.1016/j.apcatb.2018.02.003.

[183] Valle B, Aramburu B, Benito PL, Bilbao J, Gayubo AG. Biomass to hydrogen-rich gas via steam reforming of raw bio-oil over $Ni/La_2O_3-\alpha Al_2O_3$ catalyst: Effect of space-time and steam-to-carbon ratio. *Fuel* 2018;216:445–455. https://doi.org/10.1016/j.fuel.2017.11.151.

[184] Valle B, Aramburu B, Olazar M, Bilbao J, Gayubo AG. Steam reforming of raw bio-oil over $Ni/La_2O_3-\alpha Al_2O_3$: Influence of temperature on product yields and catalyst deactivation. *Fuel* 2018;216:463–474. https://doi.org/10.1016/j.fuel.2017.11.149.

[185] Remiro A, Valle B, Aguayo AT, Bilbao J, Gayubo AG. Operating conditions for attenuating $Ni/La2O3-\alpha Al_2O_3$ catalyst deactivation in the steam reforming of bio-oil aqueous fraction. *Fuel Processing Technology* 2013;115:222–232. https://doi.org/10.1016/j.fuproc.2013.06.003.

[186] Arregi A, Lopez G, Amutio M, Artetxe M, Barbarias I, Bilbao J, et al. Role of operating conditions in the catalyst deactivation in the in-line steam reforming of volatiles from biomass fast pyrolysis. *Fuel* 2018;216:233–244. https://doi.org/10.1016/j.fuel.2017.12.002.

[187] Bimbela F, Oliva M, Ruiz J, García L, Arauzo J. Hydrogen production via catalytic steam reforming of the aqueous fraction of bio-oil using nickel-based coprecipitated catalysts. *International Journal of Hydrogen Energy* 2013;38:14476–14487. https://doi.org/10.1016/j.ijhydene.2013.09.038.

[188] Xing R, Dagle VL, Flake M, Kovarik L, Albrecht KO, Deshmane C, et al. Steam reforming of fast pyrolysis-derived aqueous phase oxygenates over Co, Ni, and Rh metals supported on $MgAl_2O_4$. *Catalysis Today* 2016;269:166–174. https://doi.org/10.1016/j.cattod.2015.11.046.

[189] Chen J, Sun J, Wang Y. Catalysts for steam reforming of bio-oil: A review. *Industrial & Engineering Chemistry Research* 2017;56:4627–4637. https://doi.org/10.1021/acs.iecr.7b00600.

[190] Rioche C, Kulkarni S, Meunier FC, Breen JP, Burch R. Steam reforming of model compounds and fast pyrolysis bio-oil on supported noble metal catalysts. *Applied Catalysis B: Environmental* 2005;61:130–139. https://doi.org/10.1016/j.apcatb.2005.04.015.

[191] Yadav AK, Vaidya PD. Reaction kinetics of steam reforming of *n*-Butanol over a Ni/hydrotalcite catalyst. *Chemical Engineering & Technology* 2018;41:890–896. https://doi.org/10.1002/ceat.201600738.

[192] Llera I, Mas V, Bergamini ML, Laborde M, Amadeo N. Bio-ethanol steam reforming on Ni based catalyst. Kinetic study. *Chemical Engineering Science* 2012;71:356–366. https://doi.org/10.1016/j.ces.2011.12.018.

[193] Vaidya PD, Rodrigues AE. Kinetics of steam reforming of ethanol over a Ru/Al_2O_3 catalyst. *Industrial & Engineering Chemistry Research* 2006;45:6614–6618. https://doi.org/10.1021/ie051342m.

[194] Arregi A, Lopez G, Amutio M, Barbarias I, Santamaria L, Bilbao J, et al. Kinetic study of the catalytic reforming of biomass pyrolysis volatiles over a commercial Ni/Al_2O_3 catalyst. *International Journal of Hydrogen Energy* 2018;43:12023–12033. https://doi.org/10.1016/j.ijhydene.2018.05.032.

[195] Santamaria L, Lopez G, Arregi A, Amutio M, Artetxe M, Bilbao J, et al. Stability of different Ni supported catalysts in the in-line steam reforming of biomass fast pyrolysis volatiles. *Applied Catalysis B: Environmental* 2019;242:109–120. https://doi.org/10.1016/j.apcatb.2018.09.081.

[196] Remón J, Broust F, Valette J, Chhiti Y, Alava I, Fernandez-Akarregi AR, et al. Production of a hydrogen-rich gas from fast pyrolysis bio-oils: Comparison between homogeneous and catalytic steam reforming routes. *International Journal of Hydrogen Energy* 2014;39:171–182. https://doi.org/10.1016/j.ijhydene.2013.10.025.

[197] Zhang S, Li X, Li Q, Xu Q, Yan Y. Hydrogen production from the aqueous phase derived from fast pyrolysis of biomass. *Journal of Analytical and Applied Pyrolysis* 2011;92:158–163. https://doi.org/10.1016/j.jaap.2011.05.007.

[198] Ramirez JA, Rainey TJ. Comparative techno-economic analysis of biofuel production through gasification, thermal liquefaction and pyrolysis of sugarcane bagasse. *Journal of Cleaner Production* 2019;229:513–527. https://doi.org/10.1016/j.jclepro.2019.05.017.

[199] Magdeldin M, Kohl T, Järvinen M. Techno-economic assessment of the by-products contribution from non-catalytic hydrothermal liquefaction of lignocellulose residues. *Energy* 2017;137:679–695. https://doi.org/10.1016/j.energy.2017.06.166.

[200] Patel M, Zhang X, Kumar A. Techno-economic and life cycle assessment on lignocellulosic biomass thermochemical conversion technologies: A review. *Renewable and Sustainable Energy Reviews* 2016;53:1486–1499. https://doi.org/10.1016/j.rser.2015.09.070.

[201] Zhang Y, Brown TR, Hu G, Brown RC. Comparative techno-economic analysis of biohydrogen production via bio-oil gasification and bio-oil reforming. *Biomass and Bioenergy* 2013;51:99–108. https://doi.org/10.1016/j.biombioe.2013.01.013.

[202] Rogers JG, Brammer JG. Estimation of the production cost of fast pyrolysis bio-oil. *Biomass and Bioenergy* 2012;36:208–217. https://doi.org/10.1016/j.biombioe.2011.10.028.

[203] Wright MM, Daugaard DE, Satrio JA, Brown RC. Techno-economic analysis of biomass fast pyrolysis to transportation fuels. *Fuel* 2010;89:S2–S10. https://doi.org/10.1016/j.fuel.2010.07.029.

[204] Zhu Y, Biddy MJ, Jones SB, Elliott DC, Schmidt AJ. Techno-economic analysis of liquid fuel production from woody biomass via hydrothermal liquefaction (HTL) and upgrading. *Applied Energy* 2014;129:384–394. https://doi.org/10.1016/j.apenergy.2014.03.053.

[205] Sarkar S, Kumar A. Large-scale biohydrogen production from bio-oil. *Bioresource Technology* 2010;101:7350–7361. https://doi.org/10.1016/j.biortech.2010.04.038.

[206] Wright MM, Román-Leshkov Y, Green WH. Investigating the techno-economic trade-offs of hydrogen source using a response surface model of drop-in biofuel production via bio-oil upgrading: Modeling and analysis: Techno-economic tradeoffs of hydrogen source in bio-oil upgrading. *Biofuels, Bioproducts and Biorefining* 2012;6:503–520. https://doi.org/10.1002/bbb.1340.

10 Free Fatty Acids and Their Role in CI Engines

P.S. Ranjit[1], Saravanan A., and Elumalai P.V.
1 Department of Mechanical Engineering,
  Aditya Engineering College, Surampalem

CONTENTS

10.1 Introduction 267
    10.1.1 Procedure to Isolate FA and Its Identification 268
    10.1.2 Method of Saponification and Lipolysis 269
        10.1.2.1 Lipolysis 269
10.2 Procedure Involved in Esterification and Silylation 270
    10.2.1 Esterification 270
    10.2.2 Silylation 271
10.3 Methods to Determine the Fatty Acids 271
    10.3.1 Chemical Methods 272
        10.3.1.1 Based on the Number of Bonds 272
        10.3.1.2 Based on the Position of Bonds 272
    10.3.2 Spectrometric Methods 273
    10.3.3 Infrared Spectroscopy 273
    10.3.4 Ultraviolet Spectroscopy 274
    10.3.5 Nuclear Magnetic Resonance Spectroscopy 274
    10.3.6 Enzymatic Methods 274
        10.3.6.1 Lipoxidases 275
        10.3.6.2 Dehydrogenases 275
        10.3.6.3 Lipases 275
10.4 Role of Free Fatty Acids in Diesel Engines 291
10.5 Conclusion 291
References 293

10.1 INTRODUCTION

Fatty acids are saturated or unsaturated aliphatic carboxylic acids. Most naturally occurring fatty acids contain straight lines with odd carbon atoms in the range of 4–28. A fatty acid is a large component (up to 70% by weight) of lipids in some

[1] psranjit1234@gmail.com

DOI: 10.1201/9781003265597-10

268   Biowaste and Biomass in Biofuel Applications

species, such as microalgae, while other organisms are found in three major ester groups: triglycerides, phospholipids, and cholesteryl esters. In 1813, Michel Eugene Chevreul proposed the idea of fatty acids (acid gras).

- Fatty acids having aliphatic tails of five carbons or less are known as short-chain fatty acids (SCFA) (for example, butyric acid).
- Fatty acids with aliphatic tails of 6 to 12 carbons are referred to as medium-chain fatty acids (MCFA) and can produce medium-chain triglycerides.
- Fatty acids having aliphatic tails of 13 to 21 carbons are referred to as long-chain fatty acids (LCFA).
- Fatty acids having aliphatic tails of 22 or more carbons are referred to as very long-chain fatty acids (VLCFA).

There are no C=C double bonds in saturated fatty acids. They all have the identical formula, $CH_3(CH_2)_nCOOH$, with minor differences in "n". Stearic acid (n = 18) is a significant saturated fatty acid.

Changes in the exclusive division and basic character strategies have uncovered significant differing qualities and complexity inside greasy acids synthesized from an assortment of vegetable fats. Different positional and geometric isomers of common ethylenic greasy acids that have been analyzed for a long time have been found and killed over the past quarter century in expansion to the recently distinguished homologs of these acids rice field. In expansion, fatty acids with an abnormal number of carbon molecules, branched chain acids, hydroxy acids, and epoxy acids, acetylene acids, and combinations of both conjugated and non-conjugated ethylene-acetylene acids, as well as cyclopropanoic corrosive and cyclopropenic corrosive have been extricated and characterized. Numerous fats comprise exceptionally small sums of uncommon acids, but other fats can be critical fixings. The discovery of furoline chromatography has released over 500 extraordinary fatty acids from plants or man-made substances. No analytical method can efficiently separate and detect all these acids. Separation and discovery of all types of acids homologs usually require combining many complementary methods. This is essential to assess the near-excessive limitations of the method of choice. Fortunately, the best evaluation strategy also requires a minimal amount of material.

10.1.1 Procedure to Isolate FA and Its Identification

Natural fatty acids are available as free or simple alkyl esters before separation and identification. This usually involves saponification or transesterification of fats, but enzymatic hydrolysis can also be used to achieve complete or selective release of fatty acid from natural fats. During production, great care is taken to prevent the loss of short-chain and polar fatty acids, prevent decomposition and artifacts by chemically unstable acids, and reduce contamination of all acids from equipment and solvents. You have to pay. I have. Polyunsaturated acids should be protected by an inert environment and antioxidants during chemical manipulation and storage [1–3].

Free Fatty Acids and Their Role in CI Engines 269

The first step in identifying fatty acids is to separate them from natural fats in a free form. Free fatty acids are more effectively changed over to numerous subsidiaries required for distinguishing proof than greasy corrosive esters.

10.1.2 Method of Saponification and Lipolysis

The capacity to take away non-acidic lipids with the aid of using extracting with a natural solvent in preference to chromatography is a crucial gain of saponification. However, a double bond switch can arise during saponification, and unconjugated polyunsaturated fatty acids may be transformed into conjugated isomers [4]. Conjugates can be polymerized, and all unsaturated acids can be autoxidized. Alkaline concentrations above 0.5N have been shown to promote polyunsaturated acid loss and reflux times above 1 hour [1,5,6]. Kates states that 15–32 mg of add up to lipid is refluxed for 1–2 hours beneath a nitrogen environment with 5 mL of 90% methanolic NaOH (0.3 N) [7]. After weakening with watery methanol, petroleum ether is utilized to expel non-saponifiable substances. Bulk greasy acids are obtained by acidifying the alcoholic division with 6 N HCI and re-extracting it with petroleum. In case short-chain acids are shown, they can be expelled after fermentation by steam refining; The buildup and steam distillate are isolated independently [8]. This hydrolysis preparation does not discharge greasy acids from amide bonds like those seen in sphingolipids. It, too, makes a difference in keeping the long-chain aldehydes within the vinyl ether joins of plasmalogens, which is valuable for planning immaculate greasy acids.

10.1.2.1 Lipolysis

A few lipases and esterases are known to free greasy acids from glycerol, cholesterol, and other liquor esters [9]. Lipolytic hydrolysis of fats happens essentially without changing the structure of acyl bunches, which is greatly useful when working with greasy acids that are unsteady to warm, acids, and alkalis. There is information on diverse rates of hydrolysis of esters containing acyl bunches with diverse chain lengths and degrees of unsaturation, as well as information on diverse rates of hydrolysis with a alter within the position of the glycerol particle. Pancreatic lipase can offer assistance with free greasy acids from the sn-1 and sn-3 areas of triacylglycerols [10]. The protein is specific for acylglycerols containing certain fatty acids [11–14], as are acids containing conjugated twofold bonds. Butyric corrosive is the shortest-chain greasy corrosive broken by lipase. Lipase from Rhizopus arrhizus moreover targets the acyl-glycerol sn-1 and sn-3 destinations, in spite of the fact that with less greasy corrosive selectivity [15]. A lipase from the bacterium Geotrichumcandidum can be utilized to specifically free normal ethylenic greasy acids from any area inside a triacylglycerol particle. This lipase hydrolyzes cis-9 18: 1 and cis,cis-9,12 18:2 more effectively than any other positional isomers of cis 18: 1 and trans-9 18: 1 [16]. Following research, it was discovered that the enzyme discriminates against the trans, trans isomer but not between the cis, trans and trans, cis isomers [17]. Another lipase that's effectively fabricated is castor bean lipase. This chemical catalyzes the hydrolysis of greasy acids from the sn-1 and sn-3 destinations of triacylglycerols. In spite of the fact that castor oil is rapidly hydrolyzed, the protein hydrolyzes triacylglycerols containing immersed greasy acids with chain lengths extending from C4 to C [18]. Sterculic corrosive represses castor bean lipase action. Phospholipase A2 from wind poison may cause a total discharge of common greasy acids from the sn-2 position [19]. This chemical hydrolyzes 1,2-diacyl-sn-glycerol-3-phosphate esters, shaping the establishment for a triacylglycerol stereospecific investigation. Natural solvents such as diethyl ether are more productive in carrying out the response [20]. Soaked fatty acids are discharged more rapidly than unsaturated greasy acids in common. Be that as it may, the rates of hydrolysis of specific immersed and unsaturated acids contrast. The chemical will discharge the acyl bunch (carbon-containing oxygen atom) from manufactured atoms in which the phosphate gathered is connected to the auxiliary hydroxyl bunch of glycerol at a slower pace [21]. The fatty acids delivered from enzymatic lipolysis are regularly sullied with the beginning materials and any middle change items. Essentially, free greasy acids discharged from cleansers amid fermentation of the saponification blend may be sullied with esters due to the halfway re-esterification of acids with alcohols in the solution. Therefore, the free greasy acids from lipolysis and saponification must be decontaminated sometime recently the subordinates are arranged. Sufficient free greasy acids can be decontaminated for gas-liquid chromatography (GLC) by lean layer chromatography (TLC) employing an unbiased lipid framework counting acidic corrosive to guarantee that all fatty acids are within the unionized state amid chromatography [22] and heptane-isopropyl ether-acetic acid 60:40:4 [23]. The fatty acids delivered from enzymatic lipolysis are frequently sullied with the beginning materials and any middle-of-the-road change items. Additionally, free greasy acids discharged from cleansers amid fermentation of the saponification blend may be sullied with esters due to the halfway re-esterification of acids with alcohols in the solution. Therefore, the free greasy acids from lipolysis and saponification must be filtered sometime recently the subordinates are arranged. Sufficient free greasy acids can be filtered for gas-liquid chromatography (GLC) by lean layer chromatography (TLC) employing an impartial lipid framework counting acidic corrosive to guarantee that all fatty acids are within the unionized state amid chromatography [24]. Particle trade chromatography may recuperate little amounts of free greasy acids from blends containing considerable sums of unbiased esters [25].

10.2 PROCEDURE INVOLVED IN ESTERIFICATION AND SILYLATION

10.2.1 ESTERIFICATION

To make a fatty acid methyl ester that is stable in heat and acid. Sulfuric acid can be used in a sealed tube at or above reflux temperature. Another good methylation reagent is dry methanol with 5% hydrogen chloride. Since triglyceride esters are insoluble in methanol, the solubility of lipids can be increased by adding an inert solvent such as benzene without affecting the outcome of the reaction [26]. Lankin et al. established calibration curves for each fatty acid to be tested by this approach and reported 97–98 percent yields of fatty acid methyl esters [27]. Utilizing boron trifluoride-methanol, small entireties of free acids may be methylated for GLC in a matter of minutes. The era of methoxy-substituted acids from conjugated unsaturated oily acids is troublesome, as is cyclopropane ring breakage [28–30]. Since of the lessened insecurity of these esters, destructive catalysis at extended temperatures has

Free Fatty Acids and Their Role in CI Engines

routinely been utilized to deliver higher-molecular-weight alcohol esters of short-chain oily acids, which modifies their management with fatty acids [31]. For tests containing a wide assortment of acids, counting those with brief chain lengths, the response of methyl iodide with silver salts of greasy acids has been supported. This technique's "on-column" alteration has demonstrated compelling for gas chroma tography-mass spectrometry [32]. At direct temperatures, the p-bromophenacyl and p-phenylphenacyl esters of C 2-C 20 acids, the benzyl esters of C 1-C 20 acids [33], and the 2-naphthacyl esters of long-chain oily acids were gotten by reacting the fitting alkyl bromides with the free oily acids inside the closeness of N,N-. The final specified esters hold UV light and may be utilized to advance oily destructive recognizing confirmation in the midst of liquid-liquid chromatography [34]. Free acids that are touchy to warm, acids, and antacids can be effectively methylated within the nearness of a small amount of methanol utilizing diazomethane [35]. It is routinely supportive of altering the free oily acids from the TLC plates on which the oily acids were separated into clear alcohol esters inside the closeness of silica gel. For this reason, the dried silica gel is collected in screw-capped (teflon-lined) vials, and adequate boron trifluoride (14 percent) in alcohol is included to cover the powder. The closed vials are warmed for 5–10 minutes at 110°C [36]. Free acids, acids, and stomach-settling agents that are warm sensitive may be expeditiously methylated inside the closeness of a little whole of methanol utilizing diazomethane. Inside the closeness of silica gel, it is as regularly as conceivable supportive of altering over the free oily acids from the TLC plates on which the oily acids were disconnected into fundamental alcohol esters. For this reason, dried silica gel is collected in screw-capped (teflon-lined) vials, and boron trifluoride (14 percent in alcohol) is included to cover the powder. The closed vials are warmed at 110°C for 5–10 minutes.

10.2.2 SILYLATION

The dry damaging blend is uncovered to a reasonable silylating reagent, such as hexamethyldisilazane and trimethylchlorosilane or bistrimethylsilylacetamide, to form trimethylsilyl (TMS) esters of sleek acids [37,38]. TMS esters are hugely dubious to clamminess and must be put truant inside the silylating reagent. The t-butyldimethylsilyl esters, which may be passed on with the proportionate silylating reagent, are distant off more unfaltering [39].

The silylating reagents also respond with any free hydroxyl bunches within the greasy acids, which is valuable for gas chromatography and mass spectrometry [37]. Weihrauch et al. made phenylhydrazine subsidiaries of keto acids [40], whereas Langenbeck et al. [41] organized quinoxalinols of a-keto acids to help in GLC and mass spectrometric division and verification. The quinoxalinols are changed into O-trimethylsilyl ethers to investigate utilizing basic or deuterated silylating reagents.

10.3 METHODS TO DETERMINE THE FATTY ACIDS

In numerous cases, chemical derivatization, spectrophotometric estimations, and enzymatic changes are required to encourage data on the structure of a greasy corrosive [42–44].

10.3.1 Chemical Methods

On the off chance that the corrosive may be a well-known part of a homologous arrangement, its recognizable proof may regularly be chemically approved if it is separated in adequate amounts and immaculateness. Markley [45] compiled a comprehensive list of the softening focuses of common greasy corrosive subsidiaries. In the event that the acid's composition or structure is obscure, it must not be as it were be decided, but it must also be orchestrated utilizing one or more indicated methods and the qualities of the confined and engineered items compared.

10.3.1.1 Based on the Number of Bonds

Quantitative catalytic hydrogenation may be a down-to-earth research facility strategy for assessing the sum of twofold bonds in a confined, greasy corrosive. It can be done on exceptionally small sums of fabric with commercially accessible microhydrogenation gear [46]. Palladium, platinum oxide, or platinum on a reasonable bolster, such as carbon or calcium carbonate, are the primary broadly utilized catalysts. Since they make double-bond development and cis-trans isomerization, these catalysts are not suited for halfway hydrogenation [1].

However, partial hydrogenation may be accomplished using hydrazine as the reducing agent [47]. Lindlar's lead-poisoned palladium catalyst has appeared to be useful for the fractional decrease of acetylenic bonds to cis twofold bonds [4]. Hydrogenation is routinely utilized with GLC to resolve ambiguities in methyl ester considers, such as the recognizing confirmation of 20: 1 ω9 and 18: 3 ω3, which cover most liquid stages and to recognize unsaturated and branched-chain acids on nonpolar columns.

10.3.1.2 Based on the Position of Bonds

The foremost broadly utilized approach for identifying the area of twofold bonds in unsaturated greasy acids is oxidative cleavage taken after by examination of the oxidation items. Potassium permanganate and ozone are predominant oxidizing pros utilized for this reason, and their application inside the consideration of unsaturated acids has been examined by Privett and Roehm and Privett [48,49].

Lemieux and von Rudloff's mixed potassium permanganate-sodium metaperiodate reagent is palatable for monounsaturated oily acids but less dependable for di- and triunsaturated oily acids [50]. GLC viably examines methyl or higher alcohol esters of medium- and long-chain monoenoic and dienoic acids conveyed from oxidation. Permanganate oxidation isn't by an expansive fitting for polyunsaturated oily acids with more than three twofold bonds since a dibasic destructive is gotten from each of the parts of the molecule between the twofold bonds as well as from the carboxy conclusion of the molecule, and consequently, more than one structure for the primary destructive may be proposed.

For the foremost portion, oily destructive methyl esters are ozonized by vaporous ozone in a nonpolar dissolvable such as pentane at uncommonly moo temperatures (for example, −70°C). Once molded, the ozonides of oily destructive methyl esters are by and huge consistent and may be separated utilizing TLC or dissolvable extraction procedures [51]. As with permanganate oxidation, the oily destructive ozonides are hydrolyzed to monobasic and dibasic acids. In any case, diminished cleavage may be chosen, with the things being aldehydes and aldehyde esters. GLC can successfully see at aldehydes, dialdehydes, and aldehyde esters.

Free Fatty Acids and Their Role in CI Engines

Reductive ozonolysis yields an unmistakable break arrange for mono- and diunsaturated sleek acids or esters, but for acids with more than two twofold bonds, more than one structure can be hypothesized since more than one dialdehyde is shaped within the middle of cleavage. On the other hand, the cleavage and examination of ozonides can be performed utilizing pyrolysis GLC, in which case the cleavage happens inside the GLC instrument's input. Roehm and Privett coupled midway hydrogenation with ozonolysis to set up the course of activity of cis and trans twofold bonds in polyunsaturated sleek acids in order to resolve issues in structure errand. After midway hydrogenation with hydrazine, the mix of monounsaturated isomers was disconnected into cis and trans components by argentation TLC. The detached isomers were, at that point, autonomously cleaved by reductive ozonolysis, and the primary polyunsaturated oily destructive structure was concluded by seeing the pieces.

A chemical procedure of investigating the geometry and position of twofold bonds in mono- and diunsaturated oily acids is the overall stereospecific hydroxylation of the compound with solvent permanganate or osmium tetroxide, taken after by change of the hydroxy compounds to their comparing isopropylidene backups. They are inspected utilizing GLC and GL-MS [52,53].

The sum of trans-corrosive in a mono- or diunsaturated greasy combination can also be decided chemically. Emken, portrayed an ester epoxidation taken after by conventional GLC procedure. After 3–4 hours of room temperature peracetic corrosive treatment, the cis and trans esters convey the comparing cis and trans epoxides [54]. The epoxides are easily disconnected on polyester columns, and the trans isomer concentration is chosen. On the other hand, an overabundance of peracid may result inside the alter of cis-epoxy destructive to hydroxy-acetoxy destructive, showing disdain toward the truth that trans epoxide remains relentless underneath these conditions. The methyl esters of trans,trans-; cis,trans-; and cis,cis-9,12-octadecadienoic acids were coordinated utilizing this approach. GLC likely separated diastereoisomers of cis,cis-diepoxide and cis,trans-diepoxide as well, yielding in a more convoluted chromatogram than found with monoenes.

10.3.2 Spectrometric Methods

Particular bunches in greasy corrosive particles assimilate electromagnetic radiation at particular vitality levels, giving critical data on chemical structure and being quantitatively valuable. The revolution of captivated light by greasy corrosive particles could be a particular instance.

10.3.3 Infrared Spectroscopy

Since of the incredible sum of CH2 and CHl bunches within the particles, all greasy acids have impressive retention within the 2750–3000 cm locale [55]. As aliphatic ring systems appear, the relative drive of the bunches related to hydrocarbon chains of particles changes when compared to non-cyclic systems. Cyclopropane oily acids have specific infrared absorption bunches at 1020 cm^{-1} owing to in-plane influencing vibrations of the methylene CH 2 assemble and at 3050 cm^{-1} due to the expanding repeat of the C-H bonds inside the cyclopropane ring. The spectra of cis and trans isomers differentiate mildly. In polyisoprenoid acids, the relative drive of bunches related to hydrocarbon chains of molecules modifies [56].

The C-H amplifies at or roughly 3020 cm^{-1} and can recognize oily destructive unsaturation. Trans twofold bonds are related to C-H mutilation at 950–1000 cm^{-1}, which is apparent inside the methyl elaidate spectra for the case. This property may be utilized to assess trans twofold bonds in oily acids, showing disdain toward the fact that the estimation is helpless to botch within the occasion that there's essential double-bond conjugation. The critical C-O amplification of the liquor gathered at 1045 cm^{-1} may well be a recognizing property of oily acids having a hydroxyl accumulation. Baumann and Ulshoefer inspected the significance of the C-O expansion of ester and hydroxyl bunches in oily acids [57].

10.3.4 ULTRAVIOLET SPECTROSCOPY

Fatty acids with one twofold bond conjugated with the carboxyl accumulate have the other maintenance most extraordinary around 208–210 m and a lower end coefficient than the bucket's conjugated kicks [45].

The maintenance bunches are brought into the accommodatingly accessible zone by the conjugation of unsaturated affiliations. As conjugation creates, so does the end. When three or more conjugated twofold bonds appear, the maintenance appears with three peaks, one essential peak and two minor maxima on either side. The peaks get more scattered and isolated as the number of twofold bonds rises. Unmistakable geometric isomers of the same destructive as well have different digestion spectra. The all-trans shape has the most prominent end coefficient, and the maxima of the cis isomers are routinely pushed to longer wavelengths. Because it is when acetylenic acids are coupled with a twofold or another triple bond, particular maintenance inside the open UV run can happen.

Acids with cis and trans isomers of conjugated polyene and polyne bunches have been well considered. A long course of action of considering declaring shinning maxima and molar absorptivity is open [58]. Spectroscopic investigation of normally happening conjugated polyene and polyeneyne acids was done [5].

10.3.5 NUCLEAR MAGNETIC RESONANCE SPECTROSCOPY

Fatty acids having one or more hilter kilter carbon particles show optical isomerism, which may be chosen by measuring how well certain destructive turns plane-polarized light. Commercial hardware with mechanized computerized readout presently offers estimations at certain wavelengths with an exactness of 0.0010 [7]. In any case, allotting supreme setup to compounds with moo optical movement could be unsafe if solvent and concentration impacts are not taken into consideration. Within the nonattendance of solvents, the foremost repeatable turns are accomplished on immaculate compounds.

10.3.6 ENZYMATIC METHODS

Enzymatic procedures can assess a few structural properties of greasy acids. Although person individuals of a homologous arrangement are seldom recognized, the number, position, and structure of useful bunches are pivotal. The straightforwardness with which the enzymatic change items may be identified or the protein action evaluated decides the effectiveness of this approach within the recognizable proof of greasy acids.

Free Fatty Acids and Their Role in CI Engines

10.3.6.1 Lipoxidases

Lipoxidases are exceptionally particular for the peroxidation of unsaturated greasy acids with the cis-1,cis-4-pentadiene setup, such as linoleic, linolenic, and arachidonic acids, but not oleic corrosive or its esters. The most item could be a cis-trans conjugated hydroperoxide that's optically dynamic [59]. The primary items of linoleic corrosive oxidation are 13-hydroperoxy-cis-9, trans-11-octadecadienoate and 9-hydroperoxy-cis-12-octadecadienoate. The 13-hydroperoxy corrosive has a place in the L arrangement, concurring with optical rotatory scattering spectroscopy [60]. The trans linoleate analogs (18:2, 9c12t; 18:2, 9t12t) are not reasonable substrates.

Numerous methylene-interrupted cis, cis isomers of linoleic destructive have been examined as substrates for perfect soybean lipoxygenase by Hamberg and Samuelsson and Holman et al. [61]. The oxidation rates of a few unsaturated greasy acids uncovered that the nearness of twofold bonds within the ω6 (and ω9) position brought about proficient oxidation.

The positional specificity of the distinctive lipoxygenases shifts to reduce oxidation rate. In this way, shelled nut lipoxygenase shifts from flaxseed lipoxygenase, which targets both areas to extents of 80% at C-13 and 20% at C-9 [62] and com lipoxygenase, which assaults for the most part (83%) the C-9 position and, to a lesser degree (17%), the C-13 position [63].

10.3.6.2 Dehydrogenases

The particular substrate and item specificity of creature and plant cell desaturation frameworks may too be used to confirm the realness of certain greasy acids. When treated with Chlorella vulgaris cells, Crying et al. found that the homologous arrangement of acids from myristic to nonadecanoic is changed to the proportionate 9-monoenoic acids. The 7-monoenoates were moreover created utilizing myristate, pentadecanoate, and palmitate [64]. Johnson et al. illustrated that hen liver arrangements desaturate greasy acids with chain lengths of C 12-C 22 to the comparing 9-monoenoates, with two maxima found, one at C 14 and the other at C 17–18 [65]. The desaturation is exceptionally cliché. Utilizing hydrogen-named stearates, examiners found that the chemical cleavage incorporates the 0–9 and 0–10 hydrogen particles, coming approximately in concurrent cis conclusion. Morris outlined that the stereo specificity of oleate to linoleate desaturation in Chlorella is the same as that of stearate desaturation [66].

10.3.6.3 Lipases

Geotrichumcandidum lipase has been recognized to target normal triacylglycerols, particularly hydrolyzing greasy acids with cis-9 and cis,cis-9,12 unsaturation. Jensen et al. uncovered that when cis-9,cis-12–18:2 was displayed within the triacylglycerol substrates and was hydrolyzed considerably, the protein debased exceptionally small of the other 14 positional isomers of oleic corrosive. There was no inclination for 9–18:1 or 18:2. The hydrolysis of isomeric 18:1 acids determined from manufactured triacylglycerols was frequently reduced than that of soaked acids. The protein besides recognizes between the cis,trans and trans,cis isomers of linoleate but not between the trans,trans and trans,cis isomers.

TABLE 10.1

Free Fatty Acids of Different Oils and Their Methyl Esters [67–77].

Name of the acid	Fatty acid	Chemical formula	Chemical structure	Crystal structure/3D conformer	% composition							
					SO Oil	Jatropha	Sunflower	Neem	Sunflower	Palm oil	Depot margine	Canola
Caproic	C6:0	C6H12O2			-	-	-	-	-	-	-	-
Enathic	C7:0	C7H14O2			-	-	0.5	-	-	0.82	-	-
Caprylic	C8:0	C8H16O2			-	-	0.24	-	1.68	0.56	1.06	-
Capric	C10:0	C10H18O2			0.2	-	0.5	-	3.79	2.43	2.84	-
Lauric	C12:0	C12H24O2			0.31	-	-	-	1.12	0.86	0.83	-

Free Fatty Acids and Their Role in CI Engines

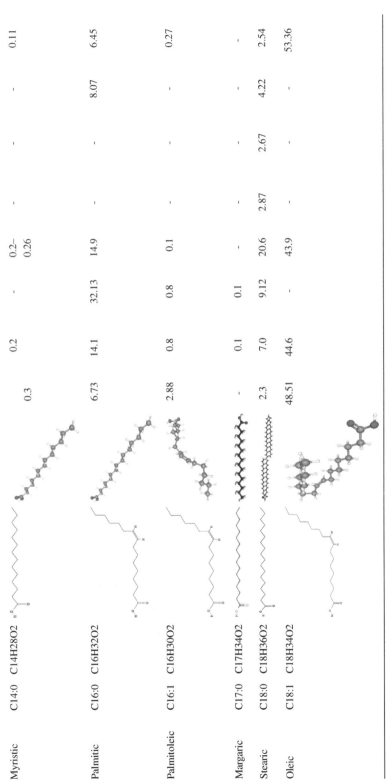

Myristic	C14:0	C14H28O2		0.3	0.2	–	0.2–0.26	–	–	–	0.11
Palmitic	C16:0	C16H32O2		6.73	14.1	32.13	14.9	–	–	8.07	6.45
Palmitoleic	C16:1	C16H30O2		2.88	0.8	0.8	0.1	–	–	–	0.27
Margaric	C17:0	C17H34O2		–	0.1	0.1	–	–	–	–	–
Stearic	C18:0	C18H36O2		2.3	7.0	9.12	20.6	2.87	2.67	4.22	2.54
Oleic	C18:1	C18H34O2		48.51	44.6	–	43.9	–	–	–	53.36

(Continued)

TABLE 10.1 *(Continued)*

Name of the acid	Fatty acid	Chemical formula	Chemical structure	Crystal structure/3D conformer	% composition							
					SO Oil	Jatropha	Sunflower	Neem	Sunflower	Palm oil	Depot margine	Canola
Linoleic	C18:2	C18H32O2			6.57	32.6	21.64	17.9	3.26	45.5	24.57	29.81
Linolenic	C18:3	C18H30O2			0.21	0.4	-	0.4	-	-	-	5.63
Arachidic	C20:0	C20H40O2			15.2	0.2	12.53	1.9	-	-	-	0.42
Gondoic	C20:1	C20H40O2		Being too flexible, Not able to draw	6.17	-	-	-	-	-	-	-

Name of the acid	Fatty acid	Chemical formula	Chemical structure	Crystal structure/3D conformer	% composition							
					Corn	Cottonseed	Hazlenut	Olive	Rapeseed	Rubberseed	Soybean	Grapeseed
Eicosadienoic	C20:2	C20H38O2		Being too flexible, Not able to draw	0.08	-	-	-	-	-	-	-
Behenic	C22:0	C22H36O2		Being too flexible, Not able to draw	0.01	-	-	-	-	-	-	0.33
Lignoceric	C24:0	C24H48O2			-	-	-	0.3	-	-	-	0.3
Caproic	C6:0	C6H12O2			-	-	-	-	-	-	-	-
Enathic	C7:0	C7H14O2			-	-	-	-	-	-	-	-
Caprylic	C8:0	C8H16O2			-	-	-	-	-	-	-	-

(*Continued*)

TABLE 10.1 *(Continued)*

Name of the acid	Fatty acid	Chemical formula	Chemical structure	Crystal structure/3D conformer	% composition							
					SO Oil	Jatropha	Sunflower	Neem	Sunflower	Palm oil	Depot margine	Canola
Capric	C10:0	C10H18O2			-	-	-	-	-	-	-	-
Lauric	C12:0	C12H24O2			-	-	-	-	-	-	-	-
Myristic	C14:0	C14H28O2			0.09	-	0.04	-	-	-	-	<0.1
Palmitic	C16:0	C16H32O2			11.17	28	5.50	5	3.49	10.2	11.75	7.2

Free Fatty Acids and Their Role in CI Engines

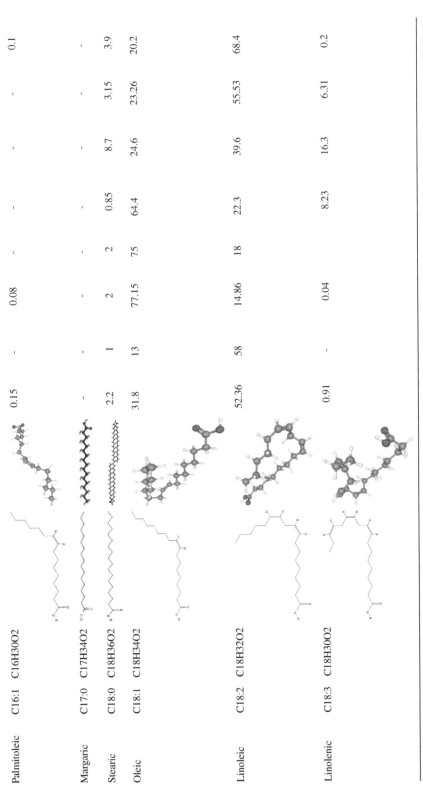

Palmitoleic	C16:1	C16H30O2		0.15	-	0.08	-	-	-	-	0.1
Margaric	C17:0	C17H34O2		-	-	-	-	-	-	-	-
Stearic	C18:0	C18H36O2		2.2	1	2	2	0.85	8.7	3.15	3.9
Oleic	C18:1	C18H34O2		31.8	13	77.15	75	64.4	24.6	23.26	20.2
Linoleic	C18:2	C18H32O2		52.36	58	14.86	18	22.3	39.6	55.53	68.4
Linolenic	C18:3	C18H30O2		0.91	-	0.04		8.23	16.3	6.31	0.2

(Continued)

TABLE 10.1 *(Continued)*

Name of the acid	Fatty acid	Chemical formula	Chemical structure	Crystal structure/3D conformer	% composition							
					SO Oil	Jatropha	Sunflower	Neem	Sunflower	Palm oil	Depot margine	Canola
Arachidic	C20:0	C20H40O2			0.4	–	0.04	–	–	–	–	–
Gondoic	C20:1	C20H40O2		Being too flexible, Not able to draw	–	–	–	–	–	–	–	<0.1
Eicosadienoic	C20:2	C20H38O2		Being too flexible, Not able to draw	0.16	–	0.04	–	–	–	–	–
Behenic	C22:0	C20H36O2		Being too flexible, Not able to draw	0.16	–	–	–	–	–	–	–

Name of the acid	Fatty acid	Chemical formula	Chemical structure	Crystal structure/3D conformer	% composition				
					Tallow	Pongamia	Ricebran	Polanga	Karanja
Caproic	C6:0	C6H12O2			-	-	-	-	-
Enathic	C7:0	C7H14O2			-	-	-	-	-
Caprylic	C8:0	C8H16O2			-	-	-	-	-
Capric	C10:0	C10H18O2			-	-	-	-	-
Lauric	C12:0	C12H24O2			-	-	-	-	-
Myristic	C14:0	C14H28O2			-	-	-	-	-

(Continued)

TABLE 10.1 (Continued)

Name of the acid	Fatty acid	Chemical formula	Chemical structure	Crystal structure/3D conformer	% composition				
					Tallow	Pongamia	Ricebran	Polanga	Karanja
Palmitic	C16:0	C16H32O2			23.3	9.8	12.5	17.9	9.8
Palmitoleic	C16:1	C16H30O2			0.1	–	–	–	–
Margaric	C17:0	C17H34O2			–	–	–	–	–
Stearic	C18:0	C18H36O2			19.3	6.2	2.1	18.5	6.2
Oleic	C18:1	C18H34O2			42.4	72.2	47.5	42.7	72.2

Name	Code	Formula							
Linoleic	C18:2	C18H32O2			2.9	11.8	35.4	13.7	11.8
Linolenic	C18:3	C18H30O2			0.9	-	1.1	2.1	-
Arachidic	C20:0	C20H40O2			-	-	0.6	-	-
Gondoic	C20:1	C20H40O2	Being too flexible, Not able to draw		-	-	-	-	-
Eicosadienoic	C20:2	C20H38O2	Being too flexible, Not able to draw		-	-	0.3	-	-
Behenic	C22:0	C20H36O2	Being too flexible, Not able to draw		-	-	0.2	2.6	-

(Continued)

TABLE 10.1 *(Continued)*

Name of the acid	Fatty acid	Chemical formula	Chemical structure	Crystal structure/3D conformer	% composition						
					POME	SOME	ROME	PONOME	LOME	JOME	COTOME
Caproic	C6:0	C6H12O2			-	-	-	-	-	-	-
Enathic	C7:0	C7H14O2			-	-	-	-	-	-	-
Caprylic	C8:0	C8H16O2			-	-	-	-	-	-	-
Capric	C10:0	C10H18O2			-	-	-	-	-	-	-
Lauric	C12:0	C12H24O2			0.115	-	-	-	-	-	-

Free Fatty Acids and Their Role in CI Engines

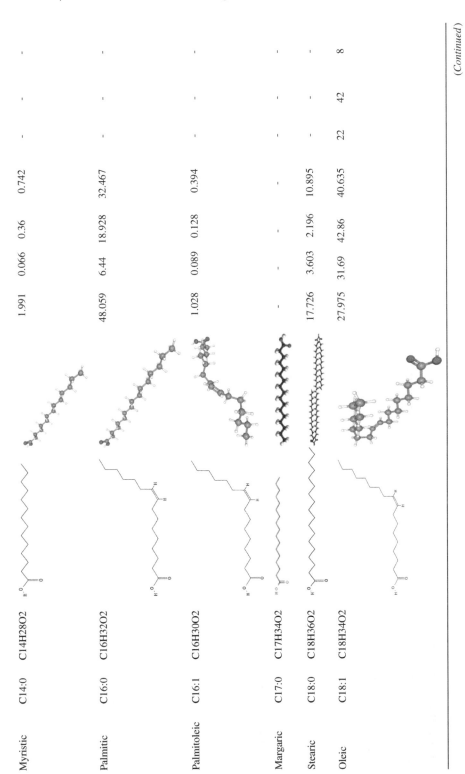

Myristic	C14:0	C14H28O2			1.991	0.066	0.36	0.742	-	-	-
Palmitic	C16:0	C16H32O2			48.059	6.44	18.928	32.467	-	-	-
Palmitoleic	C16:1	C16H30O2			1.028	0.089	0.128	0.394	-	-	-
Margaric	C17:0	C17H34O2			-	-	-	-	-	-	-
Stearic	C18:0	C18H36O2			17.726	3.603	2.196	10.895	-	-	-
Oleic	C18:1	C18H34O2			27.975	31.69	42.86	40.635	22	42	8

(Continued)

TABLE 10.1 (Continued)

Name of the acid	Fatty acid	Chemical formula	Chemical structure	Crystal structure/3D conformer	% composition						
					POME	SOME	ROME	PONOME	LOME	JOME	COTOME
Linoleic	C18:2	C18H32O2			2.309	56.737	31.919	11.134	13	30	2
Linolenic	C18:3	C18H30O2			0.078	0.035	0.594	0.238	–	–	–
Arachidic	C20:0	C20H40O2			0.524	0.231	0.844	0.834	–	–	–
Gondoic	C20:1	C20H40O2		Being too flexible, Not able to draw	0.056	0.117	0.44	0.477	–	–	–

Free Fatty Acids and Their Role in CI Engines

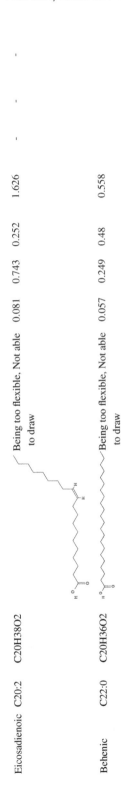

POME: Palm Oil Methyl Ester; SOME: Sunflower Oil Methyl Ester; ROME: Ricebran Oil Methyl Ester; PONOME: Pongamia Oil Methyl Ester; LOME: Linseed Oil Methyl Ester; JOME: Jatropha Oil Methyl Ester; COTOME: Coconut Oil Methyl Ester

290 Biowaste and Biomass in Biofuel Applications

TABLE 10.2

Comparison of Unsaturated FA with Saturated FA.

Description	Saturated	Mono-unsaturated (MUSA)	Poly-unsaturated (PUSA)		Total saturated	Total unsaturated
	(C18:0)	(C18:1)	(C18:2)	(C18:3)		
Rapeseed oil	0.85	64.4	22.3	8.23	0.85	86.7
Olive oil	2	75	18	-	2	93
Hazelnut oil	2	77.15	14.86	0.04	2	92.01
Grapeseed oil	3.9	20.2	68.4	0.2	3.9	88.8
Sunflower oil	3.603	31.69	56.737	0.035	3.603	88.42
Canola	2.54	53.36	29.81	5.63	2.54	83.17
Pongamia	6.2	72.2	11.8	-	6.2	84
Rubberseed oil	8.7	24.6	39.6	16.3	8.7	80.5
Soybean oil	3.15	23.26	55.53	6.31	3.15	78.79
Corn oil	2.2	31.8	52.36	0.91	2.2	84.16

It is observed from the above tables that unsaturated free fatty acids dominate over saturated fatty acids. The leading Saturated Fatty acids are unbranched, straight chains of CH_2 bunches related by carbon-carbon single bonds with one terminal carboxylic damaging amass. The term immersed outlines that the preeminent exceptional conceivable number of hydrogen particles are invigorated to each carbon interior of the particle. Different soaked sleek acids have an inconsequential or common title as well as a chemically practical capable title. The beneficial names are based on numbering the carbon particles, starting with the acidic carbon. The table gives the names and ordinary common sources of the preeminent common submerged sleek acids. In appearing to abhor toward the reality that the chains are generally between 12 and 24 carbons long, a few shorter-chain sleek acids are biochemically vital. Unsaturated Fatty acids have one or more carbon-carbon twofold bonds. The term unsaturated outlines that less than the preeminent uncommon conceivable number of hydrogen particles are braced to each carbon interior of the particle. The number of twofold bonds is shown up by the nonexclusive name: monounsaturated for particles with one twofold bond and polyunsaturated for particles with two or more twofold bonds. Oleic danger is a case of a monounsaturated sleek danger. Common agent monounsaturated oily acids at the side their names and standard sources are recorded interior the table. The prefix cis-9 interior, the effective title of palmitoleic dangerous, implies that the position of the twofold bond is between carbons 9 and 10. Two conceivable conformations, cis and trans, can be taken by the two CH_2 bunches that are absent, adjoining to the double-bonded carbons. Interior the cis course of activity, the one happening in all common unsaturated sleek acids, the two interfacing carbons [78].

10.4 ROLE OF FREE FATTY ACIDS IN DIESEL ENGINES

Sukumar Puhan et al. [79] worked on a four stroke, single cylinder, direct injection, bowl-in-piston-based combustion geometry of a Kirloskar oil engine at a constant speed of 1500 rpm at a power of 4.4 kW with three different biodiesel, like linseed oil methyl ester, *Jatropha curcas* oil methyl ester, and coconut oil methyl ester. Saturated free fatty acids of the linseed oil methyl ester, *J. curcas* oil methyl ester, and coconut oil methyl ester are 7%, 26%, and 87%, respectively, whereas their unsaturated free fatty acids are 93%, 74%, and 13%, respectively. Concerning physicochemical properties, densities vary from 860 to 890, and kinematic viscosity ranges from

The specific energy consumption of all methyl esters shown higher than conventional diesel operation is due to higher density and lower calorific value. And Linseed Oil Methyl Ester recorded higher specific energy consumption compared to other Methyl Esters [80–84]. Whereas the highest brake thermal efficiency was noticed at full load with Coconut Oil Methyl Ester. However, the lighter viscosity of *J. curcas* oil methyl ester increased its brake thermal efficiency at part load conditions. Further, it is noticed that higher content of unsaturated fatty acids leads to polymerization at higher temperatures in the presence of oxygen, causing more heat release rate after burning at higher loads [85–93]. Even the exhaust gas temperature of linseed oil methyl ester is higher compared to the other two methyl esters. When it comes to combustion, linseed oil methyl ester exhibited longer ignition delay and higher uncontrolled combustion phase compared to *J. curcas* oil methyl ester and cottonseed oil methyl ester. The longer ignition delay of these methyl esters is because of their lower cetane number, which demands higher energy in order to start the reaction. Thus, the influence of the uncontrolled combustion heat release rate phase increases the oxides of nitrogen emissions. Further, it is noticed that higher unsaturated fatty acids produce higher hydrocarbons, carbon monoxide, and smoke emissions compared to saturated fatty acids. Sara Pinzi revealed that, as unsaturation increases, peak pressure s were increased due to an increase in its double bonds [94,95]. With respect to emissions, methyl esters, being long-chain molecules, are less prone to vaporize, leading to an increase in total hydrocarbon emissions. There is a wide variety of opinions on the increase in NOx, like thermal NOx, adiabatic flame temperature, fuel NOx, cetane number, and chain length. Of course, thermal NOx is one of the major contributors out of all identified points. However, chain length is also a prominent factor in developing NOx. Even longer chain-length molecules are also responsible for the generation of smoke or particulate matter [96–100].

10.5 CONCLUSION

The comprehensive distinguishing proof of a particular greasy corrosive is eventually subordinate to its division in unadulterated shape and suitable amounts for chemical and physical characterization. This can be unfeasible for all examinations. Thus numerous strategies have been concocted to expect the exact composition of the fabric to a specific extent, with expanding exactness as the examination advances. With basic blends, it is attainable to go straight from segregation to the last instrumental investigation with exceptionally small pre-fractionation. Numerous complicated combinations require a preparatory division utilizing complementary chromatographic strategies. Sometime recently, indeed, a distinguishing theoretical proof may be fulfilled.

Various chromatographic strategies loan themselves well to consecutive applications, coming about in continuously basic greasy corrosive combinations. The particular combination of frameworks fundamental for a fitting preparatory determination of greasy acids is managed on the mixture's complexity and the study's necessities. Person GLC is the foremost common and fruitful complementary chromatographic framework combination, taken after by argentation TLC. The bulk of known acids may be recognized utilizing unsaturation classes alone. Numerous analysts have created standard TLC and GLC combinations for early distinguishing proof of greasy acids in normal blends, and this approach is presently regularly favored over repetitive calculations of hypothetical maintenance periods and fragmentary chain length gauges.

TLC-GLC is consistent with the quantitative recuperation of TLC divisions, permitting the relative extents of the constituent components of the general blend to be decided. Besides, TLC prefractionation frequently yields tall immaculate minor components that are less demanding to recoup and recognize than GLC alone. Utilizing nonpolar siloxane columns, this method moreover permits for the orderly era of greasy corrosive subfractions for GC-MS examination.

Preparative GLC on nonpolar columns, which settle the oily destructive methyl esters concurring to nuclear weight, is another profitable combination of complementary chromatographic techniques. After catching the divisions, they are rechromatographed on a polar column to recognize the individual unsaturated oily acids in each chain length. Much desire has been voiced in the past for a complementary expository GLC on polar and nonpolar fluid stages as a way of unambiguous greasy corrosive distinguishing proof. It has been built up that in essential measures blends, diverse varieties in elution terms may be seen, which can be utilized within the shape of semi-log frameworks to distinguish obscure greasy acids based on their maintenance times in polar and nonpolar fluid stages. When working with complex greasy corrosive blends, in any case, this method isn't recommended since it is difficult to distinguish which crest is which within the GLC elution designs, particularly when the relative amounts of the components are unknown.

When the crests from one or both columns are assembled, this issue is dealt with, and the points of interest inutilizing the two fluid stages are kept. Even though capillary columns perform way better for close isomer investigation, issues emerge due to destitute reproducibility and restricted recuperation of higher molecular-weight components. Total examinations of greasy corrosive esters, counting minor components, frequently require considerable chromatographic division as well as a few frames of chemical or physiochemical minor component improvement. A few enhancement strategies are amazingly particular, while others are more non-specific.

The presence of conjugated twofold and trans twofold bonds may be affirmed using bright and infrared spectroscopy separately. Essentially, infrared spectroscopy can ordinarily build up the nearness of hydroxy or keto functionalities within the greasy chain. Atomic attractive reverberation spectroscopy can give advance proof for the preparatory structure of the greasy corrosive created from chromatographic

Free Fatty Acids and Their Role in CI Engines 293

fractionations, as well as prescribe significant consequent examinations and the procedure of structure recognizable proof by chemical methods.

The distinguishing chemical proof of an obscure greasy acid's structure is basically an issue in auxiliary natural chemistry, which incorporates both ancient and present-day approaches. Numerous early examinations, as well as cutting-edge precise blends, give great occurrences of chemical union approval of greasy corrosive structures. In a few cases, recognizing the metabolic equivalency of characteristic and manufactured compounds may be required, especially if the last mentioned were produced by strategies that will have involved the reversal of deviated carbons.

The combination of GC-MS has the potential to be the foremost capable explanatory strategy for identifying greasy acids. Be that as it may, imperfections in evaluating the position of the twofold bonds, as well as their geometric structures, are found. The strategy, too, does not offer data on the stereochemical course of action of other utilitarian bunches. In any case, this may be cured by chemical derivatization and the accessibility of polar fluid stages reasonable for GC-MS work. In any case, the lion's share of well-characterized greasy acids has been distinguished in terms of atomic weight, sum, and twofold bond area, utilizing standard TLC-GLC or GC-MS strategies. Moreover, knowing the substance's source or beginning increments the certainty of distinguishing the greasy acids. As a result, exceptionally basic chromatographic strategies can routinely produce precise greasy corrosive recognizable pieces of proof. Further, higher unsaturation also influences the formation of exhaust emissions.

REFERENCES

[1] Holman, R.T. and J.J. Rahm, Analysis and characterization of polyunsaturated fatty acids. *Progress in the Chemistry of Fats and other Lipids*, 1971. **9**: pp. 13–90.

[2] Schauenstein, E., Autoxidation of polyunsaturated esters in water: chemical structure and biological activity of the products. *Journal of Lipid Research*, 1967. **8**(5): pp. 417–428.

[3] Lundberg, W.O. and P. Järvi, Peroxidation of polyunsaturated fatty compounds. *Progress in the Chemistry of Fats and other Lipids*, 1971. **9**: pp. 377–406.

[4] Kuksis, A., Separation and determination of structure of fatty acids, in *Fatty Acids and Glycerides*. 1978, Springer. pp. 1–76.

[5] Hopkins, C., Fatty acids with conjugated unsaturation. *Topics in Lipid Chemistry*, 1972. **3**: pp. 37–87.

[6] Böttcher, C., et al., Methods for the analysis of lipids extracted from human arteries and other tissues. *Recueil des Travaux Chimiques des Pays-Bas*, 1959. **78**(10): pp. 794–814.

[7] Kates, M., Technology of lipidology. *Laboratory Techniques in Biochemistry and Molecular Biology*, 1972: pp. 267–610.

[8] Hilditch, T.P. and P.N. Williams, *The Chemical Constitution of Natural Fats* (4th edition). 1964, ACS Publications.

[9] Brockerhoff, H., *Lipolytic Enzymes*. 2012, Elsevier.

[10] Luddy, F., et al., Pancreatic lipase hydrolysis of triglycerides by a semimicro technique. *Journal of the American Oil Chemists' Society*, 1964. **41**(10): pp. 693–696.

[11] Anderson, R.E., N.R. Bottino, and R. Reiser, Pancreatic lipase hydrolysis as a source of diglycerides for the stereospecific analysis of triglycerides. *Lipids*, 1967. **2**(5): pp. 440–442.

[12] Kleiman, R., et al., Retarded hydrolysis by pancreatic lipase of seed oils withTrans-3 unsaturation. *Lipids*, 1970. **5**(6): pp. 513–518.

[13] Bottino, N.R., G.A. Vandenburg, and R. Reiser, Resistance of certain long-chain polyunsaturated fatty acids of marine oils to pancreatic lipase hydrolysis. *Lipids*, 1967. **2**(6): pp. 489–493.

[14] Brockerhoff, H., Stereospecific analysis of triglycerides. *Lipids*, 1971. **6**(12): pp. 942–956.

[15] Fischer, W., E. Heinz, and M. Zeus, The suitability of lipase from Rhizopus arrhizus delemar for analysis of fatty acid distribution in dihexosyl diglycerides, phospholipids and plant sulfolipids. *Hoppe Seylers Z Physiol Chem*, 1973. **354**(9): pp. 1115–1123.

[16] Jensen, R.G., et al., Specificity of Geotrichum candidum lipase with respect to double bond position in triglycerides containing cis-octadecenoic acids. *Lipids*, 1972. **7**(11): pp. 738–741.

[17] Jensen, R.G., D.T. Gordon, and C. Scholfield, Hydrolysis of linoleate geometric isomers by Geotrichum candidum lipase. *Lipids*, 1973. **8**(5): pp. 323–325.

[18] Ory, R.L., J. Kiser, and P.A. Pradel, Studies on positional specificity of the castor bean acid lipase. *Lipids*, 1969. **4**(4): pp. 261–264.

[19] Nutter, L. and O. Privett, Phospholipase A properties of several snake venom preparations. *Lipids*, 1966. **1**(4): pp. 258–262.

[20] Wells, M.A. and D.J. Hanahan, Phospholipase A from Crotalus adamanteus venom: EC 3.1.1.4 Phosphatide acyl-hydrolase, in *Methods in Enzymology*. 1969, Elsevier. pp. 178–184.

[21] Van Deenen, L. and G.H.d. Haas, The substrate specificity of phospholipase A. *Biochimica et Biophysica Acta (BBA)-Specialized Section on Lipids and Related Subjects*, 1963. **70**: pp. 538–553.

[22] Gloster, J. and R. Fletchek, Quantitative analysis of serum lipids with thin-layer chromatography. *Clinica Chimica Acta*, 1966. **13**(2): pp. 235–240.

[23] Breckenridge, W. and A. Kuksis, Structure of bovine milk fat triglycerides. *Lipids*, 1968. **3**(4): pp. 291–300.

[24] Rodrigues de Miranda, J. and T. Eikelboom, Thin-layer chromatographic separation of free fatty acids; analysis and purification of radioactivity labelled fatty acids. *Journal of Chromatography*, 1975. **114**(1): pp. 274–279.

[25] Goodridge, A.G., Regulation of fatty acid synthesis in the liver of prenatal and early postnatal chicks: Hepatic concentrations of individual free fatty acids and other metabolites. *Journal of Biological Chemistry*, 1973. **248**(6): pp. 1939–1945.

[26] Hornstein, I., et al., Determination of free fatty acids in fat. *Analytical Chemistry*, 1960. **32**(4): pp. 540–542.

[27] Lankin, V., S. Anikeova, and A. Ananenko, Quantitative determination of serum nonesterified fatty acids by gas liquid chromatography. *Voprosy meditsinskoi khimii*, 1974. **20**(4): pp. 435–439.

[28] Morrison, W.R. and L.M. Smith, Preparation of fatty acid methyl esters and dimethylacetals from lipids with boron fluoride–methanol. *Journal of Lipid Research*, 1964. **5**(4): pp. 600–608.

[29] Koritala, S. and W. Rohwedder, Formation of an artifact during methylation of conjugated fatty acids. *Lipids*, 1972. **7**(4): pp. 274–274.

[30] Minnikin, D.E., Ring location in cyclopropane fatty acid esters by boron trifluoride-catalyzed methoxylation followed by mass spectroscopy. *Lipids*, 1972. **7**(6): pp. 398–403.

[31] Sheppard, A.J. and J.L. Iverson, Esterification of fatty acids for gas-liquid chromatographic analysis. *Selected Technical Publications*, 1975. **13**(22): pp. 352.

[32] Johnson, C. and E. Wong, Esterification and etherification by silver oxide-organic halide reaction gas chromatography. *Journal of Chromatography A*, 1975. **109**(2): pp. 403–408.

Free Fatty Acids and Their Role in CI Engines 295

[33] Cooper, M. and M. Anders, Determination of long chain fatty acids as 2-naphthacyl esters by high pressure liquid chromatography and mass spectrometry. *Analytical Chemistry*, 1974. **46**(12): pp. 1849–1852.

[34] Hintze, U., H. Röper, and G. Gercken, Gas chromatography-mass spectrometry of C1-C20 fatty acid benzyl esters. *Journal of Chromatography A*, 1973. **87**(2): pp. 481–489.

[35] Schlenk, H. and J.L. Gellerman, Esterification of fatty acids with diazomethane on a small scale. *Analytical Chemistry*, 1960. **32**(11): pp. 1412–1414.

[36] Nelson, G.J., *Quantitative Analysis of Blood Lipids*. 1972, Wiley–Interscience.

[37] Tallent, W. and R. Kleiman, Bis (trimethylsilyl) acetamide in the silylation of lipolysis products for gas-liquid chromatography. *Journal of Lipid Research*, 1968. **9**(1): pp. 146–148.

[38] Kuksis, A., O. Stachnyk, and B. Holub, Improved quantitation of plasma lipids by direct gas-liquid chromatography. *Journal of Lipid Research*, 1969. **10**(6): pp. 660–667.

[39] Phillipou, G., D. Bigham, and R. Seamark, Subnanogram detection oft-butyldimethylsilyl fatty acid esters by mass fragmentography. *Lipids*, 1975. **10**(11): pp. 714–716.

[40] Weihrauch, J., C. Brewington, and D. Schwartz, Trace constituents in milk fat: Isolation and identification of oxofatty acids. *Lipids*, 1974. **9**(11): pp. 883–890.

[41] Langenbeck, U., H.-U. Möhring, and K.-P. Dieckmann, Gas chromatography of α-keto acids as their o-trimethylsilylquinoxalinol derivatives. *Journal of Chromatography A*, 1975. **115**(1): pp. 65–70.

[42] Christie, W., Cyclopropane and cyclopropene fatty acids. *Topics in Lipid Chemistry*, 1970. **1**: pp. 1–49.

[43] Schlenk, H., Odd numbered polyunsaturated fatty acids. *Progress in the Chemistry of Fats and other Lipids*, 1971. **9**: pp. 587–605.

[44] Polgar, N., Natural alkyl-branched long-chain acids, in *Topics in Lipid Chemistry*. 1971, Logos Press. pp. 207–247.

[45] Markley, K.S., *Fatty Acids: Their Chemistry, Properties, Production, and Uses*. 1967, Interscience Publishers.

[46] Brown, C.A., Simple compact apparatus for rapid precise determination of unsaturation via hydrogenation on a micro and ultramicro scale. *Analytical Chemistry*, 1967. **39**(14): pp. 1882–1884.

[47] Aylward, F. and M. Sawistowska, Hydrazine-a reducing agent for olefinic compounds. *Chemistry & Industry*, 1962(11): pp. 484–491.

[48] Privett, O., Determination of the structure of unsaturated fatty acids via degradative methods. *Progress in the Chemistry of Fats and other Lipids*, 1971. **9**: pp. 91–117.

[49] Roehm, J. and O. Privett, Improved method for determination of the position of double bonds in polyenoic fatty acid esters. *Journal of Lipid Research*, 1969. **10**(2): pp. 245–246.

[50] Lemieux, R. and E.v. Rudloff, Periodate–permanganate oxidations: I. Oxidation of olefins. *Canadian Journal of Chemistry*, 1955. **33**(11): pp. 1701–1709.

[51] Privett, O. and E.C. Nickell, Preparation of highly purified fatty acids via liquid-liquid partition chromatography. *Journal of the American Oil Chemists Society*, 1963. **40**(5): pp. 189–193.

[52] Wood, R., GLC and TLC analysis of isopropylidene derivatives of isomeric polyhydroxy acids derived from positional and geometrical isomers of unsaturated fatty acids. *Lipids*, 1967. **2**(3): pp. 199–203.

[53] McCloskey, J.A. and M.J. McClelland, Mass spectra of O-isopropylidene derivatives of unsaturated fatty esters. *Journal of the American Chemical Society*, 1965. **87**(22): pp. 5090–5093.

[54] Emken, E., Determination of cis and trans in monoene and diene fatty esters by gas chromatography. *Lipids*, 1971. **6**(9): pp. 686–687.

[55] Fischmeister, I., Infrared absorption spectroscopy of normal and substituted long-chain fatty acids and esters in the solid state. *Progress in the Chemistry of Fats and other Lipids*, 1975. **14**: pp. 91–162.

[56] Wright, A., et al., Characterization of a polyisoprenoid compound functional in O-antigen biosynthesis. *Proceedings of the National Academy of Sciences*, 1967. **57**(6): pp. 1798–1803.

[57] Baumann, W. and H. Ulshöfer, Characteristic absorption bands and frequency shifts in the infrared spectra of naturally-occurring long-chain ethers, esters and ether esters of glycerol and various diols. *Chemistry and Physics of Lipids*, 1968. **2**(1): pp. 114–128.

[58] Bohlmann, F. and P. Hänel, Polyacetylenverbindungen, 168. Über die Polyine aus Cicuta virosa L. *Chemische Berichte*, 1969. **102**(10): pp. 3293–3297.

[59] Hitchcock, C. and B.W. Nichols, *Plant Lipid Biochemistry. The Biochemistry of Fatty Acids and Acyl Lipids with Particular Reference to Higher Plants and Algae*. 1971, Academic Press, Inc.

[60] Hamberg, M. and B. Samuelsson, On the specificity of the oxygenation of unsaturated fatty acids catalyzed by soybean lipoxidase. *Journal of Biological Chemistry*, 1967. **242**(22): pp. 5329–5335.

[61] Holman, R.T., P.O. Egwim, and W.W. Christie, Substrate specificity of soybean lipoxidase. *Journal of Biological Chemistry*, 1969. **244**(5): pp. 1149–1151.

[62] Zimmerman, D. and B. Vick, Specificity of flaxseed lipoxidase. *Lipids*, 1970. **5**(4): pp. 392–397.

[63] Gardner, H. and D. Weisleder, Lipoxygenase from Zea mays: 9-D-hydroperoxy-trans-10, cis-12-octadecadienoic acid from linoleic acid. *Lipids*, 1970. **5**(8): pp. 678–683.

[64] Howling, D., L. Morris, and A. James, The influence of chain length on the dehydrogenation of saturated fatty acids. *Biochimica et Biophysica Acta (BBA)-Lipids and Lipid Metabolism*, 1968. **152**(1): pp. 224–226.

[65] Johnson, A., et al., Fatty acid desaturase systems of hen liver and their inhibition by cyclopropene fatty acids. *Lipids*, 1969. **4**(4): pp. 265–269.

[66] Morris, L., Mechanisms and stereochemistry in fatty acid metabolism. *Biochemical Journal*, 1970. **118**(5): pp. 681.

[67] Pali, H.S., N. Kumar, and C. Mishra, *Some Experimental Studies on Combustion, Emission and Performance Characteristics of an Agricultural Diesel Engine Fueled with Blends of Kusum Oil Methyl Ester and Diesel*. 2014, SAE Technical Paper.

[68] Sharma, Y. and B. Singh, An ideal feedstock, kusum (Schleichera triguga) for preparation of biodiesel: Optimization of parameters. *Fuel*, 2010. **89**(7): pp. 1470–1474.

[69] Yadav, A.K., et al., Performance and emission characteristics of a transportation diesel engine operated with non-edible vegetable oils biodiesel. *Case Studies in Thermal Engineering*, 2016. **8**: pp. 236–244.

[70] Acharya, S.K., et al., The performance and emission characteristics of a diesel engine using preheated Kusum oil and Kusum diesel blend. *International Journal of Energy Technology And Policy*, 2011. **7**(5–6): pp. 503–518.

[71] Bringi, N.V., *Non-Traditional Oilseeds and Oils in India*. 1987, Oxford and IBH Pub. Co.

[72] Kundu, M. and C. Bandyopadhyay, Studies on some chemical aspects of kusum oil. *Journal of the American Oil Chemists Society*, 1969. **46**(1): pp. 23–27.

[73] Selvan, T. and G. Nagarajan, Combustion and emission characteristics of a diesel engine fuelled with biodiesel having varying saturated fatty acid composition. *International Journal of Green Energy*, 2013. **10**(9): pp. 952–965.

[74] Mahmudul, H., et al., Production, characterization and performance of biodiesel as an alternative fuel in diesel engines–A review. *Renewable and Sustainable Energy Reviews*, 2017. **72**: pp. 497–509.

[75] Awogbemi, O., E.I. Onuh, and F.L. Inambao, Comparative study of properties and fatty acid composition of some neat vegetable oils and waste cooking oils. *International Journal of Low-Carbon Technologies*, 2019. **14**(3): pp. 417–425.

Free Fatty Acids and Their Role in CI Engines

[76] Dabi, M. and U.K. Saha, Application potential of vegetable oils as alternative to diesel fuels in compression ignition engines: A review. *Journal of the Energy Institute*, 2019. **92**(6): pp. 1710–1726.

[77] Esteban, B., et al., Temperature dependence of density and viscosity of vegetable oils. *Biomass and Bioenergy*, 2012. **42**(0): pp. 164–171.

[78] www.britannica.com/science/lipid/Saturated-fatty-acids.

[79] Puhan, S., et al., Effect of biodiesel unsaturated fatty acid on combustion characteristics of a DI compression ignition engine. *Biomass and Bioenergy*, 2010. **34**(8): pp. 1079–1088.

[80] Ranjit, P.S., et al., Enhancement of performance and reduction in emissions of hydrogen supplemented Aleurites Fordii biodiesel blend operated diesel engine. *International Journal of Vehicle Structures and Systems*, 2022. **14**(2): pp. 174–178.

[81] Khader Basha, S., et al., Experimental investigation of diesel engine with Neem seed oil and compressed natural gas. *International Journal of Ambient Energy*, 2021: pp. 1–10.

[82] Ranjit, P., S.K. Dash, and V.V. Kamesh, Experimental investigation on influence of injection pressure on gaseous hydrogen supplemented SVO operated IDI CI engine. *Materials Today: Proceedings*, 2021. **43**: pp. 281–286.

[83] Dash, S., et al., Experimental investigation on synthesis of biodiesel from non-edible Neem seed oil: Production optimization and evaluation of fuel properties. *Materials Today: Proceedings*, 2021. **47**: pp. 2463–2466.

[84] Ranjit, P., et al., Experimental investigations on gaseous hydrogen supplemented Aleurites Fordii biodiesel in a direct injection diesel engine for performance enhancement and reduction in emissions. *Materials Today: Proceedings*, 2021. **46**: pp. 11140–11148.

[85] Ranjit, P.S., S. Pankaj Kumar, and S. Mukesh, Experimental Investigations on influence of Gaseous Hydrogen (GH_2) supplementation in in-direct injection (IDI) compression ignition engine fuelled with pre-heated straight vegetable Oil (PHSVO). *International Journal of Scientific & Engineering Research (IJSER)*, October 2014. **5**(10).

[86] Ranjit, P., et al. Experimental investigations on Schleichera Oleosa (SO) based biodiesel operated indirect injection (IDI) diesel engine for performance enhancement and reduction in emissions. in *IOP Conference Series: Materials Science and Engineering*. 2021, IOP Publishing.

[87] Ranjit, P. and V. Chintala, Impact of liquid fuel injection timings on gaseous hydrogen supplemented-preheated straight vegetable oil (SVO) operated compression ignition engine. *Energy Sources, Part A: Recovery, Utilization, and Environmental Effects*, 2020: pp. 1–22.

[88] Ranjit, P.S., et al., Studies on combustion, performance and emission characteristics of IDI CI engine with single-hole injector using SVO blends with diesel. *Asian Academic Research Journal of Multidisciplinary (AARJM)*, May 2014. **1**(21): pp. 239–248.

[89] Ranjit, P.S., et al., Studies on combustion and emission characteristics of an IDI CI engine by using 40% SVO diesel blend under different preheating conditions. *Global Journal of Research Analysis (GJRA)*, May 2014. **1**(21): pp. 43–46.

[90] Ranjit, P.S., et al., Studies on influence of turbocharger on performance enhancement and reduction in emissions of an IDI CI engine. *Global Journal of Research Analysis (GJRA)*, May 2014. **1**(21): pp. 239–248.

[91] Ranjit, P.S., et al., Studies on various performance, combustion & emission characteristics of an IDI CI engine with Multi-hole injector at different injection pressures and using SVO-diesel blend as fuel. *International Journal of Emerging Technology and Advanced Engineering (IJETAE)*, April 2014. **4**(4): pp. 340–344.

[92] Ranjit, P., et al., Experimental investigations on Hydrogen supplemented Pinus Sylvestris oil-based diesel engine for performance enhancement and reduction in emissions. *FME Transactions*, 2022. **50**(2): pp. 313–321.

298   Biowaste and Biomass in Biofuel Applications

[93] Ranjit, P., et al., Direct utilisation of straight vegetable oil (SVO) from Schleichera Oleosa (SO) in a diesel engine–a feasibility assessment. *International Journal of Ambient Energy*, 2022: pp. 1–11.

[94] Pinzi, S., et al., The effect of biodiesel fatty acid composition on combustion and diesel engine exhaust emissions. *Fuel*, 2013. **104**: pp. 170–182.

[95] Ranjit, P. and V. Chintala, Direct utilization of preheated deep fried oil in an indirect injection compression ignition engine with waste heat recovery framework. *Energy*, 2022. **242**: p. 122910.

[96] Knothe, G., C.A. Sharp, and T.W. Ryan, Exhaust emissions of biodiesel, petrodiesel, neat methyl esters, and alkanes in a new technology engine. *Energy & Fuels*, 2006. **20**(1): pp. 403–408.

[97] Graboski, M., et al., *The Effect of Biodiesel Composition on Engine Emissions from a DDC Series 60 Diesel Engine*. National Renewable Energy Laboratory (Report No: NREL/SR-510-31461), 2003.

[98] Lapuerta, M., O. Armas, and J. Rodriguez-Fernandez, Effect of biodiesel fuels on diesel engine emissions. *Progress in Energy and Combustion Science*, 2008. **34**(2): pp. 198–223.

[99] Dash, S.K., et al., Biodiesel prepared from used palm oil collected from hostel mess is a promising supplement for diesel fuel, in *Advances in Mechanical and Materials Technology*. 2022, Springer. pp. 841–850.

[100] Ranjit, P., et al., Use of Schleichera Oleosa biodiesel blends with conventional diesel in a compression ignition engine–A feasibility assessment. *Materials Today: Proceedings*, 2021. **46**: pp. 11149–11154.

Index

A

acid number, 69
acid treatment, 148
active, 22
alkali treatment, 155
anaerobic digestion, 100
aniline point, 73

B

bio-based nanofluid, 113
biochemical, 100
biodiesel, 4
bioenergy, 96
biofuel generations, 51
biomass, 128

C

calorific value, 7
catalytic pyrolysis, 168
cetane number, 7
chip thickness, 117
classification, 21
conversion, 96
cutting temperature, 116

D

density, 7
downdraft, 98
downstream, 205

E

economic factors, 56
electrochemical, 220
emission and performance, 73
emulsification, 212
enzymatic methods, 274

F

fatty esters, 66
feedstocks, 6
fermentation, 101
first generation, 51

free fatty acids, 267
friction, 9

G

gasification, 97
grinding, 136

H

hot-water extraction, 166
hydrothermal, 99
hydrotreatment, 222

I

infrared spectroscopy, 272

J

Jatropha curcas, 36

L

lipolysis, 269
lubricant, 113

M

machining, 115
moisture content, 73
monoalkyl, 34

N

nanoparticles, 25, 37
number of bonds, 272

P

passive, 24
position of bonds, 272
pyrolysis, 128

S

second generations, 52
silylation, 271

smoke opacity, 41
solar desalination, 20
solvent addition, 205
specific gravity, 69
steam explosion, 163
steam reforming, 236
surface roughness, 118
syngas, 236
synthesis, 113

T

tallow, 36
third generations, 55
torrefaction, 141
transportation fuel, 35

U

ultraviolet
   spectroscopy, 274
updraft, 98

V

viscosity, 7

W

waste, 96
waste cooking
   oil, 5
wear, 9